IMMUNE RESPONSE ACTIVATION

Edited by **Guy Huynh Thien Duc**

Immune Response Activation
http://dx.doi.org/10.5772/57004
Edited by Guy Huynh Thien Duc

Contributors

Mohamed Labib Salem, Abdel-Aziz Zidan, Said Hammad, Karine Breckpot, Tatsuaki Tsuruyama, Jonathan Moorman, Jedidiah Griffin, Marie Moulton, Zhi Yao, Andrew Foey, Maria Ines Becker, Sergio Arancibia, Fabian Alberto Salazar, Miguel Del Campo, Alfredo De Ioannes, Louise Hafner, Danica Hickey, Trudi Collet, Ana Maria Carmona-Ribeiro, Takemi Otsuki, Suni Lee, Megumi Maeda, Hiroaki Hayashi, Hidenori Matsuzaki, Naoko Kumagai-Takei, Yasumitsu Nishimura, Kozo Urakami, Masayasu Kusaka

Published by InTech

Janeza Trdine 9, 51000 Rijeka, Croatia

Publishing Process Manager Iva Lipovic

Technical Editor InTech DTP team

Cover InTech Design team

First published May, 2014

Printed in Croatia

Additional hard copies can be obtained from orders@intechopen.com

Immune Response Activation, Edited by Guy Huynh Thien Duc

p. cm.

ISBN 978-953-51-1374-4

For EU product safety concerns:
IN TECH d.o.o., Prolaz Marije Krucifikse Kozulić 3, 51000 Rijeka, Croatia,
info@intechopen.com or visit our website at intechopen.com.

Meet the editor

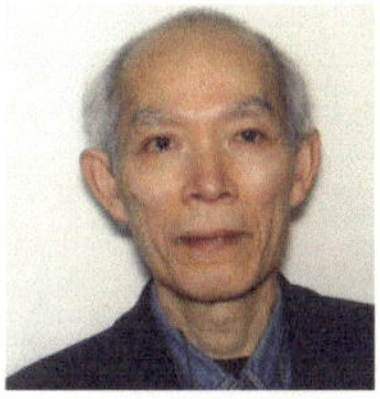

Guy Huynh Thien Duc is Research Director Emeritus from the CNRS (Centre National de la Recherche Scientifique). Medicine student and Master's degree of Science, he started his career in the Pasteur Institute and the Sorbonne, Faculty of Science in Paris, where he prepared his Ph.D in the field of Immunopathology. Thereafter, as researcher in the CNRS, he has been mainly involved in the fundamental aspects of Immunology, focusing on Transplantation Immunity and Immunomodulation. In the last two decades, his work at the University Paris XI, southern of Paris, presently inside the structure of INSERM U-1014, Groupe hospitalier Paul-Brousse-Villejuif, is essentially devoted to Immunology, its fundamental aspects and Cancer Immunotherapy.

Contents

Preface

The immune system plays a central role against pathogens that is seen further, extending beyond this context in recognizing alloantigens, modified transformed antigens expressed on tumoral cells, but unfortunately also self-antigens. As such, the immune response is involved in a large number of clinical settings, among which, protection against pathogenic organisms (bacteria, viruses), transformed tumoral cells and, finally, recognition and reaction against allergens and autoantigens. Therefore, beside the aspect relative to inducing generation of neutralizing protective antibodies and cytotoxic T lymphocytes against pathogens, there is need to consider the resistance developed by some pathogens to the traditional immune effector agents. Moreover, the immune response could also be acerbated in response to allergens and/or targeting the organism's own components leading to allergy and autoimmune diseases, respectively. Thus, along with its stimulation and activation, the immune response has to be tightly controlled and regulated. In this context, the multifaceted immune response is analyzed in the present book in several review chapters, treating a number of representative cases in which the immune response is, on one hand, activated against pathogens and, on the other hand, involved in pathologic settings, leading to allograft rejection, allergy and autoimmunity. The regulatory mechanisms in which the immune system can be modulated for rendering its effector components more efficient and not harmful to the organism is also dissected in translational purposes in cancer immunotherapy, local immunity against bacteria and viruses, as well as in allergy and autoimmunity.

In this regard, the book "Immune Response Activation", is divided into four sections related to:

Vaccines, with chapters concerning: 1) Cationic Nanostructures for Vaccines, and 2) Mollusk Hemocyanins as Natural Immunostimulants in Biomedical Applications.

Immunomodulation, with chapters: 1) Manipulating Immune Regulatory Pathways to Enhance T Cell Stimulation ; 2) Negative Immunomodulators – Blunting Immunostimulation and Facilitating Infection ; 3) Macrophages — Masters of Immune Activation, Suppression and Deviation, and 4) Immunostimulatory Effects of Triggering TLR3 Signaling Pathway — Implication for Cancer Immunotherapy.

Local Immunity, with chapters : 1) Immune Regulation of Chlamydia trachomatis Infections of the Female Genital Tract, and 2) The Roles of Invariant NKT Cells in Bowel Immunity — Suppression of Tumor Progression and Rejection of Intestinal Transplants.

Autoimmune Disregulation, with the chapter : Immunostimulation by Silica Particles and the Development of Autoimmune Dysregulation.

Guy Huynh Thien Duc
Research Director Emeritus from the CNRS
(Centre National de la Recherche Scientifique),
University Paris XI,
INSERM U-1014-Groupe Hospitalier Paul-Brousse,
France

Acknowledgments
We thank Chaobin Zhu for his assistance.

Section 1

Vaccines

Chapter 1

Cationic Nanostructures for Vaccines

Ana Maria Carmona-Ribeiro

Additional information is available at the end of the chapter

http://dx.doi.org/10.5772/57543

1. Introduction

Cationic lipid bilayers, particles, polysaccharides and a variety of hybrid nanostructures provide adequate matrixes for supporting antigens such as peptides, proteins, DNA or oligonucleotides on model surfaces (latex, silica, silicon wafers, self-assembled monolayers, metals, polymers, insoluble drugs, biological cells and viruses).Particulate vaccines are currently an area receiving a high level of attention [1-3]. Particles deliver both antigen and adjuvant into the same population of antigen presenting cells limiting both the systemic distribution of the adjuvant and its potential toxicity [1]. Biological particlesrepresented by live or attenuated bacterial vacines, engineered biological vectors and virus-like particles are often less safe than synthetic particulates for which quality control and validation in vaccine development and production are more rapid [2]. While developing novel particulate vaccines, particle size and charge do matter [2]. Virus-sized particles (20–200 nm) are usually taken up by endocytosis via clathrin-coated vesicles, caveolae or their independent receptors [4], and preferentially ingested by dendritic cells (DC). Larger sized particles such as bacteria (500–5000 nm) are predominantly taken up by phagocytosis, and primarily ingested by macrophages. All particles used in vaccine formulations are consequently internalized efficiently by antigen presenting cells by one or a combination of the quoted mechanisms [5, 6]. Particles with diameters smaller than 500 nm, in particular the nanometric ones with sizes in the 40–100 nm range are more eficient to promote CD8 and CD4 type 1 T cell responses than those with diameters above 500 nm, although the latter could induce good type 2 and antibody responses [5]. Cationic microparticles are effectively taken up both by macrophages and dendritic cells since electrostatic attraction promotes particle binding and subsequent internalization. Cationized polymeric particles carrying antigen significantly enhanced both antibody production and cytotoxic T cells at low antigen dose [7] and induced maturation of dendritic cells [8, 9]. As a consequence particles for vaccines should be positive and available over a range of sizes. Cationic particles of aluminium compounds, identified as having immunostimulatory properties more than 70 years ago, remain the only type of adjuvant licensed world-wide [3]. Oil-in-water emulsions or virosomes were licensed in some countries in compositions for influenza [10] or hepatitis B vaccines [11]. However, both of these adjuvants are characterised by inducing humoral immune response and are thus effective in elevating serum antibody titers whereas their ability to elicit cell-mediated immune response is limited [12]. For vaccines against influenza, malaria and HIV, the induction of a humoral response is insufficient and a substantial complementary cell-mediated immune response is necessary for adequate protection. For vaccines against tuberculosis, a cellular response seems to be the sole effector mechanism required for protection [13]. Among the cationic compounds used to produce cationic nanostructures to present antigens for vaccines formulations, some cationic compounds appear to be of special relevance.They are the cationic and synthetic lipid named dioctadecyldimethylammonium bromide (DODAB), the cationic polysaccharide named chitosan (CH) and its derivatives with pH-independent positive charge and the biocompatible cationic polymeric nanostructures.This chapter presents and critically evaluates these three types of cationic nanostructures.

2. Cationic nanostructures based on DODAB

DODAB is a cationic lipid which can be dispersed ultrasonically in aqueous solution using a macrotip probe [14]. Thereby, bilayer vesicles are simultaneously obtained and disrupted yielding nano-sized bilayer disks or cationic bilayer fragments (BF) stabilized by electrostatic repulsion at low ionic strength [14,15].DODAB BF have previously been used as antimicrobial agents [16] or in the production of lipid-covered particles such as bilayer-coated silica [17] or latex [18]. These cationic, bilayer-covered latex or silica particles where the bilayer is solely composed of DODAB were recently employed to present antigens to the immune system with better results than alum as adjuvants for induction of cellular immune responses [19, 20]. The open DODAB BF in aqueous dispersions are different from their mother vesicles presenting the following features: (i) osmotic non-responsiveness of the dispersion indicative of absence of inner vesicle compartment [21]; (ii) discoidal shape with disks exhibiting one bilayer thickness as visualised by means of transmission electronic microscopy (TEM) after electronic staining the nanostructures [22]; (iii) cryo-TEM micrographs performed without any staining [23]; (iv) fluid and solid state coexistence and complex formation with oppositely charged surfactant [24]; (v) solubilization of hydrophobic drugs at the borders of DODAB bilayer fragments, which does not occur for DODAB closed bilayer vesicles [25]. These bilayer fragments have more fluid environments at their edges that are absent in closed bilayer systems such as vesicles or liposomes. Due to its cylindrical molecular shape, DODAB molecules self-assemble in aqueous solutions as bilayers instead of micelles as shown in the seventies by transmission electron microscopy [26]. Supramolecular assemblies of DODAB bilayer fragments by themselves or after interaction with supporting particles have been combined with different model antigens in separate and tested as immunoadjuvants. The cationic nanoadjuvants with DODAB BF are either reduced to a single-component, nanosized system-DODAB

BF-or are dispersions of cationic particles with controllable nature and size as obtained after covering silica or polystyrene sulfate latex (PSS) with a cationic DODAB bilayer (Figure 1).

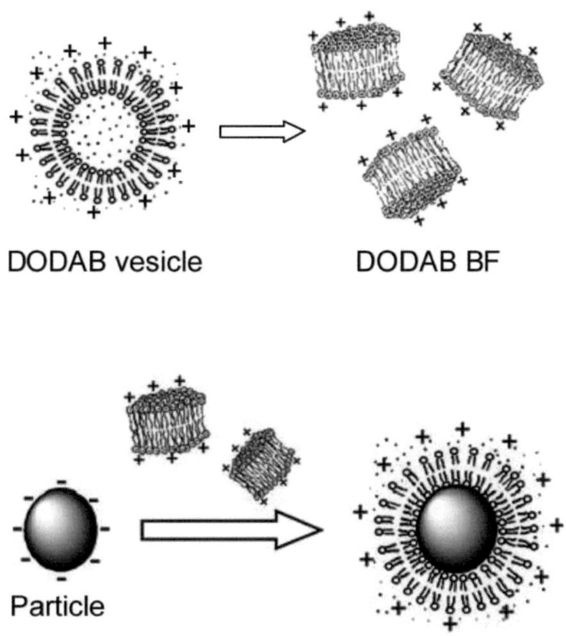

Figure 1. Cationic nanostructures and particles based on the cationic lipid DODAB useful to present antigens (reproduced with permission from [27]).The DODAB bilayer fragments are usually obtained at low ionic strength by sonication with a macrotip.Particles acting as supports for the cationic bilayer can be organic or inorganic. Reprinted from Vaccine, 27/42, Nilton Lincopan,Noelí M. Espíndola,Adelaide J. Vaz,Maria Helena B. da Costa,Eliana Faquim-Mauro,Ana M. Carmona-Ribeiro, Novel immunoadjuvants based on cationic lipid: Preparation, characterization and activity *in vivo*, 5760-5771.Copyright 2009, with permission from Elsevier.

DODAB BF may interact with proteins both via the hydrophobic effect and the electrostatic attraction at low ionic strength. This interaction has been properly characterized by means of dynamic light scattering for sizing, zeta-potential analysis and evaluation of immunoadjuvant activity *in vivo*. The model antigens employed with DODAB-based cationic nanostructures were bovine serum albumin (BSA), purified 18 kDa/14 kDa antigens from *Taenia crassiceps* cysticerci (18/14-*Tcra*) or a recombinant heat-shock protein from *Mycobacterium leprae* [27]. Antigen choices were due to different reasons. BSA adsorption at interfaces [28] and, specifically, onto large DODAB vesicles [29] is well described and has been useful to prevent nonspecific binding in immunoassays, biosensing and proteomics applications [28,30].The purified 18 kDa/14 kDa antigens from *Taenia crassiceps* cisticerci are proteins specific for this parasite found as circulating antigens and often employed in immunodiagnosis;they can be obtained from *in-vitro* cultures of *T. crassiceps* cysticerci in hybridoma media from vesicles budding from cysts contain the excretory/secretory (ES) antigens [31,32]. Human and pig infections by *T. solium* and *crassiceps*, respectively, represent an important health problem, with socio-economical repercussions affecting many countries in Latin America, Asia and Africa

[31]. The 18 kDa-hsp protein is a heat-shock protein of *M. leprae* displaying pronounced immunogenicity and considered able to induce proliferation of peripheral blood mononuclear cells and T-cell lines from *M. leprae* vaccinated subjects [33] andavailable at large amounts for studies on vaccine formulation; its overexpression and scaling-up in *Saccharomyces cerevisae* have already been described and the recombinant protein can be produced in large scale [34,35]. Nanostructured cationic adjuvant/antigen complexes based on DODAB were characterized over a range of adjuvant and antigen concentrations. Figure 2 shows the effect of antigen and adjuvant concentration on physical properties of the dispersions. Stable cationic nanostructures are available over a limited range of adjuvant and antigen concentrations which clearly depend on antigen nature and are different for different antigens.

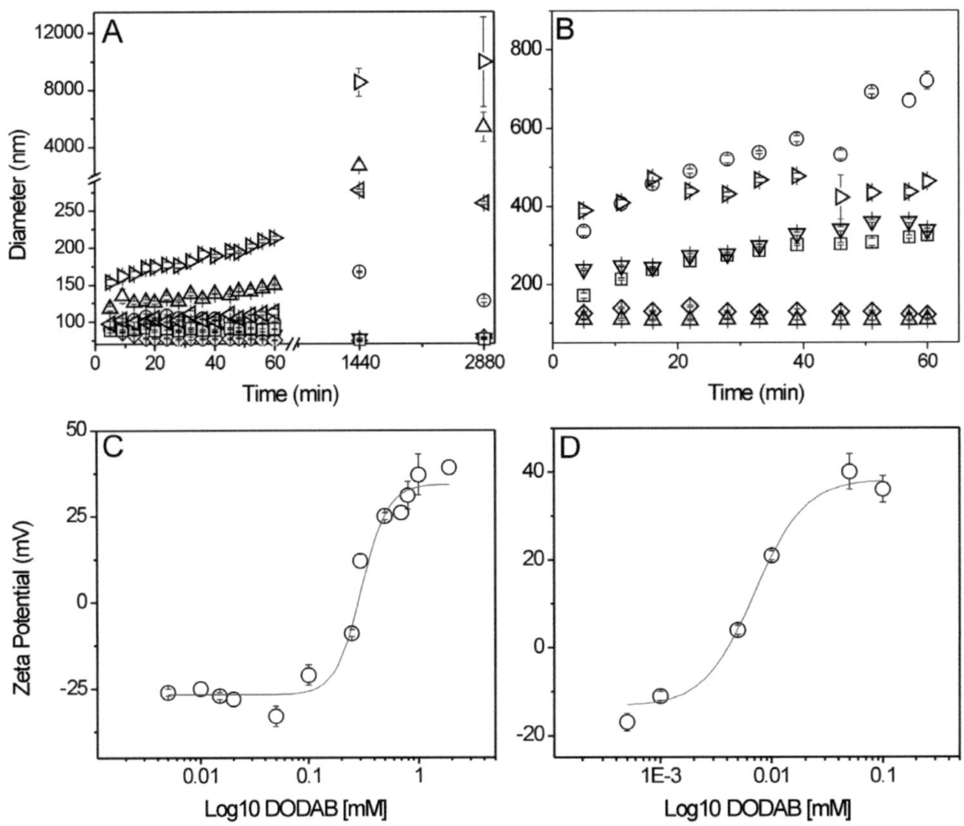

Figure 2. Effect of time and DODAB concentration on the zeta-average diameter of DODAB/BSA (A) or DODAB BF/ 18/14-Tcra complexes (B). In (A), the kinetics were obtained upon adding DODAB BF at a final concentration of 0.005 ((▷), 0.01 (△), 0.02 (◁), 0.05 (○), 0.5 (◇), 0.8 (□), and 1.0 mM DODAB (◁) to 0.5 mg/mL BSA. In (B), the kinetics were obtained upon adding DODAB BF at a final concentration of 0.0005 (□), 0.001 (○), 0.005 (▷), 0.01(▽), 0.05(◇), and 0.1 mM DODAB (△) to 0.05 mg/mL 18/14-Tcra. The effect of [DODAB] on zeta-potential of complexes with 0.5 mg/mL BSA (C) or 0.05 mg/mL 18/14-Tcra (D) were obtained after 1 h interaction at 25 °C in 1 mM NaCl.Reproduced with permission from reference [27].Reprinted from Vaccine, 27/42, Nilton Lincopan,Noelí M. Espíndola,Adelaide J. Vaz,Maria Helena B. da Costa,Eliana Faquim-Mauro,Ana M. Carmona-Ribeiro,Novel immunoadjuvants based on cationic lipid: Preparation, characterization and activity in vivo,5760-5771.Copyright 2009, with permission from Elsevier.

The humoral and cellular immune responses induced by stable cationic adjuvant/antigen complexes were evaluated in mice from determination of antigen-specific-IgG antibody in serum by ELISA, delayed type hypersensitivity (DH) reactions from footpad swelling tests and cytokines analysis. The results evidence the good colloid stability of the complexes, complete absence of toxicity in mice (i.e. local or general reactions) and their potential utility to induce Th 1 immune response at reduced doses of cationic and toxic DODAB lipid. Possibly due to its chemical stability and low cost when compared to other natural or synthetic lipids, DODAB use as an immunoadjuvant started more than forty years ago [36,37]. This was well before the bilayer nature of DODAB self-assembly in water solution had been described [26]. DODAB as an effective immunoadjuvant has been intensively investigated aiming at subunit vaccine design [38-41]. A major problem of liposomal formulations based on DODAB has been the usually high concentration employed, namely 1-10 mM DODAB [38-41]. DODAB is a cationic lipid and as such, cytotoxic [14-16] requiring dose minimization for administration in vivo. Using the DODAB bilayer fragments to present antigens only 0.1 mM DODAB was employed [27]. The large cellular imune response achieved might be related to the total surface area available for antigen association, which is much larger in the BF dispersion than in closed, large and sometimes multibilayered liposomes. Moreover, the hydrophobic interaction possibly available from BF edges could be an additional and powerful driving force for antigen adsorption and presentation. The second advantage of the bilayer fragments besides their large surfaces area is their size. Depending on sonication power and time plus composition of the dispersing medium, which determine colloid stability, DODAB BF/antigens complexes may have their sizes reduced to and stabilized at a few tenths of nanometers acting similarly to solid inert beads of nanometric size (40-50 nm). These beads turned out to be effective for antigen delivery to antigen-presenting cells (APC), generating potent and combined humoral and CD8+T cell immunity [3]. They are also expected to be optimal for dendritic cells uptake since their size is inside the range of particle diameters (500 nm and below) for optimal dendritic cells uptake of antigens and elicitation of an adequate cellular response [2,5,42]. In reconstituted pig gastric mucus, sub-200 nm particulates from poly (D, L-lactic-co-glycolic) acid and DODAB condensing DNA on particles surface exhibited improved transport rates, stability in mucus, and ability to transfect cells [43]. Silica/DODAB, latex/DODAB and DODAB BF (Figure 1) are available over the sub-200 nm range of sizes thus presenting potential also for design of mucosal vaccines. The third advantage of the bilayer fragments is the absence of depots at the injection site [27]. These depots have been reported for other DODAB formulations at concentrations much higher than 0.1 mM [37,41,44].

Consistently with electrostatic forces between negatively charged antigens and positively charged DODAB BF, cationic bilayer fragments readily adsorb BSA, 18-14/*Tcra* and the hsp-18 kDa recombinant protein.Rapid and extensive adsorption of BSA, anti-BSA or ovalbumin onto large DODAB liposomes was indeed reported previously [29,45,46].On the other hand, bacteria, fungus and eukaryotic cells were also found to adsorb DODAB vesicles and bilayer fragments with high affinity at low ionic strength [14-16], so that cationic DODAB liposomes readily adsorb antigen, such as ovalbumin, and bind avidly to dendritic cells [41], thereby enhancing antigen uptake. Delivery of antigen to cells by immediate contact with the cell surface via electrostatic interaction followed by the induction of active uptake seems to be the mechanism behind the ability of DODAB liposomes or bilayer fragments to act as immunoadjuvants. Sizes and zeta-potentials for assemblies of antigen and cationic lipid based adjuvants depend on cationic lipid and antigen concentrations. Adjuvant-antigen stability around sizes that are close to the one of adjuvants themselves indicates that the proteins readily adsorb and stabilize them. The adjuvants also stabilized the proteins acting as important dispersing nanocarriers able to induce remarkable degree of protein disaggregation by attaching the proteins either electrostatically or hydrophobically to their structure. At [DODAB] $\leq$ 0.1 mM and 0.001-0.05 mg/mL of antigen concentration, DODAB based adjuvant /antigen assemblies are cationic, well-dispersed, colloidally stable and immunogenic combining the advantages of low DODAB dose, low cost, controllable sizes for optimal dendritic cells uptake, high chemical stability, ability to incorporate multiple antigens and minimization of toxicity. Their performance is remarkably superior to the one of alum as adjuvant regarding Th1 mediated responses. In contrast to alum or cationic liposomes at 1-10 mM of cationic lipid, local or systemic adverse effects in mice were completely absent at 0.1-0.01mM DODAB.

An important component of the early innate immune response to viruses and bacteria is the secretion of cytokines, which mediate many of the effector functions of innate immunity. IL-10 is an inhibitor of activated macrophages and dendritic cells and is an example of negative feedback regulation because it is produced by macrophages to inhibit their function. This cytokine also inhibits the production of IL-12 and expression of class II major histocompatibility (MHC) molecules. IL-12 is also secreted by macrophages and dendritic cells inducing T cells differentiation into Th1 and natural killer (NK) cells with increased IFN-gamma synthesis and cytotoxic activity. IL-12 and IFN-gamma are the most important cytokines in innate responses to intracellular bacteria such as *Mycobacterium leprae* or tuberculosis [13]. Figure 3 shows the high levels of IL-12 and IFN-gamma induced by the novel cationic adjuvants while presenting the hsp-18 kDa of *M. leprae* to lymphonode cells suggesting a possible application of the novel adjuvants for the design of subunit vaccines against intracelular bacteria. As in DH, adaptive immunity against intracellular bacteria is principally cell mediated and consists of activation of macrophages by CD4+T cells as well as killing of infected cells by CD8+cytotoxic T lymphocytes (CTL).

On basis of IL-12 enhancement of IFN-gamma production and development of Th1 cells, this interleukin itself has been used as a vaccine adjuvant for many infections that are combated by cell-mediated immunity, e.g. leishmaniasis [47]. Subunit vaccines against protozoa that survive within macrophages require as principal defense mechanism cell-mediated immunity, particularly directed to macrophage activation by Th1 cell-derived cytokines. Leishmaniasis mucocutaneous and disseminated is caused by *Leishmania donovani* and CD4+Th1 cells are required to activate macrophages to kill phagocytosed parasites. Resistance to the infection is associated with activation of Leishmania-specific Th1 CD4+T cells which produce IFN-gamma and thereby activate macrophages to destroy intracellular parasites. Conversely, activation of Th2 cells by the protozoan results in increased parasite survival and exarcerbation of lesions because of the macrophage-suppressive actions of Th2 cytokines [47]. Other significant example is the protective role played by CD8+T cells in immunity to the hepatic stages of malaria. These effects may be mediated by direct killing of sporozoite-infected hepatocytes or indirectly by the secretion of IFN-gamma and activation of hepatocytes to produce nitric oxide and other agents that kill parasites. IL-12 induces resistance to sporozoite challenge in rodents and nonhuman primates, presumably by stimulating IFN-gamma production [48].

In viral infections, Il-12 enhances the cytotoxic activity of natural killer cells so that NK cell-mediated killing of virus-infected cells eliminates the reservoir of infection. In this respect, vaccination against the dengue virus is urgently needed in tropical or neotropical regions of the planet and some recombinant DNA vaccines expressing membrane and envelope of viral proteins have been proposed [49]. Possibly the cationic adjuvants available from our group would properly enhance the required Th-1 response for a more effective vaccination against dengue.

Another possible application for the novel adjuvants might be in immunotherapy for tumors. This approach is based in augmentation of host immunity to tumors with tumor vaccines. Immune responses that are able of killing tumor cells consist of CTLs, NK cells, and activated macrophages and these may be actively enhanced by vaccination with tumor cells or antigens, administration of tumors modified to express high levels of cytokines that stimulate T cell proliferation and differentiation, and systemic administration of cytokines [49]. The induction of T cell responses in tumors depends on processing and presentation of tumor antigens to T cells by professional antigen-presenting cells (APCs) which might internalize the tumor antigen adsorbed onto the novel cationic adjuvants. These APCs may stimulate CD8+T cells and CD4+helper T lymphocytes to differentiate for recognition and killing of tumor cells.

Naïve CD4+T cells may differentiate into distinct subsets, such as Th1 and Th2 cells in response to different antigens. For example, the enhancement in production of IL-10 and Il-13 by lymphonode cells elicited by the antigens of *Taenia crassiceps* presented by the DODAB BF adjuvant can be appreciated in Figure 3 [27]. These cytokines are typically associated with responses to allergens and parasites such as helminths and mediate differentiation of CD4+-T cells into Th2 cells [50]. Consistently, low levels of these cytokines were elicited by the *M. leprae* antigen presented by the novel adjuvants (Figure 3). Responses were indeed different for the helminthes and the bacteria antigens and very antigen-specific as they should be [27].

The size, charge and hydrophobic features of DODAB BF led to novel applications in solubilization of hydrophobic drugs [25,51,52], production of biomimetic particles from bilayer coverage of silica [17] or polystyrene particles [53] and design of vaccines [27].Recently, BF was also combined with oligonucleotides [54]. Since synthetic oligonucleotides can inhibit the replication of the Rous sarcoma virus [55], antisense oligonucleotides have been considered a great promise as therapeutic agents and several oligonucleotide-based formulations have reached the clinical trial phase [56,57]. Antisense oligonucleotides have also been extensively used in research on gene expression and function [58-60], vaccine formulation [61], allergy [62] and cancer therapeutics [63].Major obstacles as their degradation by nucleases and poor delivery to the target cells [60,64] suggest the essential role of suitable carriers able to protect oligonucleotides in the biological milieu [60,63–65].There are peculiar features for the interaction between BF and oligonucleotides in comparison to other electrolytes.Effects of salt, dAMP or poly (dA) concentration on BF size and zeta-potential are shown on Figure 4 taken from reference [54]. From 0 to 0.25 mM salt, Dz and zeta-potentials decreased with salt concentration possibly due to massive phosphate anion binding. From 0.25 to 2.5 mM of divalent salt, Dz increased but zeta-potential remained approximately constant and low (Fig. 4A and D).Dz and zeta-potential decreased with dAMP concentration (0– 2.5 mM) (Fig. 4B and E). At 0.05 mM poly (dA) and 0.5 mM DODAB, extensive BF aggregation and/or fusion took place as depicted from large Dz (N 500 nm) (Fig. 4C) and zero of zeta-potential (Fig. 4F). The screening of DODAB

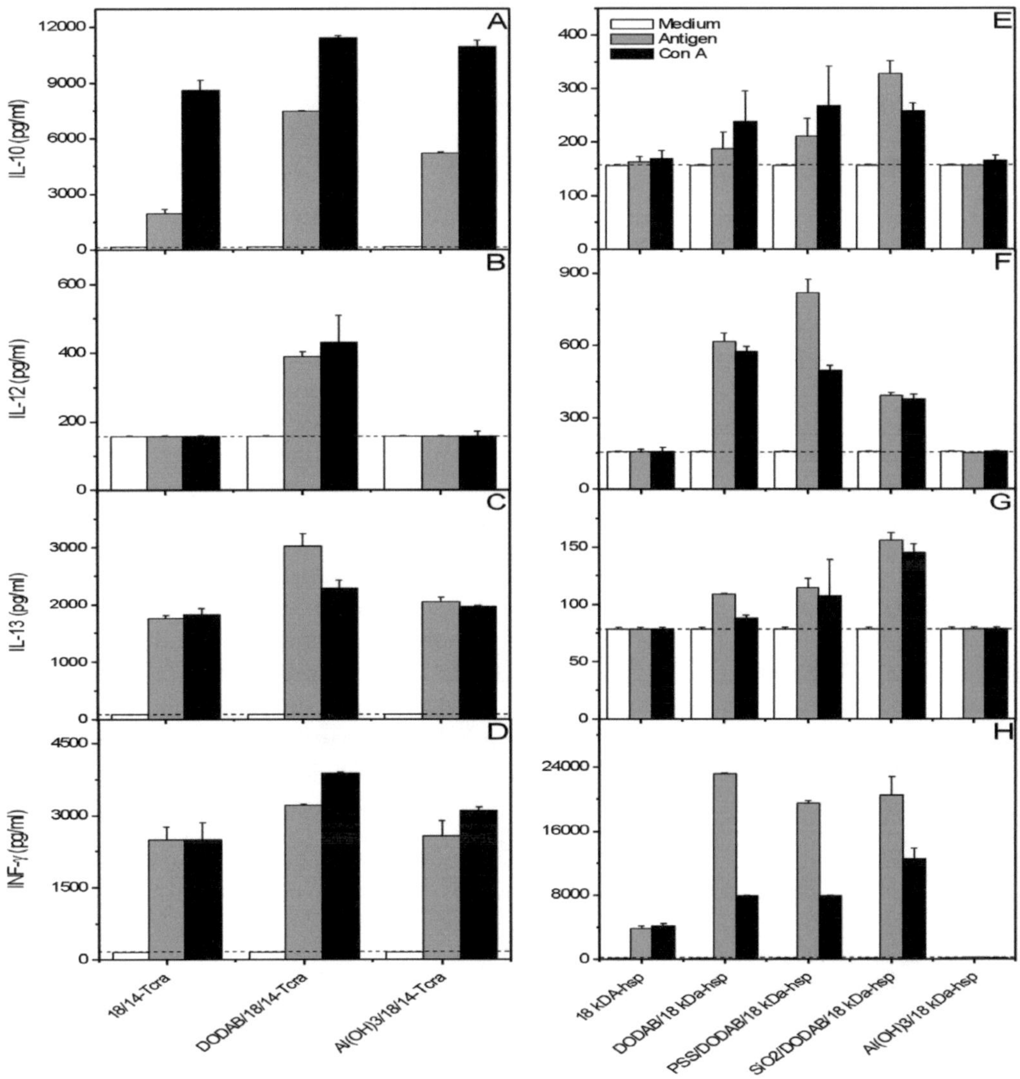

Figure 3. Quantitative analysis of cytokines secreted by lymph node cells from DODAB/18/14-Tcra and Al(OH)3/18/14-Tcra immunized mice (on the left column, A-D) or from 18kDa-hsp, DODAB/18kDa-hsp, PSS/DODAB/18kDa-hsp, SiO_2/DODAB/18 kDa-hsp and $Al(OH)_3$/18kDa-hsp immunized mice (on the right column, E-F). Cells from lymph nodes of BALB/c mice previously immunized with 10 µg of 18/14-*Tcra* administered alone, in DODAB BF or in $Al(OH)_3$ were *in vitro* stimulated with medium, 160 µg/ml of 18/14-*Tcra* or 2.5 µg/mL of ConA for 48 hours and the supernatants collected for cytokine analysis by sandwich kit enzyme-linked immunosorbent assay (ELISA). The results were expressed as mean of the cytokine concentration of two distinct assays ± standard deviation. Limits of detection are shown as horizontal dashed lines. Similarly, cells from lymph nodes of BALB-c mice previously immunized with 15 µg of 18 kDa-hsp from *M. leprae* administered alone or in DODAB BF, PSS/DODAB, silica/DODAB or Al $(OH)_3$ were *in vitro* stimulated with medium, 250 µg/ml of 18 kDa-hsp or 2.5 µg/mL of ConA for 48 hours before following cytokines analysis as above (reproduced with permission from reference [27]). Reprinted from Vaccine, 27/42, Nilton Lincopan, Noelí M. Espíndola, Adelaide J. Vaz,Maria Helena B. da Costa, Eliana Faquim-Mauro, Ana M. Carmona-Ribeiro, Novel immunoadjuvants based on cationic lipid: Preparation, characterization and activity *in vivo*, 5760-5771.Copyright 2009, with permission from Elsevier.

charges by Na_2HPO_4, followed by a decrease in electrostatic repulsion between fragments, could be responsible for DODAB BFs aggregation and/or fusion. DLS data also showed that diameters increase upon addition of Na_2HPO_4 concentrations above 0.5mM (Figure 4A), and this diameter increase up to 400 nm is related to a decrease in the zeta-potential of the fragments (Figure 4D). The charge screening of DODAB charged heads by Na_2HPO_4 explains the decrease in zeta-potential (Figure 4D) as well as the tighter bilayer packing represented by higher mean phase transition temperature for the bilayer [54]. Addition of dAMP leads to a decrease in diameter and zeta-potential of the assemblies (Figures 4B and E). It was shown that DODAB bilayer fragments are able to order dAMP molecules on their surface, causing the dAMP bases to stack [68]. In this case, bulky moieties of dAMP would be exposed at the fragments surface representing a steric hindrance to fragments aggregation and/or fusion which would also contribute to colloid stabilization in dispersion. For polynucleotides such as poly(dA), charge neutralization leads to flocculation whereas charge overcompensation upon increasing poly(dA) concentration leads to colloidal restabilization due to electrostatic repulsion (Figures 4C and F) [54]. This behavior has been often described for polyelectrolytes interacting with particles of opposite charge [67,68]. Beyond the neutralization point, the system regains stability due to charge overcompensation. This phenomenon was observed only for the electrolyte poly (dA) and not for the electrolytes Na_2HPO_4 and dAMP, which are unable to completely neutralize the bilayer [54], as shown in Figure 4. Colloid instability induced by oligonucleotide or salt could be associated with bilayer fusion [54]. In contrast, mononucleotide neither reduced colloid stability over the low range of concentrations tested nor caused BF fusion [54].

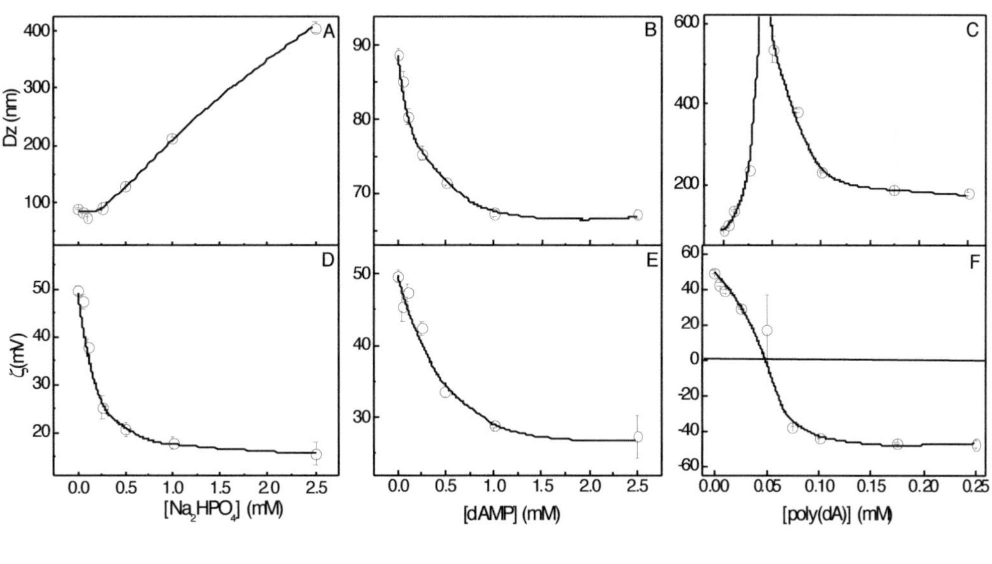

Figure 4. Effect of [Na_2HPO_4], [dAMP] or [poly (dA)] concentrations on the zeta-average diameter (A, B and C) and zeta-potential of DODAB BF at 0.5 mM DODAB (D, E and F).Reprinted from reference [54].Reprinted from Biochimica et Biophysica Acta (BBA)-Biomembranes, 1808/3, Julio H.K. Rozenfeld,Tiago R. Oliveira,M. Teresa Lamy,Ana M. Carmona-Ribeiro, Interaction of cationic bilayer fragments with a model oligonucleotide, 649-655.Copyright 2011, with permission from Elsevier.

Particles are finding a large variety of biomedical and pharmaceutical applications since their size scale can be similar to that of biomacromolecules (e.g., proteins, DNA) and structures (e.g., bacteria and viruses). Their utility for imaging, gene and drug delivery, and vaccine design is undeniable [69,70].Particulate systems are naturally targeted to antigen presenting cells (APC) so that particles deliver antigens to APC more efficiently than soluble antigen [71,72].Positively charged particles with diameters of 500 nm and below were shown to be optimal for dendritic cells uptake [42].DODAB bilayers electrostatically combine with a vast variety of negatively charged biomolecules or biological structures [14]. Silica [17], latex [21,73,74] or hydrophobic drug particles [51,75] have been coated with DODAB with optimal bilayer deposition on particles achieved by coalescence of bilayer fragments at an adequate ionic strength [17,76]. Figure 5 shows how DODAB can cover oppositely charged polystyrene nanoparticles modifying their charge as shown in reference [19]. These cationic nanoparticles contrast with alum regarding their small size and very low polydispersity as shown in Table 1 taken from reference [19]. The optimal bilayer coverage of polystyrene sulfate (PSS) nanoparticles with a DODAB bilayer produces homodisperse particles that successfully present a mixture of purified 18/14 *Taenia crassiceps* proteins (18/14-Tcra) to the immunological system [19].

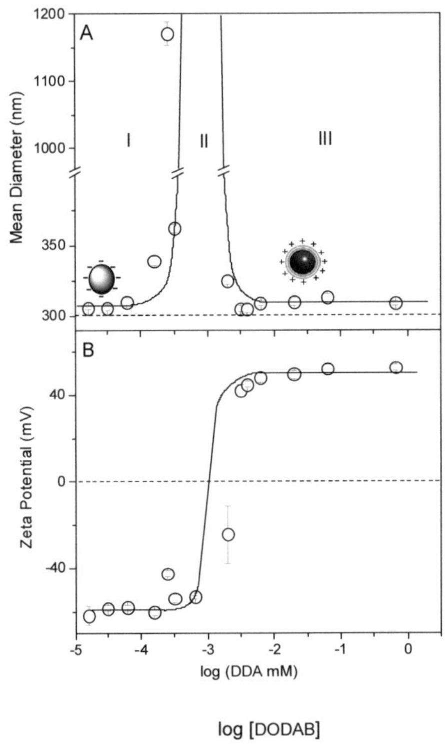

Figure 5. Effect of [DODAB] (in mM) on mean z-average diameter (A) and zeta-potential (B) of PSS particles at 5 x 10^9 particles/mL, 25 °C, in 1 mM NaCl. Bare particle diameter is 301 ± 2 nm. Regions I, II and III define particle charge, which is negative, zero and positive, respectively, from reference [19]. Reprinted from International Journal of Pharmaceutics, 340 / 1–2, N. Lincopan, N.M. Espíndola, A.J. Vaz, A.M. Carmona-Ribeiro, Cationic supported lipid bilayers for antigen presentation, 216-222.Copyright 2007, with permission from Elsevier.

Dispersion	[DODAB] (mM)	[Ag] (μg/mL)	Mean diameter (nm)	Zeta-Potential (mV)	Polydispersity
PSS	-	-	301 ± 2	-60 ± 1	0.064 ± 0.020
DODAB	2.00	-	81 ± 1	45 ± 2	0.230 ± 0.006
PSS/DODAB	0.01	-	309 ± 2	48 ± 2	0.040 ± 0.010
18/14-*Tcra*	-	25	310 ± 5	-52 ± 1	0.214 ± 0.030
DODAB/18/14-*Tcra*	0.01	25	295 ± 3	6 ± 6	0.167 ± 0.023
PSS/DODAB/18/14-*Tcra*	0.01	25	328 ± 3	11 ± 8	0.060 ± 0.020
$Al(OH)_3$	-	-	883 ± 29	28 ± 3	0.381 ± 0.013
$Al(OH)_3$/18/14-*Tcra*	-	25	9574 ± 2361	-23 ± 1	0.525 ± 0.030

Table 1. Physical properties of particles, DODAB dispersion, DODAB-covered particles, proteins and proteins/DODAB-covered particles at 1 mM NaCl.Particles concentration is 5 x 10^9 particles /mL; PSS particle diameter from transmission electron microscopy is 301±2 nm.The $Al(OH)_3$ and PSS were tested at final concentration of 0.05 and 0.075 mg/mL, respectively,from reference [19]. Reprinted from International Journal of Pharmaceutics, 340 / 1–2, N. Lincopan, N.M. Espíndola, A.J. Vaz, A.M. Carmona-Ribeiro, Cationic supported lipid bilayers for antigen presentation, 216-222. Copyright 2007, with permission from Elsevier.

Several cationic agents have been employed for DNA compaction such as cationic peptides and proteins [77], cationic lipids [78], cationic polyelectrolytes, cationic surfactants, or iron (III) [79].DNA compaction has also been used to model chromatin structure and its influence on gene expression. The self-assembled complex of basic histone proteins wrapped by approximately two turns of DNA is a nucleosome, which is the building block in the chromatin structure where DNA of lengths on the order of meters suffers compaction into an~10 μm diameter cell nucleous. Phage DNA, for example, is remarkable for its density of packing. In solution the 40 kbp T7 genome with its contour length of 13.6 μm might span a space several micrometers across and in an infected bacterium, ~1 μm across. Thus, confinement to a 55 nm capsid represents a compaction marked by a density increase by a factor of ~10^4 [80]. Systematic studies on the physical chemistry of the association between cationic nanoparticles and DNA yield rather complex phase diagrams as a function of particle size and concentration [81,82].The way in which positively charged nanoparticles tie up DNA is not obvious, and mechanisms change dramatically with particle size [83]. Only the smallest (10 nm) particles allowed transcription to occur at intermediate loading densities. Larger particles shut transcription down rather abruptly [81]. Cationic nanoparticles have found many uses such as efficient cell transfection agents *in vitro* [84-86] and complexation with long-chained DNA as a simple model of chromatin for transcription studies [81, 87].The compaction of long duplex DNA by cationic nanoparticles (NP) used as a primary model of histone core particles has been systematically studied regarding the effect of salt concentration, particle size, and particle charge by means of single-molecule observations from fluorescence and transmission electron microscopy [87]. DNA compaction proceeds through the formation of beads-on-a-string structures of various morphologies with DNA adsorbed amount per particle depending weakly on NP concentration but increasing with particle size and being optimal at an intermediate salt concentration [87]. Three different complexation mechanisms were proposed: free DNA adsorption onto NP surface, DNA wrapping around NP, and NP collection on DNA chain [87]. On the other hand, particle size has been recognized as an important parameter that determines the mechanism of particle entry into cells. Particles with a diameter of 200 nm or less enter cells almost exclusively via the clathrin-coated pathway whereas particles with a larger diameter penetrate cells via caveolae-mediated endocytosis [88,89].Cationic biomimetic particles produced from adsorption of dioctadecyldimethylammonium bromide (DODAB) bilayers onto polystyrene sulfate (PSS) microspheres have been described by our group since 1992 [18,73,76,90].These cationic bilayer-covered particles exhibit a narrow size distribution and can be produced at any desired size ranging from 70-500 nm of mean hydrodynamic diameter [90]. Polystyrene sulfate (PSS) particles with different sizes were covered by a dioctadecyldimethylammonium bromide (DODAB) bilayer yielding the so-called cationic biomimetic particles (PSS/DODAB). These cationic particles are highly organized, present a narrow size distribution and were obtained over a range of particle sizes [53,90].Thereafter, upon adding λ, T5 or T2-DNA to PSS/DODAB particles, supramolecular assemblies PSS/DODAB/DNA were obtained and characterized over a range of DNA concentrations and particle sizes (80-700 nm). Over the low DNA concentration range, PSS/DODAB/DNA assemblies were cationic, colloidally stable with moderate polydispersity and high cytotoxicity against *E. coli*. From the DNA concentration corresponding to charge neutralization, neutral or anionic supramolecular assemblies PSS/DODAB/DNA exhibited low colloid stability, high polydispersity and moderate cytotoxicity [53]. Some nucleosome mimetic assemblies were observed by atomic force microscopy (AFM) at charge neutralization (zeta-potential equal to zero) [55].Figure 6 shows how cationic nanoparticles can induce DNA compaction [53].

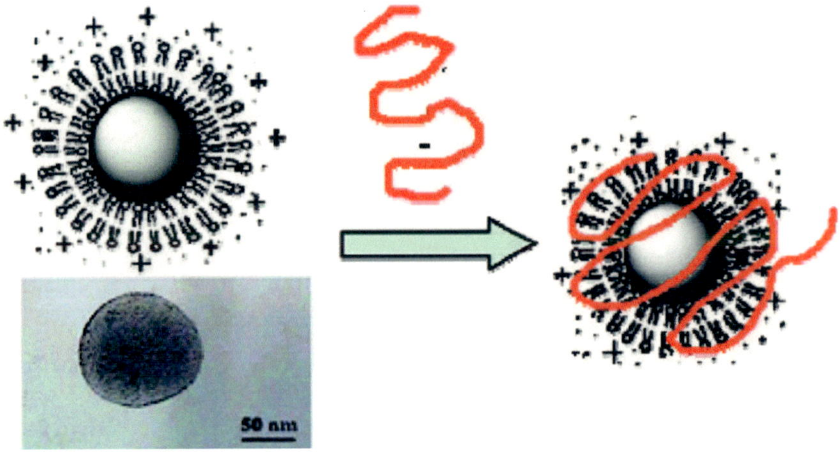

Figure 6. DNA compaction by biomimetic cationic particles of polystyrene microspheres covered by a DODAB cationic bilayer from reference [53].Adapted with permission from Rosa H, Petri DF, Carmona-Ribeiro AM.Interactions between bacteriophage DNA and cationic biomimetic particles. J Phys Chem B. 2008; 112(51):16422-30.Copyright (2008) American Chemical Society.

DNA sequences containing unmethylated CpG dinucleotide are recognized as danger signals by the immune system since they are typical of bacteria and viruses but rare in vertebrates [91, 92]. Natural or synthetic sequences containing unmethylated CpG motifs activate cells that express Toll-like receptor 9 to induce an innate immune response characterized by the production of Th1 and proinflammatory cytokines [92]. Hence, CpG has been extensively used in the induction of cellular immune responses against cancer [63, 93], intracellular infections by pathogens [94, 95] and allergies [62,96]. Both CpG [92] and DODAB BF [27] were reported to improve Th1 responses against antigens when used separately. Recently, DODAB BF and CpG were combined in a single assembly aiming at the comparison between the small, stable and cationic DODAB BF carrying ovalbumin (OVA) and the small, stable and anionic DODAB BF/OVA/CpG assemblies of very similar sizes but opposite charges [97]. Both adjuvants produced similar enhanced Th1 immune responses despite their opposite charges emphasizing the novel concept that particle charge does not matter. In comparison with the traditional alum, the size minimization for the cationic assemblies elicited different responses: alum drove the Th2 whereas DODAB BF/OVA/CpG and DODAB BF/OVA drove the Th1 response. The effects of DODAB BF or DODAB BF/CpG adjuvants with opposite charges but very similar sizes showed that the charge is not important but the size is [97]. Table 2 shows the physical properties of the assemblies. A comparison between mean hydrodynamic diameter (Dz), zeta-potentials and polydispersities for DODAB BF/OVA/CpG and $Al(OH)_3$/OVA/CpG as reproduced from reference [97]. At 20 μM CpG and 0.1 mg/mL $Al(OH)_3$, the dispersion was characterized by a low colloidal stability (large Dz, low zeta-potential (ζ) and high polydispersity). OVA stabilized both $Al(OH)_3$ or $Al(OH)_3$/CpG to a certain extent (Table 2). However, sizes were still larger than those determined for assemblies based on DODAB BF (Table 2). In particular, polydispersity for DODAB BF/OVA/CpG was notably low (0.150) and well below the one obtained for DODAB BF only (0.251), suggesting that OVA/CpG induced stabilization of the DODAB BF dispersion (Table 2).

Dispersion	Dz ± δ (nm)	ζ ± δ (mV)	Polydispersity ± δ
DODAB BF	67 ± 0	47 ± 1	0.251 ± 0.006
DODAB BF/ OVA	274 ± 2	21 ± 0	0.291 ± 0.008
DODAB BF/ OVA/ CpG	245 ± 1	-26 ± 1	0.150 ± 0.020
$Al(OH)_3$	3147 ± 197	16 ± 2	0.415 ± 0.018
$Al(OH)_3$/ OVA	916 ± 17	-29 ± 1	0.231 ± 0.020
$Al(OH)_3$/ CpG	3584 ± 74	9 ± 1	0.407 ± 0.026
$Al(OH)_3$/ OVA/ CpG	570 ± 19	-35 ± 2	0.210 ± 0.020

Table 2. Physical properties of alum or DODAB BF dispersions combined with ovalbumin (OVA) and/or CpG oligonucleotide. Concentrations are 0.1mg/mL OVA, 0.1mM DODAB BF, 0.1mg/mL $Al(OH)_3$ and 20μM CpG. Reprinted from reference [97]. Reprinted from Journal of Controlled Release, 160/2, Julio H.K. Rozenfeld, Sandriana R. Silva, Priscila A. Ranéia, Eliana Faquim-Mauro, Ana M. Carmona-Ribeiro, Stable assemblies of cationic bilayer fragments and CpG oligonucleotide with enhanced immunoadjuvant activity *in vivo*, 367-373.Copyright 2012, with permission from Elsevier.

At 0.1 mg/mL OVA, the dependence of DODAB BF/OVA size and zeta-potential on time and [DODAB] established 0.1 mM DODAB as suitable for obtaining stable and cationic DODAB BF/ OVA assemblies [97]. At 0.1 mM DODAB, 0.1 mg/mL OVA and 0.006 mM CpG, the zeta-potential is zero showing charge neutralization [97]. At [CpG]> 0.006 mM, good colloidal stability for the anionic assemblies due to charge overcompensation was observed whereas at 0.020 mM CpG, these DODAB BF/OVA/CpG assemblies turned out to be highly effective *in vivo* generating responses similar to those elicited by the stable and cationic DODAB BF/OVA. The anti-OVA delayed-type hypersensitivity (DTH) reaction and the secretion of IFN-gamma and IL-12 resulted 6, 42 and 9 times larger for the DODAB BF/OVA/CpG-immunized mice than the same responses by OVA-immunized mice, respectively [97].Figure 7 A and B illustrate the colloidal stability of the assemblies over a range of DODAB concentrations.

The delayed-type hypersensitivity reaction (DTH) is an important *in vivo* response mediated by cells that can be quantified from the footpad sweelling test [44]. Mice immunized with OVA alone or with DODAB BF/CpG or with OVA / $Al(OH)_3$ exhibited a footpad swelling equal to the one observed for naive mice [97]. The largest increase in footpad swelling was observed for DODAB BF/OVA/CpG mice immunization, which was about 6 times larger than the one observed for naive mice and 1.3 times larger than the one observed for DODAB BF/OVA [97]. Figure 7 C shows the improved DTH response in mice induced by the assemblies as adapted from reference [97].

Since OVA isoelectric point is 4.5 [98], this protein is negatively charged at 6.3, the pH of water. Thus, OVA adsorption onto DODAB BF is initially electrostatically driven.The OVA titration with DODAB BF determined ranges of DODAB concentration for occurrence of stable DODAB BF/OVA assemblies as illustrated in Figure 7 A and B. Similar results had been previously described also for DODAB BF/ bovin serum albumin or DODAB BF/ purified antigens from *Taenia crassiceps* [27].When the net charge of the assemblies is zero (at charge neutralization), maximal aggregation was observed for the assemblies. Further increasing DODAB concentration, stabilized them to a certain extent (Figure 7 B). However, sizes and polydispersities were still higher than those of DODAB BF in absence of OVA. Optimal colloidal stability was only achieved upon CpG addition to the system yielding high and negative zeta-potentials plus remarkably small polydispersity [98]. Oligonucleotides with less than 20 nucleotide residues usually behave as rigid charged rods in solution [99]. CpG would also adsorb as rigid charged rods on vacant positive sites of DODAB BF/ OVA assemblies inducing charge overcompensation and recovery of colloidal stability as previously described for a model oligonucleotide above charge neutralization [56].

Figure 7 also illustrates the improvement in the cellular OVA-specific response from the analysis of cytokines secreted by lymph node cells of mice as adapted from reference [97]. IFN-γ and IL-12 production is associated to the Th1 response whereas IL-10 and IL-13 production reflects the Th2 response. Levels of IFN-γ and IL-12 secretion observed in cell cultures of mice immunized with OVA or $Al(OH)_3$/ OVA were low and close to the detection limit for these cytokine assays (Figure 7). For mice immunized with OVA/CpG or DODAB BF/OVA assemblies, the secretion of IFN-γ and IL-12 substantially increased in comparison to secretion from cultured cells of OVA-immunized mice [97]. For the DODAB BF/OVA/CpG immunized mice, the secretion of IFN-γ and IL-12 increased by 33 and 49 %, respectively when compared to DODAB BF/OVA-immunized mice group and 52% and 35% when compared to OVA/CpG-group. In contrast, the highest secretion of IL-10 and IL-13 was observed in cultures of cells from mice that were immunized with Al(OH)3 /OVA whereas all other assemblies resulted in poor production of these cytokines [97]. Immune responses were similar for anionic DODAB BF/OVA/CpG and cationic DODAB BF/OVA of similar sizes showing that the charge is not important but the size is. The adsorption of antigen on the surface of DODAB large vesicles was shown to stimulate active antigen capture and presentation by dendritic cells (DCs) [41]. Administration of antigen adsorbed on DODAB large vesicles (LV) resulted in formation of an antigen depot at the site of injection which hampered the rapid clearance of antigen that takes place in absence of a carrier [100]. In contrast to DODAB LV, the small DODAB BF/antigen assemblies did not result in any observable depot effect [27, 97]. Furthermore, since the depot was absent for DODAB BF/CpG/OVA the immunostimulatory effect must have occurred via direct effect of the assemblies on the lymphonode antigen presenting cells [97]. Only nanoparticles can specifically target lymph node-resident cells [101]. CpG combined with DODAB BF yielded improved cellular Th1 response [97] possibly due to the appropriate targeting of DODAB BF/CpG/antigen to DCs in charge of expressing endosomal toll like receptor 9 (TLR9) in the lymph nodes [102]. The enhanced Th1 response by anionic DODAB BF/OVA/CpG relative to OVA alone was evidenced by the 6 times increase in DTH reaction, the 42 times increase in IFN-γ secretion by lymph node cells in culture and the 9 times increase in IL-12 secretion also by lymph node cells in culture (Figure 7) [97].

Other delivery systems based on anionic [103] or cationic lipid bilayer [41,44,100,104,105] have also been successful for improving Th1 response against important antigens such as those of influenza [103], hepatitis A and B [103,104], and fungal infections [105]. In general, cationic lipids are known for the production of a large inflammatory response [41, 44].However, for small cationic bilayer fragments as immunoadjuvants, this adverse reaction is absent [27, 97]. The small and anionic DODAB BF/OVA/CpG assemblies [97] also did not elicit adverse reactions similarly to other anionic assemblies [103]. There was no depot effect for these small assemblies [97] and their net negative charge ensured the absence of the adverse reactions observed previously for the large cationic liposomes and vesicles [100]. Recently, based on cross reactivity with *Neisseria lactamica* outer membrane vesicles (OMV) antigens, DODAB BF were combined with OMV to develop a vaccine against *Neisseria meningitidis* in young children [106]. Complexes of 25 μg of OMV in 0.1 mM of DODAB BF were colloidally stable, exhibiting optimal physical properties for efficient antigen presentation [106].

3. Cationic nanostructures based on chitosan and other biocompatible polymers

Chitin is a long-chain polymer of N-acetylglucosamine, a derivative of glucose which can be deacetylated to yield chitosan as shown in Figure 8.

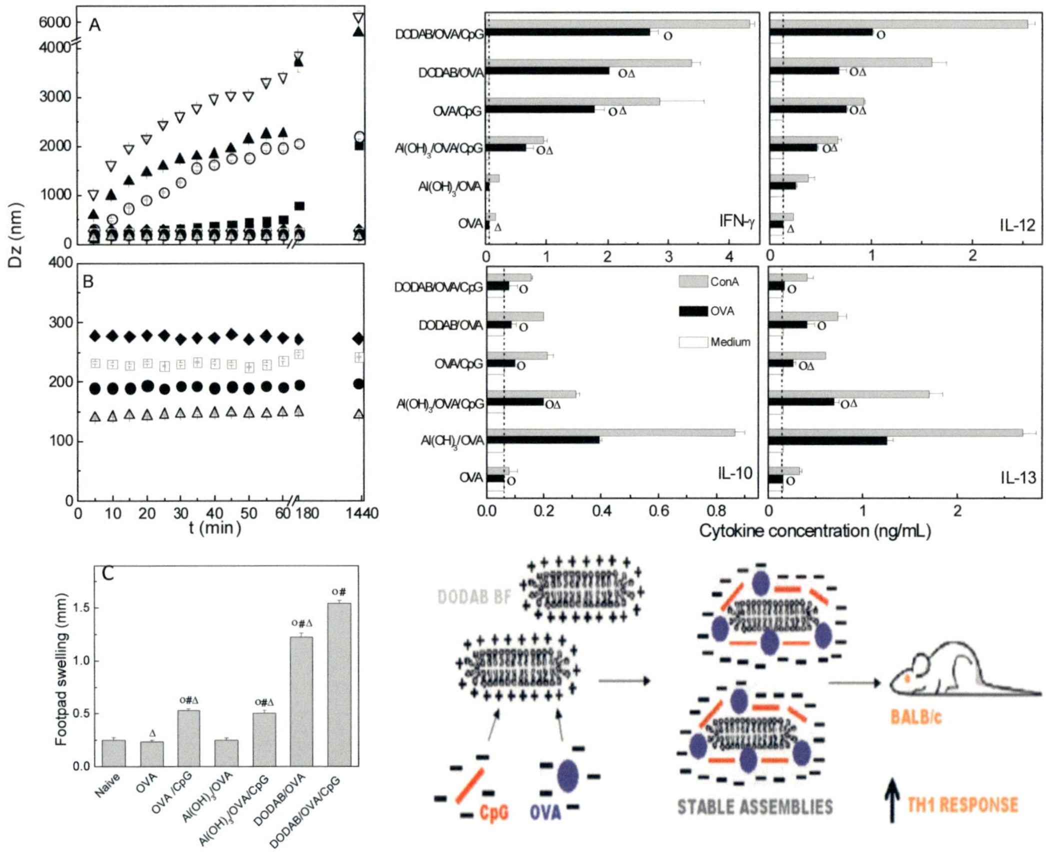

Figure 7. Nanostructures of cationic bilayer fragments and CpG oligonucleotide with enhanced immunoadjuvant activity *in vivo*. In (A), the effect of time and DODAB concentration on zeta-average diameter of DODAB BF/OVA assemblies is seen from the kinetics obtained after adding DODAB BF at a final concentration of 0.005 (■); 0.01 (○); 0.02 (▲); 0.05 (▽); 0.1 (◆); 0.2 (□); 0.5 (●) and 1mM DODAB (△) to 0.1mg/mL OVA. In (B), kinetical data are detailed for the larger DODAB BF concentrations.Assemblies were prepared in 1mM NaCl.In (C), delayed-type hypersensitivity response for BALB/c mice immunized with OVA in different adjuvant formulations determined from the footpad swelling (nm) ± standard error of the mean. Final concentrations are 0.1mM DODAB BF, 20μM CpG and 0.1mg/mL $Al(OH)_3$ and 0.1mg/mL OVA. $p< 0.05$ compared to naive (○), $p< 0.05$ compared to OVA/$Al(OH)_3$ (#) and $p< 0.05$ compared to OVA/DODAB/CpG (△) from reference [97].Adapted from Journal of Controlled Release, 160/2, Julio H.K. Rozenfeld, Sandriana R. Silva, Priscila A. Ranéia, Eliana Faquim-Mauro, Ana M. Carmona-Ribeiro, Stable assemblies of cationic bilayer fragments and CpG oligonucleotide with enhanced immunoadjuvant activity *in vivo*, 367-373.Copyright 2012, with permission from Elsevier.

Since they are biocompatible, biodegradable by deacetylases, mucoadhesive, and nontoxic, with antimicrobial, antiviral, and adjuvant properties, chitin, chitosan and their derivatives have been widely applied in medicine, pharmacy and vaccine design [107, 108]. Chitosan is soluble in diluted acids but is insoluble in water due to deprotonation of its amino moiety [109]. The poor solubility of chitosan at the pH of water represents a serious limitation for its applications as an immunoadjuvant in the clinics [107]. Several chitosan derivatives have been obtained to circumvent this limitation.For example, by attaching galactose moieties to the

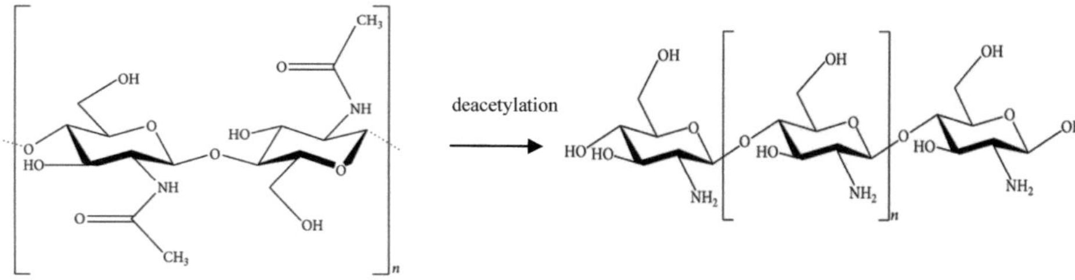

Figure 8. Chitin yielding chitosan by deacetylation.

chitosan molecules, a new water-soluble compound, glycated chitosan (GC), was synthesized [109,110]. GC is a non-toxic biodegradable product used in laser immunotherapy (LIT) which combines local laser irradiation and local administration of GC at primary or metastatic cancers where the tumoral antigens of the irradiated tumor cells combined with GC elicit a potent immune response against the cancer [111,112]. After the first step involving tumor irradiation with a laser beam that causes swelling and disruption of tumor cells by thermal effect, the local injection of GC as immunoadjuvant would lead to the capture of the tumoral antigens by dendritic cells and migration to the lymph nodes where the antigens would be presented to T cells, thus activating cytotoxic T-lymphocytes [113-115]. LIT using GC induced regression of primary and secondary tumours in rats and caused resistance to repeated challenges with tumours of the same type [116]. Furthermore, rats developed immunity could be adoptively transferred [116].

Chitosan nanoparticles have been obtained by ionotropic gelation, complex coacervation, emulsion and microemulsion techniques, and self-assembly of hydrophobically modified chitosan [117]. Ionotropic gelation consists of the ionic crosslinking of chitosan with multivalent counter-ions such as sodium tripolyphosphate (TPP) by adding a dilute chitosan acid solution to a solution of TPP or vice versa, with stirring [118]. Chitosan particles of nanometric size were obtained for chitosan concentrations up to 2.8 g L^{-1} and TPP concentrations from 0.21 to 0.43 g L^{-1}. The size and surface charge of particles can be modified by varying the ratio of chitosan and stabilizer. The main problematic aspects of the technique are the poor colloidal stability of the dispersion which may require the addition of stabilizers, and the need of using very dilute solutions which may be inconvenient when large amounts of nanoparticles are required [117]. Complex coacervation is achieved by mixing two oppositely charged polyelectrolytes. The polyelectrolyte or coacervate complex is structured as nanoparticles. Chitosan–poly (acrylic acid) (PAA) nanoparticles carrying a positive charge with sizes from 50 to 400 nm were obtained by the dropwise addition of dilute chitosan solutions [119]. Carboxymethylcellulose and alginate have also been complexed with chitosan to prepare nanoparticles. Chitosan–carboxymethylcellulose nanoparticles were subsequently coated with plasmid DNA (pDNA) [120]. Chitosan–alginate nanoparticles were loaded with insulin [121]. Nanoparticles have also been obtained in which the polyanion is the active principle itself as for example heparin or DNA or even siRNA. Chitosan–heparin nanoparticles crosslinked with TPP were described [122]. Figure 9 shows on the left a scanning electron micrograph of chitosan– heparin nanoparticles adapted from reference [117] and, on the right, an atomic force micrograph of chitosan-carboxymethylcellulose nanoparticles [123] prepared by complex coacervation without using without using any organic solvent or crosslinker. These coacervates have the interesting property of combining with cisplatin [123] but can also be combined with peptides, proteins and DNA and therefore are potentially useful for vaccine design.

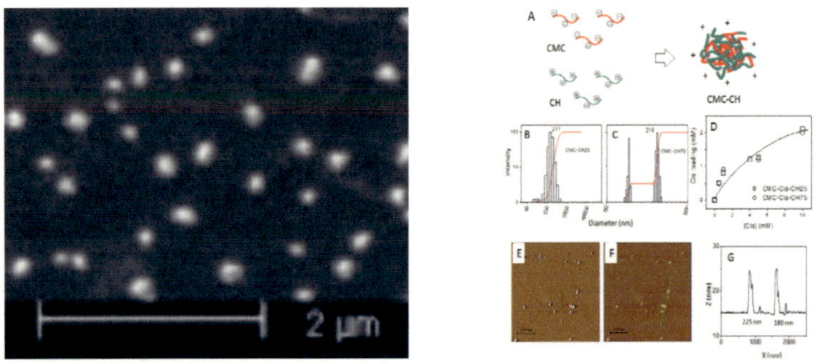

Figure 9. Nanoparticles obtained by complex coacervation of oppositely charged polyelectrolytes: chitosan-heparin on the left [117] and chitosan-carboxymethylcellulose on the right [123].On the left, adapted with permission from Peniche H, Peniche C. Polym Int. Chitosan nanoparticles: a contribution to nanomedicine.2011; 60:883–889. DOI: 10.1002/pi.3056, http://onlinelibrary.wiley.com/doi/10.1002/pi.3056/abstract. Copyright 2011, John Wiley and Sons.On the right, adapted with permission from Vieira DB, Kim V, Petri DFS, Menck CFM, Carmona-Ribeiro AM. Supra-molecular assemblies of cisplatin and polyelectrolytes: preparation, characterization and activity against cancer cells. In: Laudon M, Romanowicz B. (eds.) Nanotech Conference & Expo 2012: An Interdisciplinary Integrative Forum on Nanotechnology, Microtechnology, Biotechnology and Cleantechnology, Santa Clara, CA, United States, June 18-21, 2012 (2012), 3, 182-185. Publisher: (CRC Press, Boca Raton, FLA) ISBN 978-1-4665-6287-5.

Other interesting chitosan derivatives have been synthesized and used for the preparation of nanoparticles such as N-trimethylchitosan (TMC) and mono-N-carboxymethyl chitosan (MCC) [124]. In general, mucosal applications of antigens result in poor immune responses. Therefore, mucoadhesive adjuvants are required to enhance the immune response by improving both antigen protection and its cellular uptake. Nanoparticles of TMC or MCC were prepared using the ionic gelation method and loaded with tetanus toxoid (TT) exhibiting high loading efficacy (>90% m/m), sizes within the range of 40-400nm and negative or positive surface charge for MCC and TMC, respectively [124]. The structural integrity of the TT in the formulations was confirmed by SDS-PAGE electrophoresis and the intranasal application in mice elicited high serum IgG titres [124].Figure 10 illustrates the excellent uptake by macrophages of these nanoparticles labeled with a green fluorescent marker as adapted from [124].

Due to the positive charge of chitosan and TMC, and the negative charge of TT, the antigen loading is driven by the electrostatic attraction. There is also a superior association and internalization of chitosan or chitosan derivatives nanoparticles with cells due to their mucoadhesive character [125-127]. CS nanoparticles have a higher association and internalisation with gastrointestinal tissue cells due to electrostatic interactions compared to polystyrene nanoparticles [125].More recently, hybrid nanoparticles based on the complexation between oppositely charged chitosan derivatives (positively charged TMC and negatively

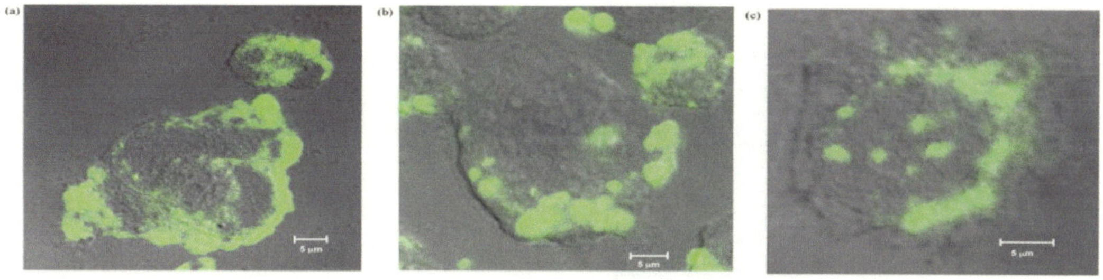

Figure 10. Uptake of chitosan (a), TMC (b) and MCC nanoparticles loaded with bovine serum albumin and labeled with a green fluorescent marker adapted from reference [124].Reprinted from International Journal of Pharmaceutics, 363/1–2, B. Sayın, S. Somavarapu, X.W. Li, M. Thanou, D. Sesardic, H.O.Alpar, S. Şenel, Mono-N-carboxymethyl chitosan (MCC) andN-trimethyl chitosan (TMC) nanoparticles for non-invasive vaccine delivery, 139-148. Copyright 2008, with permission from Elsevier.

charged MCC) without using any organic solvent or crosslinker yielded results similar to those described for the non hybrid nanoparticles [128].

A very promising approach is the development of vaccines based on the initiation of immune response by transfecting dendritic cells (DC) with DNA encoding tumor-associated antigens or immunostimulatory molecules such as cytokines or chemokines [129].Although unmodified chitosan may not be a good gene delivery carrier for DCs because of its low transfection efficiency, some modified chitosans showed improved behavior in delivering genes into DCs. IL-12 gene was delivered to DCs *in vivo* using mannosylated chitosan (MC) via mannose receptor-mediated endocytosis [130,131]. MC not only has good physicochemical properties and low cytotoxicity, but also transfect DCs with much higher efficiency than do the unmodified chitosan particles *in vitro* [130]. *In vivo*, intratumoral injection of MC /plasmid encoding murine IL-12 complex into BALB/c mice bearing CT-26 carcinoma cells clearly suppressed tumor growth and angiogenesis, and significantly induced cell cycle arrest and apoptosis [131]. Mannose-bearing chitosan nanoparticles were also synthesized to entrap complexes of DNA with polyethyleneimine (PEI) and improve the delivery of DNA into antigen-presenting cells (APCs) after intramuscular (i.m.) injection [132]. Compared with the traditional chitosan microspheres, these nanoparticles targeted the DCs (which express a high density of mannose receptors when they are immature) and released their PEI/DNA cargo inside them. After i.m. immunization, the MC/PEI/DNA nanospheres induced significantly enhanced serum antibody and cytotoxic T lymphocyte (CTL) responses in comparison to naked DNA [132]. Figure 11 shows the MC/PEI/DNA nanoparticles and superior cumulative DNA release *in vitro* of these nanoparticles in PBS buffer as adapted from reference [132].

In recent years, DC vaccines, especially DNA-based DC vaccines, have been the focus of attention in immunotherapy against cancer [129]. Genetically engineered DCs previously modified *in vitro* can then be implanted *ex vivo* and activate the tumor-specific CTL response for the killing of cancer cells [129]. Most of these immunotherapy approaches based on DCs genetic modification for the treatment of melanoma [133,134], renal carcinoma [135] and other malignant diseases [136] are in phase I/II clinical trials. However, in many of these clinical trials adenovirus vector is the carrier still employed for DCs modification [137].Since the major

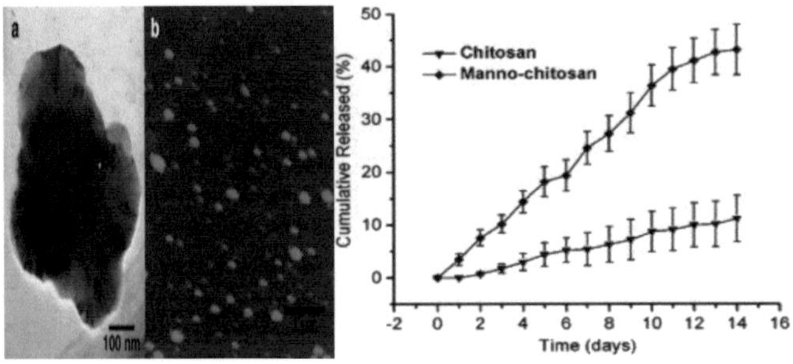

Figure 11. Atomic force micrograph of MC nanoparticles. Release profiles of chitosan and MC nanoparticles as determined from 10 mg of nanoparticles suspended in 1 ml of PBS at pH 7.4 (120mM NaCl, 2.7mM KCl, 10mM PBS) at 37 °C under stirring. At predetermined time intervals, the suspension was centrifuged and replaced with the same volume of fresh medium. The DNA concentration in the supernatant was determined by absorbance at 260nm.Adapted with permission from reference [132]. Reprinted from Journal of Controlled Release, 121 /3, Xianfeng Zhou, Bin Liu, Xianghui Yu, Xizhen Zhang, Yu Chen, Xueyun Wang, Yinghuan Jin, Yongge Wu, Yue Chen, Yaming Shan, Yan Chen, Junqiu Liu, Wei Kong, Jiacong Shen, Controlled release of PEI/DNA complex from mannose-bearing chitosan microspheres as a potent delivery system to enhance immune response to HBV DNA vaccine, 200-207. Copyright 2007, with permission from Elsevier.

barrier for the use of nonviral carriers is their low transfer efficiency compared with viral vectors, the design of novel and efficient nonviral carriers remains a most warranted area of research. Recently, CpG was combined with chitosan in order to enhance the Th1 and Th17-cell polarizing cytokines representing a convenient strategy to elicit cell-mediated immunity [138].Alum, aluminium phosphate and calcium phosphate adjuvants, as well as biodegradable PLG microparticles, inhibited the secretion of bioactive IL-12 by DCs.Thus many of the most widely used adjuvants in preclinical and clinical use exert a specific inhibitory effect on the secretion of IL-12 by DCs. In contrast, chitosan does not inhibit IL-12 secretion and CpG-chitosan is a potent stimulus for the induction of pro-inflammatory T-cell responses [138]. CpG-chitosan [138] behaved similarly to DODAB BF/CpG [98].

The design of DC-based vaccines depends strongly on the generation of effective DCs, so that technologies are needed that produce high antigen expression as a result of delivering DNA encoding antigen into the nucleus of DCs. Barriers to gene delivery into cells start with cell adhesion and uptake, escape from endosomes to the cytoplasm prior to fusion with the lysosomes, trafficking to the nucleus and uptake by the nucleus [139].In particular, large foreign molecules such as proteins and genes are mostly unable to enter the nucleus of non-dividing cells. An interesting strategy has been the combination of cationic nanoparticles with a nuclear localization signal (NLS) which enhanced pDNA delivery to the nucleus of DCs when combined with electroporation [140].

There is a consensus in the literature that additional immunostimulation provided by LPS, CpG and other molecules are required to improve the Th1 response of cationic chitosan or quaternized trimethylchitosan (TMC) [138,141].These nanoparticles containing ovalbumin as a model antigen (TMC/OVA nanoparticles) and an immunopotentiator (TMC/OVA/immunopotentiator nanoparticles) were recently evaluated [141]. The selection of immunopotentiators included Tolllike receptor (TLR) ligands lipopolysaccharide (LPS), PAM3CSK4 (PAM), CpG

DNA, the NOD-like receptor 2 ligand muramyl dipeptide (MDP) and the GM1 ganglioside receptor ligand, cholera toxin B subunit (CTB). The TMC/OVA/immunopotentiator nanoparticles were characterised regarding their immunogenicity by determining the serum IgG, IgG1, IgG2a titres and secretory IgA levels in nasal washes after intradermal and nasal vaccination in mice. After nasal vaccination, TMC/OVA nanoparticles containing LPS or MDP elicited higher IgG, IgG1 and sIgA levels than non-adjuvanted TMC/OVA particles, whereas nanoparticles containing CTB, PAM or CpG did not. After intradermal vaccination, the TMC/OVA/CpG and TMC/OVA/LPS nanoparticles provoked higher IgG titres than plain TMC/OVA particles [141]. Co-encapsulation of the antigen and an additional immunopotentiator into TMC nanoparticles improved the immunogenicity of the vaccine [141].

Nanoparticles of Fe_3O_4 coated with glutamic acid plus PEI were used to encapsulate DNA encoding a potent antigen of *Mycobacterium tuberculosis* (Ag85A-ESAT-6) plus IL-21 generating a strong immune response and marked growth inhibition of *M. tuberculosis* in mice [142]. More importantly, compared with using DNA vaccine Ag85A-ESAT-6-IL-21 alone, the nanoparticle-based DNA vaccine Ag85A-ESAT-6-IL-21 showed a statistically significant increase in the protective efficacy against *M. tuberculosis* infection in the immunized mice [142]. The expression of both the fusion protein of Ag85A-ESAT-6 and secreted IL-21 protein was confirmed by western blot [142]. Cationic poly(lactide-co-glycolide) (PLGA) nanoparticles were obtained by coating the PLGA nanoparticles with chitosan and used as an intranasal delivery vehicle as a means of administering foot and mouth disease virus (FMDV) DNA vaccine encoding the FMDV capsid protein and the bovine IL-6 gene as a means of enhancing mucosal and systemic immune responses in animals [143]. Guinea pigs and rats were intranasally vaccinated with the respective chitosan-coated PLGA nano/microparticles-loaded FMDV DNA vaccine formulations; the IL-6 gene was important as an additional immunoestimulator [143].

Cationized gelatin nanoparticles (GNPs) were used as carriers to improve delivery of immunostimulatory CpG oligonucleotides (CpG ODN) both *in vitro* and *in vivo* [144]. Gelatin nanoparticles were prepared according to the two step desolvation method including further optimization [145].Briefly, 1.25 g gelatin was dissolved in 25 ml highly purified water (5%w/w) at 50oC under constant stirring (700 rpm). The first desolvation step was initiated by quick addition of 25 ml acetone. After discarding the supernatant containing low molecular weight fractions of gelatin, the sediment was redissolved in 25 ml water under constant stirring at 50 oC. Depending on the desired particle size, the pH was then adjusted to a value between 2.3 (approx.resulting particle size: 150 nm) and 3.0 (approx. resulting particle size: 300 nm).Subsequently, the second desolvation step was initiated by drop-wise addition of 50 ml acetone (during constant stirring at 700 rpm) and resulted in the formation of nanoparticles. The nanoparticles were stabilized by cross-linking with glutaraldehyde (150 ml of a 25% solution) under stirring. After 12 h the particles were purified from non-reacted glutaraldehyde by centrifugation and redispersion in water. Cationization of the nanoparticles was achieved through introduction of a quaternary amino group by covalent coupling of cholaminechloride hydrochloride onto the particles surface.The delivery by cationic gelatin nanoparticles strongly increased the imunostimulatory effects of CpG oligonucleotides [144].

The effects of CpG are not restricted to modulation of immune responses in vaccine adjuvants. CpG itself has been considered for the treatment of asthma and other allergic diseases [62]. CpG oligonucleotides (CpG–ODN, resembling bacterial DNA) engage TLR-9 on B-cells, dendritic cells and other cell types, resulting in a cascade that includes induction of Th1-type and T-regulatory-type immune responses. Preclinical models of asthma have demonstrated that CpG–ODN are potent inhibitors of atopic responses, suppressing Th2 cytokine and, reducing airway eosinophilia, systemic levels of IgE, and bronchial hyperreactivity-in short the critical attributes of the asthmatic phenotype. In models of chronic allergen exposure, CpG–ODN are also effective at preventing the development of airway remodeling. In established asthma, CpG–ODN can reverse manifestations of disease, both when used alone or in combination with allergen immunotherapy. Early clinical trials have had mixed results, including a significant benefit when CpG–ODN were conjugated to ragweed allergen in an allergic rhinitis immunotherapy study, but only limited efficacy seen when administered prior to allergen challenge in asthmatics [145]. Further study of CpG–ODNs for the treatment of asthma and other atopic disorders is warranted by existing data.Figure 12 summarizes the cellular trafficking of CpG [62].

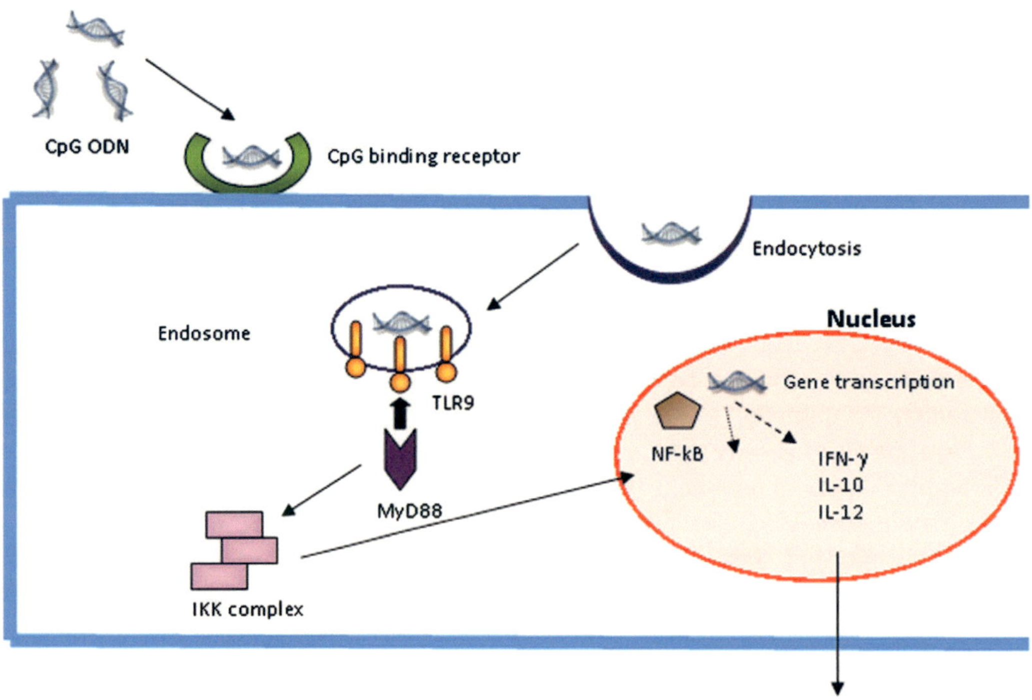

Figure 12. CpG–ODNs are bound by CpG binding protein at the cell surface. The oligonucleotide then undergoes endocytosis where it is bound by TLR9 in the endosome. TLR9 then interacts with MyD88 and the IKK complex and is translocated to the cell nucleus. Once in the cell nucleus, the CpG ODNs activate NF-kB and initiate the induction of cytokines and chemokines.Reproduced with permission from reference [62].Reprinted from Advanced Drug Delivery Reviews, 61 / 3, David E. Fonseca, Joel N. Kline, Use of CpG oligonucleotides in treatment of asthma and allergic disease, 256-272. Copyright 2009, with permission from Elsevier.

Polymer-based nanoscale assemblies based on cationic polymers have been intensively searched for biomedical applications [146-148]. Poly(2-aminoethyl methacrylate) (PAEM) cationic homopolymers with defined chain length and narrow molecular weight distribution were synthesized using atom transfer radical polymerization (ATRP), and PAEM/plasmid DNA polyplexes interaction with DCs showed its potential for DNA vaccines [149]. PAEM of different chain lengths (45, 75, and 150 repeating units) showed varying strength in condensing plasmid DNA into narrowly dispersed nanoparticles with very low cytotoxicity. Longer polymer chain length resulted in higher levels of overallcellular uptake and nuclear uptake of plasmid DNA, but shorter polymer chains favored intracellular and intranuclear release of free plasmid from the polyplexes [149]. When a model antigen-encoding ovalbumin plasmid was used, transfected DCs stimulated the activation of naïve CD8 (+) T cells to produce high levels of interferon-γ. The efficiency of transfection, DC maturation, and CD8 (+) T cell activation showed varying degrees of polymer chain-length dependence [149].These structurally defined cationic polymers may have much potential as efficient DNA vaccine carriers and immunoadjuvants.

Other strategies involve the production of hybrid nanoparticles. For example, biocompatible polymeric particles of poly caprolactone were coated with chitosan for effective immunization against influenza using recombinant Influenza A virus (A/California/07/2009) H1N1 hemagglutinin (HA) protein, for the induction of humoral, cellular and mucosal immunity [150]. CS-PCL nanoparticles (cationic nanoparticles) produced humoral (both systemic and mucosal) and cellular immune responses upon nasal administration demonstrating high potential for their use as a carrier adjuvant for nasal administered influenza antigens [150]. Other example is represented by biocompatible core-shell cationic nanoparticles, composed of an inner hard core of poly(methylmethacrylate) (PMMA) and a hydrophilic tentacular shell bearing positively charged groups and poly(ethyleneglycol) chains covalently bound to the core prepared by emulsion polymerization and characterized *in vitro* and *in vivo* for DNA vaccine applications [151]. The nanoparticles reversibly adsorbed large amounts of DNA, mainly through electrostatic interactions, preserved its functional structure, efficiently delivered it intracellularly, and were not toxic *in vitro* or *in mice* [151]. Furthermore, two intramuscular (i.m.) immunizations (4 weeks apart) with a very low dose (1 microg) of the plasmid pCV-tat delivered by these nanoparticles followed by one or two protein boosts induced significant antigen-specific humoral and cellular responses and greatly increased Th1-type T cell responses and CTLs against HIV-1 Tat [151].

Chitosan-based DNA vaccines against Japanese encephalitis virus using transdermal immunization were prepared by using the associative feature of cationic chitosan and anionic DNAs which formed nanoscale complexes [152]. The expression of green fluorescent protein (GFP) reporter gene was observable and traceable in epidermis and spleen over 3 days. The expressions of GFP and the activation of dendritic cells (DCs) were evident and co-localized in hair follicles and epidermis. Mice immunized with the developed chitosan-JEV DNA vaccines elicited desired JEV specific antibodies, whereby the mice maintained high survival rates against 50xLD(50) JEV challenge. The low-pressure-gene-gun mediated chitosan-based JEV

DNA vaccines have proven to be convenient and efficacious, thereby with high capacity in deployment for future prophylaxis against JEV outbreaks [152].

Pullulan, a fungal exopolysaccharide produced from starch is a water soluble, neutral linear biopolymer consisting of α-1,6-linked maltotriose residues. Recently, a cationic cholesteryl group-bearing pullulan (cCHP) derivative was used to obtain self-assembled nanogels for administering an intranasal vaccine containing a non-toxic subunit fragment of *Clostridium botulinum* type-A neurotoxin BoHc/A (cCHP-BoHc/A) which continuously adhered to the nasal epithelium and was effectively taken up by mucosal dendritic cells after its release from the cCHP nanogel. Vigorous botulinum-neurotoxin-A-neutralizing serum IgG and secretory IgA antibody responses were induced without co-administration of mucosal adjuvant. Importantly, intranasally administered cCHP-BoHc/A did not accumulate in the olfactory bulbs or brain. Moreover, intranasally immunized tetanus toxoid with cCHP nanogel induced strong tetanus-toxoid-specific systemic and mucosal immune responses suggesting that cCHP nanogel can be used as a universal protein-based antigen-delivery vehicle for adjuvant-free intranasal vaccination [153].Recently, the same system was used to deliver a vaccine against pneumonia [154]. This pneumococcal vaccine combined the advantages of pneumococcal surface protein A (PspA) with a nontoxic intranasal vaccine delivery system based on a nanometer-sized hydrogel cCHP. The efficacy of the nanogel-based PspA nasal vaccine (cCHP-PspA) was tested in murine pneumococcal airway infection models. Intranasal vaccination with cCHP-PspA provided protective immunity against lethal challenge with Streptococcus pneumoniae Xen10, reduced colonization and invasion by bacteria in the upper and lower respiratory tracts, and induced systemic and nasal mucosal Th17 responses, high levels of PspA-specific serum immunoglobulin G (IgG), and nasal and bronchial IgA antibody responses. Moreover, there was no sign of PspA delivery by nanogel to either the olfactory bulbs or the central nervous system after intranasal administration showing the effectiveness and safety of the nanogel-based PspA nasal vaccine system as a universal mucosal vaccine against pneumococcal respiratory infection.

Lipid-biopolymer hybrid systems have long been described for incorporation of pDNA [155].Cationic liposomes mixed with pDNA that had been pre-condensed with a polycation (e.g.protamine) yielded the LPD formulation or lipid-polymer-DNA (DOTAP, protamine, pDNA) [156]. As compared to conventional lipoplexes, the double bilayer of LPD confers greater stability and structural homogeneity to the assemblies [156]. Strong antitumor immunity could be generated when a peptide antigen was incorporated into LPD (cationic liposome-polycation-pDNA) nanoparticles [155, 156]. In another study, both the cationic liposome and DNA were shown to be required for the full immunostimulation activity of LPD [157]. The unique ability of LPD to readily move into local lymphoid tissues and to activate antigen-presenting cells might be responsible for its strong immunostimulatory activity [157]. Moreover, cationic liposome stimulates the expression of CD80/CD86 on dendritic cells (DCs), but not the release of TNF-alpha from DCs, suggesting the existence of a NF-kappa B-independent immunostimulation pathway for cationic lipids such as DOTAP [157].The LPD complexes were nanoparticles with less than 100 nm of mean diameter due to the compaction of DNA induced by the polycation [158].

Similarly, cationic maltosylated PEI (mPEI) was electrostatically complexed to a plasmid encoding the human papillomavirus (HPV) type 16L1 protein (pHPV16L1), and further complexed to a maltose binding protein (MBP)-fused human papilloma virus type 16L1 fusion protein (HPV16L1-MBP) [159]. The intracellular co-delivery of protein and plasmid DNA vaccines was significantly higher for mPEI-based triple nanocomplexes than for a simple physical mixture of the proteins and DNA [160]. The high expression levels were comparable to those obtained using dual complexes of mPEI and the plasmid DNA. In vivo, co-immunization of mice with HPV16L1-MBP/mPEI/pHPV16L1 nanocomplexes triggered the highest levels of humoral immune responses among various vaccination groups and there was a significant increase in the number of interferon-γ producing CD8 (+) T cells compared with the use of mixed proteins and plasmid DNA. This approach could enhance the immunogenicity of HPV16L1 vaccines [159].

Platelet-derived growth factor-bb (PDGF-BB) and fibroblast growth factor-2(FGF-2) are known to induce chemotaxis, proliferation, differentiation, and matrix synthesis so that growth factor therapy is an emerging treatment modality that enhances tissue vascularization, promotes healing and regeneration and can treat a variety of inflammatory diseases or promote healing of chronic wounds [160]. Chitosan was combined with PDGF-BB and FGF-2 genes to induce the therapeutic expression of these genes in mice. The percentage of the residues that are glucosamine is called the degree of deacetylation (DDA). PDGF-BB and FGF-2 genes were amplified from human tissues by RT-PCR. To increase the secretion of FGF-2, a recombinant 4sFGF-2 was constructed bearing eight amino-acid residues of the signal peptide of FGF-4. PCR products were inserted into the expression vector pVax1 to produce recombinant plasmids pVax1-4sFGF2 and pVax1-PDGF-BB, which were then injected into BALB/C mice in the format of polyelectrolyte nanocomplexes with specific chitosans of controlled DDA and molecular weight, including 92-10, 80-10, and 80-80(DDA-number average molecular weight or M(n) in kDa) [160]. ELISA assays on mice sera showed that recombinant FGF-2 and PDGF-BB proteins were efficiently expressed and specific antibodies to these proteins could be identified in sera of injected mice, but with levels that were clearly dependent on the specific chitosan used [160]. High DDA low molecular weight chitosans were efficient protein expressors with minimal or no generation of neutralizing antibodies, while lowering DDA resulted in greater antibody levels and correspondingly lower levels of detected recombinant protein. Histological analyses corroborated these results by revealing greater inflammatory infiltrates in lower DDA chitosans, which produced higher antibody titers [160]. The subcutaneous delivery of the plasmids was more efficient than the one by intramuscular injection [160]. Certain chitosans can be efficient, non-toxic and therapeutic protein delivery systems or vectors for DNA vaccines [160]. The recent advances that have led to a more rational design of chitosan polyplexes has recently been reviewed [161]. Recent progress in preparation and characterisation of chitosan based polyplexes has enabled coupling analysis of chitosans structural parameters that has led to increased transfection efficiency by tailoring of chitosan's structure in accordance with a more rational design of chitosan polyplexes [161].

Genetic vaccination against leishmaniasis has been intensively pursued by Rafati´s group [162-166]. Leishmaniasis is a major health problem in many tropical and sub-tropical countries and development of a safe and easily-available vaccine has high priority. Several antigens potentially capable of inducing protective immunity have been studied like cathepsin L-like cysteine proteinases (CPs) and type Iand II CPs used in a heterologous prime-boost vaccination regime for experimental visceral leishmaniasis in dogs. Due to the promising results of the mentioned vaccination regime, cationic solid lipid nanoparticles (cSLNs) for in vitro delivery of these antigens were used as a cocktail DNA vaccine to deliver immunogenic CP genes efficiently. Briefly, the cationic lipid DOTAP (0.4% w/v) was dissolved in hot aqueous phase which was then added to the melted cetyl palmitate and cholesterol (5.1%w/v) phase containing tween 80 as a nonionic surfactant at 3.2:1molar ratio. Emulsification was carried out by stirring the mixture at 2000 rpm for 10 min at 90°C. Samples were then homogenized using a high shear homogenizer at 18,000 g for 15 min and the cSLN dispersion was obtained by direct cooling of hot O/W microemulsion on an ice-bath while stirring at 1000 rpm. The cSLNs were washed by centrifugation (6000 g, 10 min, three times) using 100 kDa ultra centrifugal filters to purify the suspension from the excess of surfactant. Efficiency/cytotoxicity ratio of cSLN-pDNAs formulations was comparable to linear PEI-25KD-pDNAs polyplexes while exhibiting significantly lower cytotoxicity [162].In addition, C-terminal domain deletion in CPs enhanced the protective activity of cpa/cpb loaded solid lipid nanoparticles against *Leishmania major* in BALB/c mice [163]. cSLN's were able to boost immuneresponse magnitude of cpa/cpb(-CTE) cocktail vaccination against leishmaniasis so that the average parasite inhibition percent could be increased significantly [163].The cSLNs were used to formulate three pDNAs encoding *L. major* cysteine proteinase type I (cpa), II (cpb) and III (cpc)\[164]. BALB/c mice were immunized twice with a 3-week interval, with SLN-pcDNA-cpa/b/c, pcDNA-cpa/b/c, SLN, SLN-pcDNA and PBS.Footpad assessments, parasite burden, cytokine and antibody responses were evaluated. Mice vaccinated with SLN-pcDNA-cpa/b/c significantly ($p<0.05$) showed higher protection levels with specific Th1 immune response development compared to other groups [164]. This was the first report demonstrating cSLNs as a nanoscale vehicle boosting immune response quality and quantity [164].

Very fundamental questions regarding size and charge of nanoscale cationic assemblies and their role in adjuvanticity have seldom been asked and properly answered [167-169]. The role of surface charge density in cationic liposome-promoted dendritic cell maturation and vaccine-induced immune responses was recently evaluated for a series of DOTAP/DOPC cationic liposomes with different surface densities by incorporating varying amounts of DOPC (a neutrallipid) into DOTAP (a cationic lipid) [167]. The liposomes with a relatively high charge density, such as DOTAP/DOPC 5:0 and 4:1 liposomes, potently enhanced dendriticcell maturation, ROS generation, antigen uptake, as well as the production of OVA-specific IgG2a and IFN-γ [167]. In contrast, low-charge liposomes, such asDOTAP/DOPC 1:4 liposome, failed to promote immune responses even at highconcentrations, confirming that the immunoregulatory effect of cationic liposomes is mostly attributable to their surface charge density. Moreover, the DOTAP/DOPC 1:4 liposome suppressed anti-OVA antibody responses *in vivo*. Overall, maintaining an appropriate surface charge is crucial for optimizing the adjuvant effect of cationic liposomes and enhancing the efficacy of liposome-based vaccines.

Recently, the high-pressure extrusion method was used to obtain cationic liposomes entrapping pDNA over a range of sizes [168]. This is a well-known sizing method for liposomes, but had not been applied for liposomes that are already loaded with pDNA. Liposomes composed of egg PC, DOTAP, and DOPE with entrapped pDNA were prepared by the dehydration-rehydration method and subjected to various extrusion cycles, comparing different membrane pore sizes and extrusion frequencies [168]. At optimized extrusion conditions, liposome diameter and polydispersity were reduced from 560 nm and 0.56 to 150 nm and 0.14, respectively, and 35% of the pDNA was retained [168]. Importantly, gel electrophoresis and transfection experiments with pDNA extracted from these extruded liposomes demonstrated the preservation of the structural and functional integrity of the pDNA. The reduction in size resulted in enhanced transfection of HeLa cells, as detected by functional expression of the fluorescent protein, eGFP. In addition, these liposomes were able to stimulate Toll-like receptor 9, indicating efficient endosomal uptake and release of the included pDNA. In conclusion, high-pressure extrusion is a suitable technique to size cationic liposomes with entrapped pDNA and allows preparation of well-defined nanosized pDNA-liposomes, with preserved pDNA integrity [168]. Their improved transfection efficiency and ability to activate an important pattern-recognition receptor are favorable properties for DNA vaccine delivery vehicles [168].

The formulation of DNA into both liposomal and polymeric cationic nanoparticles was found to block completely vaccination-induced antigen expression in mice and ex vivo human skin [169].This detrimental effect of cationic nanoparticle formulation was explained by immobilization of the nanoparticles in the extracellular matrix, caused by electrostatic interactions of the cationic nanoparticles with negatively charged extracellular matrix components [169]. Shielding the surface charge of the nanoparticles by PEGylation improved *in vivo* antigen expression more than 55 fold [169]. Furthermore, this shielding of cationic surface charge resulted in antigen-specific T cell responses that were similar as those induced by naked DNA for the two lipo-and polyplex DNA carrier systems tested [169]. Charge shielding should be generally applied for the development of intradermal vaccine formulations [169].

Various aspects that could be decisive in the formulation of efficient and stable carrier system(s) for the development of malaria vaccine have recently been reviewed [170]. The capacity of multi subunit DNA vaccine encoding different stage *Plasmodium* antigens to induce CD8+cytotoxic T lymphocytes and interferon-γ responses in mice, monkeys and humans has been observed [170]. Moreover, genetic vaccination may be capable of eliciting both cell mediated and humoral immune responses. The cytotoxic T cell responses are categorically needed against intracellular hepatic stage and humoral response with antibodies targeted against antigens from all stages of malaria parasite life cycle. Therefore, the key to success for any DNA based vaccine is to design a vector able to serve as a safe and efficient delivery system. Also against malaria the development of non-viral DNA-mediated gene transfer techniques based on artificial vectors such as liposomes, virosomes, microspheres and nanoparticles is strongly warranted [170].

4. Conclusions

Cationic nanostructures from lipids, biocompatible polymers, hybrid lipid-polymer or organic-inorganic systems efficiently combine with important biomolecules such as proteins, DNA, epitopes and enhancers of the immune response, most of them negatively charged. Their growing importance for vaccine design becomes evident from the examination of the works briefly described in this overview.

Acknowledgements

Financial support from Conselho Nacional de Desenvolvimento Científico e Tecnológico (CNPq) and research grant 2011/00046-5 to AMC-R from Fundação de Âmparo à Pesquisa do Estado de São Paulo (FAPESP) are gratefully acknowledged.

Author details

Ana Maria Carmona-Ribeiro*

Address all correspondence to: amcr@usp.br

Biocolloids Laboratory, Instituto de Química, Universidade de São Paulo, São Paulo SP, Brazil

References

[1] O'Hagan DT, Singh M. Microparticles as vaccine adjuvants and delivery systems.Expert Rev Vaccines.2003; 2:269-83.

[2] Xiang SD, Scholzen A, Minigo G, David C, Apostolopoulos V, Mottram PL, Plebanski M. Pathogen recognition and development of particulate vaccines: Does size matter? Methods 2006; 40:1-9.

[3] Caputo A, Sparnacci K, Ensoli B, Tondelli, L. Functional Polymeric Nano/Microparticles for Surface Adsorption and Delivery of Protein and DNA Vaccines. Curr Drug Delivery 2008; 5:230-42.

[4] Pelkmans L. Secrets of caveolae-and lipid raft-mediated endocytosis revealed by mammalian viruses. Biochim Biophys Acta, Mol Cell Res 2005; 1746:295-304.

[5] Fifis T, Gamvrellis A, Crimeen-Irwin B, Pietersz GA, Li, J, Mottram PL, McKenzie I FC, Plebanski M. Size-Dependent Immunogenicity: Therapeutic and Protective Properties of Nano-Vaccines against Tumors. J Immunol 2004; 173:3148-54.

[6] O'Hagan DT, MacKichan ML, Singh M.Recent developments in adjuvants for vaccines against infectious diseases. Immunol Infectious Dis Biomol Eng 2001; 18:69-85.

[7] Singh M, Briones M, Ott G, O'Hagan D. Cationic microparticles: A potent delivery system for DNA vaccines. Proc Natl Acad Sci U S A. 2000; 97(2):811-6.

[8] Thiele L, Rothen-Rutishauser B, Jilek S, Wunderli-Allenspach H, Merkle HP, Walter E. Evaluation of particle uptake in human blood monocyte-derived cells in vitro. Does phagocytosis activity of dendritic cells measure up with macrophages? J Control Release 2001; 76:59-71.

[9] Little SR, Lynn DM, Ge Q, Anderson DG, Puram SV, Chen J, Eisen HN, Langer R.Poly-beta amino ester-containing microparticles enhance the activity of nonviral genetic vaccines. Proc Natl Acad Sci U S A. 2004; 101(26):9534-9.

[10] O'Hagan DT. MF59 is a safe and potent vaccine adjuvant that enhances protection against influenza virus infection. Expert Rev Vaccines 2007; 6:699–710.

[11] Gluck R, Moser C, Metcalfe IC.Influenza virosomes as an efficient system for adjuvanted vaccine delivery. Expert Opin Biol Ther 2007; 4:1139–45.

[12] McMichael AJ, Gotch F, Cullen P, Askonas B, Webster RG.The human cytotoxic T cell response to influenza A vaccination.Clin Experim Immunol.1981; 43:276–84.

[13] North RJ, Jung Y-J.Immunity to tuberculosis.Annual Rev. Immunol.2004; 22:599-623.

[14] Carmona-Ribeiro AM.Lipid bilayer fragments and disks in drug delivery.Curr Med Chem.2006; 13:1359-70.

[15] Carmona-Ribeiro AM.Biomimetic particles in drug and vaccine delivery.J Liposome Res.2007; 17:165-72.

[16] Carmona-Ribeiro AM.Bilayer-forming synthetic lipids: drugs or carriers? Curr Med Chem.2003; 10:2415-46.

[17] Moura SP, Carmona-Ribeiro AM.Cationic Bilayer Fragments on Silica at Low Ionic Strength: Competitive Adsorption and Colloid Stability.Langmuir.2003; 19:6664-67.

[18] Carmona-Ribeiro AM, Lessa MM.Interactions between bilayer vesicles and latex.Colloids Surf A.1999; 153:355-61.

[19] Lincopan N, Espíndola NM, Vaz AJ, Carmona-Ribeiro AM.Cationic supported lipid bilayers for antigen presentation. Int J Pharm. 2007; 340(1-2):216-22.

[20] Lincopan N, Santana MRA, Faquim-Mauro E, da Costa MHB, Carmona-Ribeiro AM.Silica-based cationic bilayers as immunoadjuvants. BMC Biotechnol.2009; 9:5.

[21] Carmona-Ribeiro AM.Synthetic amphiphile vesicles.Chem Soc Rev.1992; 21:207-13.

[22] Carmona-Ribeiro AM, Castuma CE, Sesso A, Schreier S.Bilayer structure and stability in dihexadecyl phosphate dispersions.J Phys Chem US 1991; 95:5361-6.

[23] Hammarstroem L, Velikian I, Karlsson G, Edwards K. Cryo-TEM evidence: sonication of dihexadecyl phosphate does not produce closed bilayers with smooth curvature.Langmuir.1995; 11:408-10.

[24] Cocquyt J, Olsson U, Olofsson G, van der Meeren, P. Temperature quenched DODAB dispersions: fluid and solid state coexistence and complex formation with oppositely charged surfactant. Langmuir.2004; 20:3906-12.

[25] Vieira DB, Carmona-Ribeiro AM.Synthetic bilayer fragments for solubilization of amphotericin B. J Colloid Interface Sci.2001; 244:427-31.

[26] Kunitake T, Okahata Y, Tamaki K, Kumamaru F, Takayanagi M.Formation of the bilayer membrane from a series of quaternary ammonium salts.Chem Lett.1977; 6: 387-90.

[27] Lincopan N, Espíndola NM, Vaz AJ, da Costa MH, Faquim-Mauro E, Carmona-Ribeiro AM. Novel immunoadjuvants based on cationic lipid: Preparation, characterization and activity in vivo.Vaccine. 2009; 27(42):5760-71.

[28] Gray JJ.The interaction of proteins with solid surfaces.Curr Opin Struct Biol.2004; 14:110-15.

[29] Carvalho LA, Carmona-Ribeiro AM.Interactions between cationic vesicles and serum proteins.Langmuir.1998; 14:6077-81.

[30] Bodzon-Kulakowska A, Bierczynska-Krzysik A, Dylag T, Drabik A, Suder P, Noga M, Jarzebinska J, Silberring J. Methods for samples preparation in proteomic research.J Chromatogr B Analyt Technol Biomed Life Sci.2007; 849:1-31.

[31] Espíndola NM, Vaz AJ, Pardini AX, Fernandes I. Excretory/secretory antigens (ES) from in-vitro cultures of *Taenia crassiceps* cysticerci, and use of an anti-ES monoclonal antibody for antigen detection in samples of cerebrospinal fluid from patients with neurocysticercosis.Ann Tropical Med Parasitol.2002; 96:361-68.

[32] Espindola NM, Iha AH, Fernandes I, Takayanagui OM, dos Ramos Machado L, Livramento JA, Maia AAM, Peralta JM, Vaz AJ.Cysticercosis immunodiagnosis using 18-and 14-kilodalton proteins from *Taenia crassiceps* cysticercus antigens obtained by immunoaffinity chromatography. J Clin Microbiol.2005; 43:3178-84.

[33] Mustafa AS, Lundin KE, Oftung F.Human T cells recognize mycobacterial heat shock proteins in the context of multiple HLA-DR molecules: studies with healthy subjects vaccinated with *Mycobacterium bovis* BCG and *Mycobacterium leprae*. Infect Immun. 1993; 61:5294-5301.

[34] Pinho JR, Cardi BA, Andrade HF Jr, Barr PJ, Bathurst IC, Vicente EJ, Schenberg AC. Immunogenic properties of the *Mycobacterium leprae* recombinant 18-kDa antigen pu-

rified from *Saccharomyces cerevisiae*; enhancement of delayed-type hypersensitivity after gamma-irradiation. Int J Lepr Other Mycobact Dis.1995; 63:381-390.

[35] Costa MHB, Ueda C, Sato RA, Liberman C, Raw I. Procedures for scaling up the recombinant 18 kDa-hsp lepra protein production. Biotechnol Tech. 1995; 9:527-32.

[36] Gall D.The adjuvant activity of aliphatic nitrogenous bases. Immunology.1966; 11:369-86.

[37] Snippe H, Belder M, Willers JM. Dimethyl diotadecyl ammonium bromide as adjuvant for delayed hypersensitivity in mice. Immunology.1997; 33:931-36.

[38] Klinguer C, Beck A, De-Lys P, Bussat MC, Blaecke A, Derouet F, Bonnefoy JY, Nguyen TN, Corvaïa N, Velin D.Lipophilic quaternary ammonium salt acts as a mucosal adjuvant when co-administered by the nasal route with vaccine antigens. Vaccine 2001; 19:4236–44.

[39] Davidsen J, Rosenkrands I, Christensen D, Vangala A, Kirby D, Perrie Y, Agger EM, Andersen PA. Characterization of cationic liposomes based on dimethyldioctadecylammonium and synthetic cord factor from M. tuberculosis (trehalose 6,6V-dibehenate)—A novel adjuvant inducing both strong CMI and antibody responses.Biochim Biophys Acta. 2005; 1718:22-31.

[40] Vangala A, Kirby D, Rosenkrands I, Agger EM, Andersen P, Perrie Y. A comparative study of cationic liposome and niosome-based adjuvant systems for protein subunit vaccines: characterisation, environmental scanning electron microscopy and immunisation studies in mice. J Pharm Pharmacol.2006; 58:787-99.

[41] Korsholm KS, Agger EM, Foged C, Christensen D, Dietrich J, Andersen CS, Geisler C, Andersen P.The adjuvant mechanism of cationic dimethyldioctadecylammonium liposomes. Immunology.2007; 121:216–26.

[42] Foged C, Brodin B, Frokjaer S, Sundblad A.Particle size and surface charge affect particle uptake by human dendritic cells in an in vitro model. Int J Pharm.2005; 298: 315-22.

[43] Dawson M, Krauland E, Wirtz D, Hanes J. Transport of polymeric nanoparticle gene carriers in gastric mucus. Biotechnol Progress.2004; 20:851-57.

[44] Hilgers LA, Snippe H. DDA as an immunological adjuvant. Res Immunol.1992; 143: 494–503.

[45] Tsuruta LR, Quintilio W, Costa, MHB, Carmona-Ribeiro AM. Interactions between cationic liposomes and an antigenic protein: the physical chemistry of the immunoadjuvant action.J Lipid Res.1997; 38:2003–11.

[46] Brgles M, Jurasin D, Sikirić MD, Frkanec R, Tomasić J. Entrapment of ovalbumin into liposomes-Factors affecting entrapment efficiency, liposome size, and zeta potential. J Liposome Res.2008; 18:235-48.

[47] Sacks D, Noben-Traut N. The immunology of susceptibility and resistance to Leishmania major in mice. Nature Rev Immunol.2002; 2:845-58.

[48] Good MF, Xu H, Wykes M, Engwerda CR. Development and regulation of cell-mediated immune responses to the blood stages of malaria: implications for vaccine research. Annual Rev Immunol.2005; 23:69-99.

[49] De Paula SO, Lima DM, França RFO, Gomes-Ruiz AC, Fonseca BAL. A DNA vaccine candidate expressing dengue-3 virus prM and E proteins elicits neutralizing antibodies and protects mice against lethal challenge.Arch Virol.2008; 153:2215–23.

[50] Abbas AK, Lichtman AH, Pillai S. Cellular and Molecular Immunology 6th Ed. 2006, Saunders Elsevier.

[51] Pacheco LF, Carmona-Ribeiro AM.Effects of synthetic lipids on solubilization and colloid stability of hydrophobic drugs. J Colloid Interface Sci. 2003; 258(1):146-54.

[52] Vieira DB, Pacheco LF, Carmona-Ribeiro AM.Assembly of a model hydrophobic drug into cationic bilayer fragments. J Colloid Interface Sci. 2006; 293(1):240-7.

[53] Rosa H, Petri DF, Carmona-Ribeiro AM.Interactions between bacteriophage DNA and cationic biomimetic particles. J Phys Chem B. 2008; 112(51):16422-30.

[54] Rozenfeld JH, Oliveira TR, Lamy MT, Carmona-Ribeiro AM. Interaction of cationic bilayer fragments with a model oligonucleotide. Biochim Biophys Acta.2011; 1808(3): 649-55.

[55] Zamecnik PC, Stephenson ML. Inhibition of Rous sarcoma virus replication and cell transformation by a specific oligodeoxynucleotide. Proc Natl Acad Sci U S A.1978; 75(1):280-4.

[56] Flaherty KT, Stevenson JP, O'Dwyer PJ. Antisense therapeutics: lessons from early clinical trials. Curr Opin Oncol. 2001; 13(6):499-505.

[57] Tamm I, Dörken B, Hartmann G. Antisense therapy in oncology: new hope for an old idea? Lancet.2001; 358(9280):489-97.

[58] De Backer MD, Nelissen B, Logghe M, Viaene J, Loonen I, Vandoninck S, de Hoogt R, Dewaele S, Simons FA, Verhasselt P, Vanhoof G, Contreras R, Luyten WH.An antisense-based functional genomics approach for identification of genes critical for growth of *Candida albicans*. Nat Biotechnol. 2001; 19(3):235-41.

[59] Dean NM. Functional genomics and target validation approaches using antisense oligonucleotide technology.Curr Opin Biotechnol. 2001; 12(6):622-5.

[60] Juliano R, Alam MR, Dixit V, Kang H. Mechanisms and strategies for effective delivery of antisense and siRNA oligonucleotides. Nucleic Acids Res. 2008; 36(12):4158-71.

[61] Liu L, Zhou X, Liu H, Xiang L, Yuan Z. CpG motif acts as a 'danger signal' and provides a T helper type 1-biased microenvironment for DNA vaccination.Immunology. 2005; 115(2):223-30.

[62] Fonseca DE, Kline JN.Use of CpG oligonucleotides in treatment of asthma and allergic disease. Adv Drug Deliv Rev. 2009; 61(3):256-62.

[63] Kuramoto Y, Nishikawa M, Hyoudou K, Yamashita F, Hashida M. Inhibition of peritoneal dissemination of tumor cells by single dosing of phosphodiester CpG oligonucleotide/cationic liposome complex.J Control Release. 2006; 115(2):226-33.

[64] Shi F, Hoekstra D. Effective intracellular delivery of oligonucleotides in order to make sense of antisense. J Control Release.2004; 97(2):189-209.

[65] Felgner PL, Barenholz Y, Behr JP, Cheng SH, Cullis P, Huang L, Jessee JA, Seymour L, Szoka F, Thierry AR, Wagner E, Wu G. Nomenclature for synthetic gene delivery systems. Hum Gene Ther. 1997; 8(5):511-2.

[66] Nantes IL, Correia FM, Faljoni-Alario A, Kawanami AE, Ishiki HM, Amaral AT,Carmona-Ribeiro AM.Nucleotide conformational change induced by cationic bilayers. Arch Biochem Biophys. 2003; 416(1):25-30.

[67] Kabanov VA, Yaroslavov AA. What happens to negatively charged lipid vesicles upon interacting with polycation species? J Control Release. 2002; 78(1-3):267-71.

[68] Sybachin AV, Efimova AA, Litmanovich EA, Menger FM, Yaroslavov AA.Complexation of polycations to anionic liposomes: composition and structure of the interfacial complexes. Langmuir. 2007; 23(20):10034-9.

[69] O'Hagan DT, Singh M, Ulmer JB.Microparticles for the delivery of DNA vaccines. Immunol Rev. 2004; 199:191-200.

[70] El-Sayed IH, Huang X, El-Sayed MA. Surface plasmon resonance scattering and absorption of anti-EGFR antibody conjugated gold nanoparticles in cancer diagnostics: applications in oral cancer. Nano Lett. 2005; 5(5):829-34.

[71] Kovacsovics-Bankowski M, Clark K, Benacerraf B, Rock KL. Efficient major histocompatibility complex class I presentation of exogenous antigen upon phagocytosis by macrophages. Proc Natl Acad Sci U S A. 1993; 90(11):4942-6.

[72] Vidard L, Kovacsovics-Bankowski M, Kraeft SK, Chen LB, Benacerraf B, Rock KL.Analysis of MHC class II presentation of particulate antigens of B lymphocytes. J Immunol. 1996; 156(8):2809-18.

[73] Carmona-Ribeiro AM, Midmore BR.Synthetic bilayer adsorption onto polystyrene microspheres. Langmuir.1992; 8:801-6.

[74] Carmona-Ribeiro AM.Bilayer vesicles and liposomes as interface agents.Chem Soc Rev.2001; 30:241-7.

[75] Lincopan N, Carmona-Ribeiro AM. Lipid-covered drug particles: combined action of dioctadecyldimethylammonium bromide and amphotericin B or miconazole. J Antimicrob Chemother.2006; 58(1):66-75.

[76] Pereira EMA, Vieira DB, Carmona-Ribeiro AM.Cationic bilayers on polymeric particles: effect of low NaCl concentration on surface coverage. J Phys Chem B. 2004; 108:11490-5.

[77] Li W, Suez I, Szoka FC Jr. Reconstitution of the M13 major coat protein and its transmembrane peptide segment on a DNA template.Biochemistry. 2007; 46(29):8579-91.

[78] Luo D, Saltzman WM. Synthetic DNA delivery systems. Nat Biotechnol. 2000; 18(1): 33-7.

[79] Gaweda S, Morán MC, Pais AA, Dias RS, Schillén K, Lindman B, Miguel MG.Cationic agents for DNA compaction. J Colloid Interface Sci. 2008; 323(1):75-83.

[80] Cerritelli ME, Cheng N, Rosenberg AH, McPherson CE, Booy FP, Steven AC.Encapsidated conformation of bacteriophage T7 DNA. Cell.1997; 91(2):271-80.

[81] Zinchenko AA, Luckel F, Yoshikawa K. Transcription of giant DNA complexed with cationic nanoparticles as a simple model of chromatin. Biophys J. 2007; 92(4):1318-25.

[82] Zinchenko AA, Yoshikawa K, Baigl D. Compaction of single-chain DNA by histone-inspired nanoparticles.Phys Rev Lett. 2005; 95(22):228101.

[83] Lindsay S. Chromatin control of gene expression: the simplest model. Biophys J. 2007; 92(4):1113.

[84] Kneuer C, Sameti M, Bakowsky U, Schiestel T, Schirra H, Schmidt H, Lehr CM.A nonviral DNA delivery system based on surface modified silica-nanoparticles can efficiently transfect cells *in vitro*. Bioconjug Chem. 2000; 11(6):926-32.

[85] Thomas M, Klibanov AM.Conjugation to gold nanoparticles enhances polyethylenimine's transfer of plasmid DNA into mammalian cells. Proc Natl Acad Sci U S A. 2003; 100(16):9138-43.

[86] Roy I, Ohulchanskyy TY, Bharali DJ, Pudavar HE, Mistretta RA, Kaur N, Prasad PN. Optical tracking of organically modified silica nanoparticles as DNA carriers: a nonviral, nanomedicine approach for gene delivery. Proc Natl Acad Sci U S A. 2005; 102(2):279-84.

[87] Zinchenko AA, Sakaue T, Araki S, Yoshikawa K, Baigl D. Single-chain compaction of long duplex DNA by cationic nanoparticles: modes of interaction and comparison with chromatin. J Phys Chem B. 2007; 111(11):3019-31.

[88] Rejman J, Oberle V, Zuhorn IS, Hoekstra D. Size-dependent internalization of particles via the pathways of clathrin-and caveolae-mediated endocytosis.Biochem J. 2004;377(Pt 1):159-69.

[89] Hoekstra D, Rejman J, Wasungu L, Shi F, Zuhorn I. Gene delivery by cationic lipids: in and out of an endosome. Biochem Soc Trans. 2007; 35 (Pt 1):68-71.

[90] Tsuruta LR, Lessa MM, Carmona-Ribeiro AM. Effect of particle size on colloid stability of bilayer-covered polystyrene microspheres.J Colloid Interface Sci. 1995; 175(2): 470-5.

[91] Krieg AM, Yi AK, Matson S, Waldschmidt TJ, Bishop GA, Teasdale R, Koretzky GA,Klinman DM. CpG motifs in bacterial DNA trigger direct B-cell activation. Nature.1995; 374(6522):546-9.

[92] Vollmer J, Krieg AM.Immunotherapeutic applications of CpG oligodeoxynucleotide TLR9 agonists. Adv Drug Deliv Rev. 2009; 61(3):195-204.

[93] Manegold C, Gravenor D, Woytowitz D, Mezger J, Hirsh V, Albert G, Al-Adhami M, Readett D, Krieg AM, Leichman CG. Randomized phase II trial of a toll-like receptor 9 agonist oligodeoxynucleotide, PF-3512676, in combination with first-line taxane plus platinum chemotherapy for advanced-stage non-small-cell lung cancer.J Clin Oncol. 2008; 26(24):3979-86.

[94] Zimmermann S, Egeter O, Hausmann S, Lipford GB, Röcken M, Wagner H, Heeg K. CpG oligodeoxynucleotides trigger protective and curative Th1 responses in lethal murine leishmaniasis.J Immunol. 1998; 160(8):3627-30.

[95] Thompson AJ, Colledge D, Rodgers S, Wilson R, Revill P, Desmond P, Mansell A, Visvanathan K, Locarnini S. Stimulation of the interleukin-1 receptor and Toll-like receptor 2 inhibits hepatitis B virus replication in hepatoma cell lines *in vitro*. Antivir Ther. 2009; 14(6):797-808.

[96] Simons FE, Shikishima Y, Van Nest G, Eiden JJ, HayGlass KT. Selective immune redirection in humans with ragweed allergy by injecting Amb a 1 linked to immunostimulatory DNA. J Allergy Clin Immunol. 2004; 113(6):1144-51.

[97] Rozenfeld JH, Silva SR, Ranéia PA, Faquim-Mauro E, Carmona-Ribeiro AM.Stable assemblies of cationic bilayer fragments and CpG oligonucleotide with enhanced immunoadjuvant activity *in vivo*.J Control Release.2012; 160(2):367-73.

[98] Beeley JA, Stevenson SM, Beeley JG. Polyacrylamide gel isoelectric focusing of proteins: determination of isoelectric points using an antimony electrode.Biochim Biophys Acta. 1972; 285(2):293-300.

[99] Walker HW, Grant SB. Influence of surface charge and particle size on the stabilization of colloidal particles by model polyelectrolytes.Colloids Surf A.1998; 135,123-133.

[100] Henriksen-Lacey M, Bramwell VW, Christensen D, Agger EM, Andersen P, Perrie Y.Liposomes based on dimethyldioctadecylammonium promote a depot effect and enhance immunogenicity of soluble antigen.J Control Release. 2010; 142(2):180-6.

[101] Manolova V, Flace A, Bauer M, Schwarz K, Saudan P, Bachmann MF. Nanoparticles target distinct dendritic cell populations according to their size. Eur J Immunol. 2008; 38(5):1404-13.

[102] Krieg AM.Therapeutic potential of Toll-like receptor 9 activation.Nat Rev Drug Discov.2006; 5(6):471-84.

[103] Joseph A, Louria-Hayon I, Plis-Finarov A, Zeira E, Zakay-Rones Z, Raz E, Hayashi T, Takabayashi K, Barenholz Y, Kedar E. Liposomal immunostimulatory DNA sequence (ISS-ODN): an efficient parenteral and mucosal adjuvant for influenza and hepatitis B vaccines. Vaccine. 2002; 20(27-28):3342-54.

[104] Mitchell LA, Joseph A, Kedar E, Barenholz Y, Galun E. Mucosal immunization against hepatitis A: antibody responses are enhanced by co-administration of synthetic oligodeoxynucleotides and a novel cationic lipid. Vaccine.2006; 24(25):5300-10.

[105] Mayorga O, Muñoz JE, Lincopan N, Teixeira AF, Ferreira LC, Travassos LR,Taborda CP.The role of adjuvants in therapeutic protection against paracoccidioidomycosis after immunization with the P10 peptide. Front Microbiol.2012; 3:154.

[106] Gaspar EB, Rosetti AS, Lincopan N, De Gaspari E. *Neisseria lactamica* antigens complexed with a novel cationic adjuvant. Hum Vaccin Immunother.2013; 9(3). [Epub ahead of print] PubMed PMID: 23296384.

[107] Li X, Min M, Du N, Gu Y, Hode T, Naylor M, Chen D, Nordquist RE, Chen WR. Chitin, chitosan, and glycated chitosan regulate immune responses: the novel adjuvants for cancer vaccine. Clin Dev Immunol. 2013; 2013:387023.

[108] Jarmila V, Vavríková E.Chitosan derivatives with antimicrobial, antitumour and antioxidant activities-a review. Curr Pharm Des.2011; 17(32):3596-607.

[109] Pillai CKS, Paul W, Sharma CP. Chitin and chitosan polymers: chemistry, solubility and fiber formation. Progress in Polymer Science.2009; 34(7):641–678.

[110] Chung YC, Yeh JY, Tsai CF. Antibacterial characteristics and activity of water-soluble chitosan derivatives prepared by the Maillard reaction. Molecules.2011; 16(10): 8504-14.

[111] Song S, Zhou F, Nordquist RE, Carubelli R, Liu H, Chen WR.Glycated chitosan as a new non-toxic immunological stimulant Glycated chitosan immunological stimulant.Immunopharmacol Immunotoxicol. 2009; 31(2):202–208.

[112] Li X, Ferrel GL, Guerra MC, Hode T, Lunn JA, Adalsteinsson O, Nordquist RE,Liu H, Chen WR.Preliminary safety and efficacy results of laser immunotherapy for the treatment of metastatic breast cancer patients.Photochem Photobiol Sci. 2011; 10(5): 817-21.

[113] Chen WR, Korbelik M, Bartels KE, Liu H, Sun J, Nordquist RE.Enhancement of laser cancer treatment by a chitosan-derived immunoadjuvant. Photochem Photobiol.2005; 81(1):190-5.

[114] Yoon TJ, Kim JY, Kim H, Hong C, Lee H, Lee CK, Lee KH, Hong S, Park SH.Anti-tumor immunostimulatory effect of heat-killed tumor cells. Exp Mol Med. 2008; 40(1):130-44.

[115] Jäger E, Jäger D, Knuth A.Antigen-specific immunotherapy and cancer vaccines.Int J Cancer.2003; 106(6):817-20.

[116] Wu F, Zhou L, Chen WR. Host antitumour immune responses to HIFU ablation. Int J Hyperthermia. 2007; 23(2):165-71.

[117] Chen WR, Jeong SW, Lucroy MD, Wolf RF, Howard EW, Liu H, Nordquist RE.Induced antitumor immunity against DMBA-4 metastatic mammary tumors in rats using laser immunotherapy. Int J Cancer. 2003; 107(6):1053-7.

[118] Peniche H, Peniche C. Chitosan nanoparticles: a contribution to nanomedicine.Polym Int. 2011; 60:883–889.

[119] Calvo P, Remuñán-López C, Vila-Jato JL, Alonso MJ, Novel hydrophilic chitosan–polyethylene oxide nanoparticles as protein carriers.J Polym Sci.1997;63:125–132.

[120] Hu Y, Jiang X, Ding Y, Ge H, Yuan Y, Yang C.Synthesis and characterization of chitosan-poly(acrylic acid) nanoparticles.Biomaterials. 2002; 23(15):3193-201.

[121] Cui Z, Mumper RJ.Chitosan-based nanoparticles for topical genetic immunization.J Control Release. 2001; 5(3):409-19.

[122] Sarmento B, Ribeiro AJ, Veiga F, Ferreira DC, Neufeld RJ.Insulin-loaded nanoparticles are prepared by alginate ionotropic pre-gelation followed by chitosan polyelectrolyte complexation.J Nanosci Nanotechnol.2007; 7(8):2833-41.

[123] Vila AI, Suárez S, Alonso MJ. Chitosan and heparin nanoparticles. Spanish Patent. 2007; WO/2007/042572.

[124] Vieira DB, Kim V, Petri DFS, Menck CFM, Carmona-Ribeiro AM. Supramolecular assemblies of cisplatin and polyelectrolytes: preparation, characterization and activity against cancer cells. In: Laudon M, Romanowicz B. (eds.) Nanotech Conference & Expo 2012: An Interdisciplinary Integrative Forum on Nanotechnology, Microtechnology, Biotechnology and Cleantechnology,18-21 June 2012, Santa Clara, CA, United States.Boca Raton, Fla: CRC Press, 2012.

[125] Sayin B, Somavarapu S, Li XW, Thanou M, Sesardic D, Alpar HO, Senel S.Mono-N-carboxymethyl chitosan (MCC) and N-trimethyl chitosan (TMC) nanoparticles for non-invasive vaccine delivery.Int J Pharm. 2008; 363(1-2):139-48.

[126] Behrens I, Pena AI, Alonso MJ, Kissel T. Comparative uptake studies of bioadhesive and non-bioadhesive nanoparticles in human intestinal cell lines and rats: the effect of mucus on particle adsorption and transport. Pharm Res. 2002; 19(8):1185-93.

[127] Huang M, Khor E, Lim LY.Uptake and cytotoxicity of chitosan molecules and nanoparticles: effects of molecular weight and degree of deacetylation. Pharm Res. 2004; 21(2):344-53.

[128] Chowdary KP, Rao YS.Mucoadhesive microspheres for controlled drug delivery. Biol Pharm Bull.2004; 27(11):1717-24.

[129] Sayin B, Somavarapu S, Li XW, Sesardic D, Senel S, Alpar OH.TMC-MCC (N-trimethyl chitosan-mono-N-carboxymethyl chitosan) nanocomplexes for mucosal delivery of vaccines. Eur J Pharm Sci. 2009; 38(4):362-9.

[130] Chen YZ, Yao XL, Tabata Y, Nakagawa S, Gao JQ.Gene carriers and transfection systems used in the recombination of dendritic cells for effective cancer immunotherapy. Clin Dev Immunol. 2010; 2010:565643.

[131] Kim TH, Nah JW, Cho MH, Park TG, Cho CS. Receptor-mediated gene delivery into antigen presenting cells using mannosylated chitosan/DNA nanoparticles.J Nanosci Nanotechnol. 2006; 6(9-10):2796-803.

[132] Kim TH, Jin H, Kim HW, Cho MH, Cho CS. Mannosylated chitosan nanoparticle-based cytokine gene therapy suppressed cancer growth in BALB/c mice bearing CT-26 carcinoma cells.Mol Cancer Ther. 2006; 5(7):1723-32.

[133] Zhou X, Liu B, Yu X, Zha X, Zhang X, Chen Y, Wang X, Jin Y, Wu Y, Chen Y, Shan Y, Chen Y, Liu J, Kong W, Shen J. Controlled release of PEI/DNA complexes from mannose-bearing chitosan microspheres as a potent delivery system to enhance immune response to HBV DNA vaccine. J Control Release.2007;121(3):200-7.

[134] Engell-Noerregaard L, Hansen TH, Andersen MH, Thor Straten P, Svane IM.Review of clinical studies on dendritic cell-based vaccination of patients with malignant melanoma: assessment of correlation between clinical response and vaccine parameters.Cancer Immunol Immunother. 2009; 58(1):1-14.

[135] Smits EL, Anguille S, Cools N, Berneman ZN, Van Tendeloo VF.Dendritic cell-based cancer gene therapy. Hum Gene Ther. 2009; 20(10):1106-18.

[136] Frankenberger B, Regn S, Geiger C, Noessner E, Falk CS, Pohla H, Javorovic M, Silberzahn T, Wilde S, Buchner A, Siebels M, Oberneder R, Willimsky G, Pezzutto A, Blankenstein T, Schendel DJ. Cell-based vaccines for renal cell carcinoma: genetically-engineered tumor cells and monocyte-derived dendritic cells. World J Urol. 2005; 23(3):166-74.

[137] Antonia SJ, Mirza N, Fricke I, Chiappori A, Thompson P, Williams N, Bepler G, Simon G, Janssen W, Lee JH, Menander K, Chada S, Gabrilovich DI.Combination of

p53 cancer vaccine with chemotherapy in patients with extensive stage small cell lung cancer. Clin Cancer Res. 2006; 12(3 Pt 1):878-87.

[138] Xiong W, Candolfi M, Liu C, Muhammad AK, Yagiz K, Puntel M, Moore PF, Avalos J, Young JD, Khan D, Donelson R, Pluhar GE, Ohlfest JR, Wawrowsky K, Lowenstein PR, Castro MG. Human Flt3L generates dendritic cells from canine peripheral blood precursors: implications for a dog glioma clinical trial.PLoS One. 2010; 5(6):e11074.

[139] Mori A, Oleszycka E, Sharp FA, Coleman M, Ozasa Y, Singh M, O'Hagan DT, Tajber L, Corrigan OI, McNeela EA, Lavelle EC. The vaccine adjuvant alum inhibits IL-12 by promoting PI3 kinase signaling while chitosan does not inhibit IL-12 and enhances Th1 and Th17 responses. Eur J Immunol. 2012; 42(10):2709-19.

[140] Yang Z, Sahay G, Sriadibhatla S, Kabanov AV. Amphiphilic block copolymers enhance cellular uptake and nuclear entry of polyplex-delivered DNA. Bioconjug Chem. 2008; 19(10):1987-94.

[141] Kanazawa T, Takashima Y, Murakoshi M, Nakai Y, Okada H. Enhancement of gene transfection into human dendritic cells using cationic PLGA nanospheres with a synthesized nuclear localization signal. Int J Pharm. 2009; 379(1):187-95.

[142] Bal SM, Slütter B, Verheul R, Bouwstra JA, Jiskoot W. Adjuvanted, antigen loaded N-trimethyl chitosan nanoparticles for nasal and intradermal vaccination: adjuvant-and site-dependent immunogenicity in mice. Eur J Pharm Sci. 2012; 45(4):475-81.

[143] Yu F, Wang J, Dou J, Yang H, He X, Xu W, Zhang Y, Hu K, Gu N.Nanoparticle-based adjuvant for enhanced protective efficacy of DNA vaccine Ag85A-ESAT-6-IL-21 against *Mycobacterium tuberculosis* infection. Nanomedicine.2012; 8(8):1337-44.

[144] Wang G, Pan L, Zhang Y, Wang Y, Zhang Z, Lü J, Zhou P, Fang Y, Jiang S.Intranasal delivery of cationic PLGA nano/microparticles-loaded FMDV DNA vaccine encoding IL-6 elicited protective immunity against FMDV challenge. PLoS One.2011; 6(11):e27605.

[145] Zwiorek K, Bourquin C, Battiany J, Winter G, Endres S, Hartmann G, Coester C.Delivery by cationic gelatin nanoparticles strongly increases the immunostimulatory effects of CpG oligonucleotides.Pharm Res. 2007; 25(3):551-62.

[146] Coester CJ, Langer K, van Briesen H, Kreuter J. Gelatin nanoparticles by two step desolvation--a new preparation method, surface modifications and cell uptake.J Microencapsul. 2000; 17(2):187-93.

[147] Doll TAPF, Raman S, Dey R,Burkhard P. 2013 Nanoscale assemblies and their biomedical applications. J R Soc Interface 10: 20120740.

[148] Carmona-Ribeiro AM, de Melo Carrasco LD.Cationic antimicrobial polymers and their assemblies. Int J Mol Sci. 2013; 14(5):9906-46.

[149] Carmona-Ribeiro AM. Biomimetic nanoparticles: preparation, characterization and biomedical applications. Int J Nanomedicine.2010; 5:249-59.

[150] Ji W, Panus D, Palumbo RN, Tang R, Wang C.Poly(2-aminoethyl methacrylate) with well-defined chain length for DNA vaccine delivery to dendritic cells.Biomacromolecules. 2011; 12(12):4373-85.

[151] Gupta NK, Tomar P, Sharma V, Dixit VK. Development and characterization of chitosan coated poly-ε-caprolactone nanoparticulate system for effective immunization against influenza.Vaccine. 2011; 29(48):9026-37.

[152] Castaldello A, Brocca-Cofano E, Voltan R, Triulzi C, Altavilla G, Laus M,Sparnacci K, Ballestri M, Tondelli L, Fortini C, Gavioli R, Ensoli B, Caputo A. DNA prime and protein boost immunization with innovative polymeric cationic core-shell nanoparticles elicits broad immune responses and strongly enhance cellular responses of HIV-1 tat DNA vaccination.Vaccine. 2006; 24(29-30):5655-69.

[153] Huang HN, Li TL, Chan YL, Chen CL, Wu CJ.Transdermal immunization with low-pressure-gene-gun mediated chitosan-based DNA vaccines against Japanese encephalitis virus.Biomaterials. 2009; 30(30):6017-25.

[154] Nochi T, Yuki Y, Takahashi H, Sawada S, Mejima M, Kohda T, Harada N, Kong IG,Sato A, Kataoka N, Tokuhara D, Kurokawa S, Takahashi Y, Tsukada H, Kozaki S,Akiyoshi K, Kiyono H.Nanogel antigenic protein-delivery system for adjuvant-free intranasal vaccines.Nat Mater. 2010;9(7):572-8.

[155] Kong IG, Sato A, Yuki Y, Nochi T, Takahashi H, Sawada S, Mejima M, Kurokawa S,Okada K, Sato S, Briles DE, Kunisawa J, Inoue Y, Yamamoto M, Akiyoshi K, KiyonoH. Nanogel-based PspA intranasal vaccine prevents invasive disease and nasal colonization by *Streptococcus pneumoniae*.Infect Immun. 2013; 81(5):1625-34.

[156] Vangasseri DP, Han SJ, Huang L. Lipid-protamine-DNA-mediated antigen delivery.Curr Drug Deliv.2005; 2(4):401–6.

[157] Watson DS, Endsley AN, Huang L. Design considerations for liposomal vaccines: influence of formulation parameters on antibody and cell-mediated immune responses to liposome associated antigens.Vaccine. 2012; 30(13):2256-72.

[158] Cui Z, Han SJ, Vangasseri DP, Huang L.Immunostimulation mechanism of LPD nanoparticle as a vaccine carrier. Mol Pharm. 2005; 2(1):22-8.

[159] Gao X, Huang L. Potentiation of cationic liposome-mediated gene delivery by polycations.Biochemistry.1996; 35(3):1027-36.

[160] Cho HJ, Han SE, Im S, Lee Y, Kim YB, Chun T, Oh YK.Maltosylated polyethylenimine-based triple nanocomplexes of human papillomavirus 16L1 protein and DNA as a vaccine co-delivery system.Biomaterials. 2011; 32(20):4621-9.

[161] Jean M, Smaoui F, Lavertu M, Méthot S, Bouhdoud L, Buschmann MD, Merzouki A.Chitosan-plasmid nanoparticle formulations for IM and SC delivery of recombi-

nant FGF-2 and PDGF-BB or generation of antibodies.Gene Ther. 2009; 16(9): 1097-110.

[162] Buschmann MD, Merzouki A, Lavertu M, Thibault M, Jean M, Darras V. Chitosans for delivery of nucleic acids. Adv Drug Deliv Rev. 2013;doi:pii:S0169-409X(13)00159-2. 10.1016/j.addr.2013.07.005. [Epub ahead of print]

[163] Doroud D, Vatanara A, Zahedifard F, Gholami E, Vahabpour R, Rouholamini Najafabadi A, Rafati S. Cationic solid lipid nanoparticles loaded by cysteine proteinase genes as a novel anti-leishmaniasis DNA vaccine delivery system: characterization and *in vitro* evaluations.J Pharm Pharm Sci. 2010;13(3):320-35.

[164] Doroud D, Zahedifard F, Vatanara A, Taslimi Y, Vahabpour R, Torkashvand F, Vaziri B, Rouholamini Najafabadi A, Rafati S.C-terminal domain deletion enhances the protective activity of cpa/cpb loaded solid lipid nanoparticles against *Leishmania major* in BALB/c mice. PLoS Negl Trop Dis.2011; 5(7):e1236.

[165] Doroud D, Zahedifard F, Vatanara A, Najafabadi AR, Taslimi Y, Vahabpour R, Torkashvand F, Vaziri B, Rafati S.Delivery of a cocktail DNA vaccine encoding cysteine proteinases type I, II and III with solid lipid nanoparticles potentiate protective immunity against Leishmania major infection.J Control Release. 2011; 153(2):154-62.

[166] Saljoughian N, Zahedifard F, Doroud D, Doustdari F, Vasei M, Papadopoulou B, Rafati S. Cationic solid lipid nanoparticles are as efficient as electroporation in DNA vaccination against visceral leishmaniasis in mice. Parasite Immunol.2013.doi: 10.1111/pim.12042. [Epub ahead of print]

[167] Mohit E, Rafati S. Biological delivery approaches for gene therapy: Strategies to potentiate efficacy and enhance specificity.Mol Immunol. 2013; 56(4):599-611.doi: 10.1016/j.molimm.2013.06.005.

[168] Ma Y, Zhuang Y, Xie X, Wang C, Wang F, Zhou D, Zeng J, Cai L.The role of surface charge density in cationic liposome-promoted dendritic cell maturation and vaccine-induced immune responses.Nanoscale. 2011; 3(5):2307-14.

[169] Carstens MG, van der Maaden K, van der Velden D, Ottenhoff TH, Melief CJ,Ossendorp F, Bouwstra JA, Jiskoot W.Evaluation of the high-pressure extrusion technique as a method for sizing plasmid DNA-containing cationic liposomes.J Liposome Res. 2011;21(4):286-95.

[170] van den Berg JH, Oosterhuis K, Hennink WE, Storm G, van der Aa LJ, Engbersen JF, Haanen JB, Beijnen JH, Schumacher TN, Nuijen B.Shielding the cationic charge of nanoparticle-formulated dermal DNA vaccines is essential for antigen expression and immunogenicity.J Control Release. 2010; 141(2):234-40.

[171] Tyagi RK, Garg NK, Sahu T.Vaccination strategies against malaria: novel carrier(s) more than a tour de force.J Control Release. 2012; 162(1):242-54.

Chapter 2

Mollusk Hemocyanins as Natural Immunostimulants in Biomedical Applications

María Inés Becker, Sergio Arancibia, Fabián Salazar,
Miguel Del Campo and Alfredo De Ioannes

Additional information is available at the end of the chapter

http://dx.doi.org/10.5772/57552

1. Introduction

Hemocyanins, the massive oxygen-transporting glycoproteins found freely dissolved in the hemolymph of some mollusks, are potent natural immunostimulants when inoculated in mammals, enhance the innate and adaptive immune response with beneficial clinical outcomes. Hemocyanins are easily purified and molecularly correspond to large multi-subunit structures, some over 10^7 Da (van Holde and Miller, 1995). Currently, hemocyanins are commonly used as carriers/adjuvants for producing antibodies against different antigens. These antigens include tumor-associated antigens (TAAs), such as glycolipid and glycoprotein (mucin-like) antigens in cutting-edge therapeutic vaccines for cancer, along with idiotypes, the most commonly used tumor antigen to prepare vaccines for nearly all non-Hodgkin lymphomas. Other therapeutic strategies using hemocyanins include their use as adjuvants to disrupt self-tolerance to tumor antigens in the generation of *ex vivo* autologous tumor cell lysate-loaded dendritic cells (DCs) to induce T-cell responses in cancer patients (Del Campo et al., 2011). Furthermore, hemocyanins can be used as non-specific immunostimulants during therapy for recurrent superficial bladder cancer after transurethral surgical resection with negligible toxic side effects, thus making them ideal for long-term on going treatments (Arancibia et al., 2012b).

Biomedical interest in hemocyanins arose in the 1960s when their remarkable immunogenicity and immunostimulatory properties in experimental animals, and in human beings, were discovered. The most popular hemocyanin, due to being the earliest discovered and the first used in biomedical studies, is purified from the giant keyhole limpet gastropod *Megathura crenulata* and is commonly known as **KLH** (keyhole limpet hemocyanin) (Harris and Markl, 1999). However, the limited resource availability and the growing demand for KLH, in addition to the biodiversity of hemocyanins, have led to a growing interest in identifying new hemocyanin candidates with either similar or improved immunological and biochemical properties. Therefore, today, there are a variety of new gastropod hemocyanins that have been purified and studied biochemically and immunologically, including *Concholepas concholepas* (**CCH**) (De Ioannes et al., 2004; Moltedo et al., 2006), *Fissurella latimarginata* (**FLH**) (Arancibia et al., 2014), *Haliotis tuberculata* (**HtH**) (Keller et al., 1999; Markl et al., 2001) and *Rapana thomasiana* (**RtH**) hemocyanins (Idakieva et al., 1993; Tchorbanov et al., 2008).

In this chapter, we reviewed what is presently known about the uses of mollusk hemocyanins as carriers/adjuvants and non-specific immunostimulants in biomedicine, with a general description of hemocyanin structure and, finally, the current knowledge on the innate and adaptive mechanisms involved in the biomedical efficacy of these colossal proteins. Various authors explain the causes of immunogenicity and immunostimulatory effects of hemocyanins in mammals as due to their extremely xenogenic complex structures, which have abundant carbohydrates, and their symmetry, which resembles an icosahedral virus capsid (D5 point group symmetry, i.e., consisting of 10 equivalent subunits). However, this explanation does not account for the mechanisms involved in the effects of hemocyanin on the mammalian immune system; our investigations have attempted to elucidate such mechanisms.

2. Structure of the mollusk hemocyanins

Mollusk hemocyanins are enormous glycoproteins (4–8 MDa) formed by an intricate arrangement of 10 subunits, approximately 350-450 kDa each, that are self-assembled into hollow cylinders 35 nm in diameter and are referred to as **decamers**. This structure is easily observed by negative staining using transmission electron microscopy, as shown in Figure 1. Each subunit consists of 7 or 8 globular folded domains known as functional units (FUs), connected by linker peptide strands of 10–15 amino acid residues. FUs vary in size from 45–55 kDa, and each of them is capable of reversibly binding one oxygen molecule through a pair of copper atoms. In gastropod hemocyanins, the hemocyanins being described in this review, the decamers may associate in pairs to form truly immense molecules called **didecamers** with molecular masses of approximately 9×10^6 Da (Decker et al., 2007; van Holde and Miller, 1995; Markl, 2013).

An additional feature of hemocyanin structures are their carbohydrate contents, which play fundamental roles in their organization and their immunological efficacy (Paccagnella et al., 2004). Gastropod hemocyanins contain variable, heterogeneous N-and O-glycosylation sites, with as high as 9% (w/w) mannose as the most abundant oligosaccharide (Hall and Wood, 1976). Some hemocyanins possess the Thomsen-Friedenreich antigen disaccharide (T antigen disaccharide Galβ1-3GalNAcα1-Ser/Thr), which, together with mannose, may play a role in the immune-related properties of hemocyanins (Geyer et al., 2005; Harris and Markl, 1999), as discussed later.

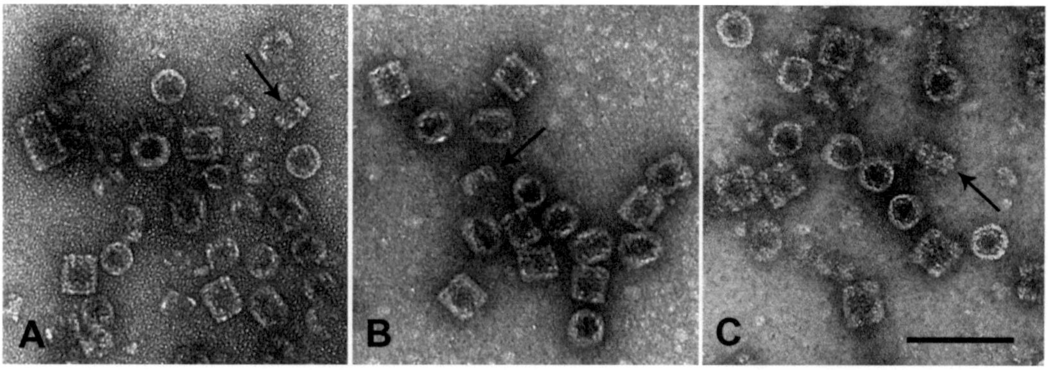

Figure 1. Electron microscopy of negatively stained purified mollusk hemocyanin molecules showing their characteristic hollow cylinder form. A. Hemocyanin from the Keyhole limpet (*Megathura crenulata*), known as KLH. B. Hemocyanin from *Concholepas concholepas,* known as CCH. C. Hemocyanin from *Fissurella latimarginata,* known as FLH. The images show the top (circles) and lateral (rectangles) views of the molecules. The side views show the characteristic didecameric forms of the protein, with subunits arranged in layers. The arrow shows decamers. The scale bar represents 100 nm.

3. Hemocyanins used in biomedicine

KLH from *Megathura crenulata* has been used for more than 40 years for biomedical and biotechnological applications. In the search for new hemocyanins that might act with similar immunostimulatory properties, the hemocyanins from *Concholepas concholepas* (CCH), *Rapana thomasiana* (RtH) and *Haliotis tuberculata* (HtH) emerge as the most promising. Surprisingly, in this search, we identified a new hemocyanin from *Fissurella latimarginata* (FLH) with superior immunogenicity compared to any other hemocyanin known to date (Arancibia et al., 2014). Background on these hemocyanins and the experimental data that support their potential use as immunostimulants is provided below and summarized in Table 1.

3.1. *Megathura crenulata* hemocyanin (KLH)

The hemocyanin from the giant keyhole limpet *Megathura crenulata,* which naturally lives on the coast of Southern California to Baja California, is a mixture of two immunologically different didecamers, named KLH1 and KLH2. In fact, diverse electrophoretic analyses have revealed that the KLH preparation is made up of two independent oligomeric isoforms that coexist in variable proportions in the animal's circulation, each composed of one type of subunit, KLH1 (350 KDa) and KLH2 (350 KDa) (Gebauer et al., 1999a; Swerdlow et al., 1996). Immunoelectrophoretic analyses using polyclonal antibodies provided insight into the antigenic individuality of these KLH isoforms, indicating that they are very different structurally (i.e., they do not display shared epitopes) (Harris and Markl, 1999). Although both KLH subunits are glycosylated, they differ in their oligosaccharide patterns: KLH1 (3.0% carbohydrate, w/w) has higher mannose content than KLH2 (3.4% carbohydrate, w/w), which has more N-acetylgalactosamine than KLH1, in addition to the presence of an O-glycosylation site

(Idakieva et al., 2004). Whether or not KLH1 and KLH2 have similar effects on the immune response has not been comprehensively analyzed. Currently, the variable proportions of KLH subunits in different preparations of the agent, in addition to its propensity to precipitate (Gathuru et al., 2005), can be problematic for some biomedical applications in which the components should be invariant and precisely defined. In addition, the KLH genes have been cloned and sequenced, and the complete amino acid sequences of its subunits are now known; however, until now, it has not been possible to express a heterologous KLH (Altenhein et al., 2002; Gatsogiannis and Markl, 2009; Markl et al., 2001).

In the 1970s, KLH was introduced in the clinic as part of a test to evaluate immunocompetence in immunosuppressed patients (Curtis et al., 1971; Curtis et al., 1970); thus, its benefits for the treatment of recurrent superficial bladder cancer were discovered serendipitously (Olsson et al., 1974), as described later. In addition, at that time, through the coupling of small molecules (or haptens, defined as substances unable to induce antibodies by themselves) to KLH, it was possible to obtain specific antibodies against them. Thereby, KLH has become, and remains to this day, the most used carrier protein to produce polyclonal and monoclonal antibodies against small molecules, including peptides, drugs, hormones, toxins, antibiotics and countless chemicals. The optimal carrier properties of KLH add to its intrinsic immunostimulatory effects, leading to its current use in the development of several therapeutic vaccines for cancer through the generation of antibodies against TAAs; these antibodies act to eliminate cancer recurrence caused by circulating tumor cells and micrometastases. Moreover, KLH, when conjugated with idiotype antibodies, can induce strong anti-idiotypic antibody responses and cell-mediated responses to tumor antigen(s) *in vivo*, which has resulted in an objective outcome in patients with B-cell lymphoma (Nelson et al., 1996). In addition, the adjuvant/immunostimulatory properties of KLH have been amply supported through its use in vaccine studies as an immunological tracer protein due to its neo-antigen character. Thus, this protein serves as a strong "surrogate" antigen and an immunogenic "marker" for immunization studies using DC-based vaccines (Shimizu et al., 2001).

3.2. *Concholepas concholepas* hemocyanin (CCH)

The hemocyanin from the edible gastropod *Concholepas concholepas*, a specie distributed on the coasts of Chile and southern Perú, is structurally distinct from traditional KLH. The decamers are formed by two subunits, named CCHA (405 KDa) and CCHB (350 kDa), which are intermingled in the molecule and form heterodecamers. Consequently, their association in pairs results in heterodidecamers (De Ioannes et al., 2004). The carbohydrate content has been determined and has demonstrated that each subunit is differently glycosylated. Thus, CCHA (3.6% carbohydrate, w/w) has N-linked and O-linked glycans; CCHB (2.5% carbohydrate, w/w) has only sugar with N-linkages, while O-linked moieties are nearly absent (Becker et al., 2009). A feature that distinguishes CCH from the remaining hemocyanins is its great stability and solubility. In fact, in contrast with other hemocyanins, after its purification from the hemolymph, the stabilization of CCH does not require additional divalent cations, such as $Ca^{2+}$and/or Mg^{2+}, in the storage media to maintain its structure (De Ioannes et al., 2004). This quality facilitates chemical coupling reactions when CCH is used as a carrier protein. Thus, CCH has been successfully used as a carrier protein to generate antibodies against hapten molecules (Becker et al., 1998; Torres et al., 1999) and peptides (Duvillie et al., 2003; Grenegard et al., 2008; Matus et al., 2007; Mura et al., 2002). Additionally, CCH has been used as carrier of a gonadotropin-releasing hormone (GnRH) in a contraceptive vaccine to control reproduction in deer, providing a longer-lasting contraceptive effect (Miller et al., 2008; Pilon et al., 2007). Furthermore, CCH has been pre-clinically evaluated in a murine experimental model of superficial bladder cancer and may be considered a safe alternative therapy to KLH (Atala, 2006; Moltedo et al., 2006), as described later.

Finally, the most important support for clinical attention to CCH in future biomedical developments includes the results of a recent study of its use as an adjuvant in a DC-based cancer vaccine for castration-resistant prostate cancer (CRPC) patients. This study demonstrated that CCH was able to induce an immune memory response, as measured by the delayed-type hypersensitivity (DTH) test, and did not produce toxic or allergic adverse reactions when administered subcutaneously in the patients. These results led to the conclusion that CCH may be considered as an alternative to KLH for providing safe and effective adjuvanticity in cancer vaccines (Reyes et al., 2013).

3.3. FLH

The hemocyanin from the black keyhole limpet *Fissurella latimarginata* (FLH) was discovered most recently (Arancibia et al., 2014). The experimental data demonstrate that FLH didecamers are composed of a single type of polypeptide with a molecular mass of approximately 350 kDa. Although the total carbohydrate content has not yet been estimated, carbohydrate staining with specific lectins has shown that FLH has exposed N-and O-linked oligosaccharides, similar to KLH (Arancibia et al., 2014). The evaluation of the humoral immune responses in different mouse strains immunized with CCH, FLH and KLH indicated that FLH is intrinsically more immunogenic than CCH and KLH and reaches titers an order of magnitude higher than those of CCH and KLH. Moreover, FLH had potent *in vivo* anti-tumor activity against melanoma in the B16F10 mouse model, delaying tumor growth and increasing the survival of mice challenged with these cells in a prophylactic setting (i.e., with the aim of preventing tumor growth). The most striking effect was observed in a therapeutic setting (specifically, therapy for established tumors in animals without previous FLH priming) (Arancibia et al., 2014). To elucidate the early immunologic mechanisms involved in this anti-tumor effect, we investigated the effect of FLH on murine DCs cultured *in vitro*. These studies demonstrated that FLH, but not CCH or KLH, is able to rapidly induce the secretion of certain pro-inflammatory cytokines, including interleukin (IL)-6, tumor necrosis factor (TNF)-α, IL-12p40 and IL-23α, a phenomenon that may explain its enhanced immunological activities (Arancibia et al., 2014).

3.4. HtH

The hemocyanin from the European abalone *Haliotis tuberculata* (**HtH**), a species under commercial aquaculture conditions, is composed of two types of didecamers that coexist in the animal's circulation, HtH1 and HtH2. Immunological analysis demonstrated that these two didecamers are closely related (Keller et al., 1999). These isoforms are formed by the HtH1 and HtH2 subunits, and each has a molecular mass of approximately 392 kDa (Altenhein et al., 2002; Lieb et al., 2000). The carbohydrate content of HtH is 4.5% (w/w); a highly heterogeneous group of structures with appreciable amounts of 3-o-methyl-d-mannose and 3-o-

Table 1. Hemocyanins available today

PROPERTIES	FEATURE	KLH	CCH	FLH	HtH	RtH
Taxonomy	Phylum	Mollusk	Mollusk	Mollusk	Mollusk	Mollusk
	Order	Gastropoda	Gastropoda	Gastropoda	Gastropoda	Gastropoda
	Family	Fissurellidae	Muricidae	Fissurellidae	Haliotidae	Muricidae
	Genus and specie	*Megathura crenulata*	*Concholepas concholepas*	*Fissurella latimarginata*	*Haliotis tuberculata*	*Rapana thomasiana*
Distribution	Habitat	Coast of California	Pacific coast of Perú and Chile	Pacific coast of Perú and Chile	Waters of the Channel Islands	Japan sea , and the East China Sea
Biochemical	Molecular weights	≈ 8 MDa	≈ 8 MDa	≈ 8 MDa	≈ 8 MDa	≈ 8 MDa
	Size of molecule	≈ 360 Å Ø 400Å height	≈ 325Å Ø 392Å height	≈350 Å Ø 370 Å height	≈ 350 Å Ø 380Å height	≈ 350 Å Ø 380Å height
	Subunits composition	2	2	1	2	2
	Subunit organization	Homodecamer	Heterodecamer	Homodecamer	Homodecamer	Homodecamer
	Stability structure in solution	Required Ca^{+2} and Mg^{+2}	Not required Ca^{+2} and Mg^{+2}	Required Ca^{+2} and Mg^{+2}	Required Ca^{+2} and Mg^{+2}	Required Ca^{+2} and Mg^{+2}
	Isoelectric point	5,7	6,0	ND	ND	ND
	% Oligosaccharides	3,2%	3,1%	ND	4,5%	2,6%
	Type of Oligosaccharides	N- and O-linked	N- and O-linked	N- and O-linked	N- and O-linked	N- and O-linked
Immunological	Immunogenicity	High	High	Very high	ND	ND
	Antitumor effects in animals models of SBC	Yes	Yes	ND	ND	ND
	Antitumor effects in animals models of melanoma	Yes	Yes	Yes	ND	ND
	Evaluated as hapten carrier	Yes	Yes	Yes	ND	ND
Biomedical uses	Used as adjuvant in DC vaccines	Yes	Yes	ND	ND	ND
	Used as immunostimulant in bladder cancer	Yes	No	No	No	No

ND: Not determinate

methyl-d-galactose has been identified in HtH (Idakieva et al., 2004; Velkova et al.). It is important to note that, although there are numerous studies on the biochemical characteristics of HtH, comprehensive studies about its immunologic and therapeutic properties are essentially absent. However, a stable preparation of abalone hemocyanin with high antiviral activity has recently been formulated and needs to be evaluated as therapeutic agent in future clinical applications (Zanjani et al., 2013).

3.5. RtH

The hemocyanin of the marine snail *Rapana thomasiana* (RtH), a species native of the China Sea and transferred to the West coast of the Black Sea, was described in the 1990s (Idakieva et al., 1993). RtH is a mixture of two hemocyanin isoforms, RtH1 and RtH2, that coexist in the animal's circulation (Gebauer et al., 1999b). Both have carbohydrate contents of 2.6% (w/w), with very similar monosaccharide compositions featuring type N-glycosylation (Idakieva et al., 2004). The biomedical applications of RtH as an adjuvant have been explored and have demonstrated that mice immunized with influenza vaccine developed a specific humoral and cellular immune response characterized by the induction of specific antibodies to viral proteins and a cytotoxic response lasting at least 5 months (Gesheva et al., 2011). Furthermore, antimicrobial activities against different strains of the genital herpes simplex virus have been reported for the RtH2 subunit (Genova-Kalou et al., 2008).

4. Hemocyanins as non-specific immunostimulants in recurrent superficial bladder cancer (SBC)

A significant decrease in the recurrence of superficial bladder cancer in 10 patients with transitional cell carcinoma (TCC) treated with KLH without toxic side effects was reported early on in the field of hemocyanin research (Olsson et al., 1974). This study was followed by tens of papers, which collectively provided encouraging support for the use of KLH and CCH as alternatives in SBC immunotherapy. The most frequently used immunotherapeutic agent to prevent recurrence of TCC is the Bacillus Calmette-Guerin (BCG) vaccine for tuberculosis (Morales et al., 1976). This attenuated form of *Mycobacterium bovis* has also been used as a therapy in other types of cancers (Edwards and Whitwell, 1974; Milas and Withers, 1976). However, despite the successful results (Nseyo and Lamm, 1997), the severe side effects of the BCG vaccine have led scientists to explore new immunostimulants (Lamm, 2003).

4.1. Experimental studies

Three different *in vivo* models have been primarily used to evaluate the therapeutic properties of hemocyanins in SBC, with the therapy being administered either subcutaneously, intraperitoneally or intravesically according to the site where the tumor was established (Lamm, 2003; Schenkman and Lamm, 2004). The mouse bladder tumor-2 cell (MBT-2) transplantable murine model of SBC was the first of these models to be developed in 1981 (Lamm et al., 1981). Mice were pre-immunized with 200 μg of KLH after a previous subcutaneous inoculation with MBT-2 and were then intralesionally immunized with 50 μg at one and seven days after implantation, leading to a significant decrease in tumor growth and a prolongation of animal survival (Lamm et al., 1981). Further studies showed that priming was essential for achieving a therapeutic effect (Lamm et al., 1993b; Lamm et al., 1982; Marsh et al., 1987). However, other researchers have studied KLH immunotherapy in the same model without promising results. The priming and transplantation of MBT-2 tumor cells, either subcutaneously or into the bladder, with immunotherapy of 50 or 200 μg of KLH did not yield different results compared to controls (Walsh et al., 1983). In a later study, the administration routes of KLH were compared. Without priming, the intralesional route was more effective than intraperitoneal administration in terms of inhibiting tumor growth (Lau et al., 1986). After that, an additive effect was observed in animals that received KLH and interferon (IFN)-α intraperitoneally without prior immunization, compared with KLH and IFN-α alone (Riggs et al., 1992). However, in a subsequent study, the presence of endotoxin in KLH preparations partially accounted for its anti-tumor effect (Lamm et al., 1993a).

The syngeneic orthotopic murine bladder cancer model MB-49 was evaluated in 1994 (Gunther et al., 1999; Swerdlow et al., 1994). Subcutaneous immunization with KLH-Immune Activator, a clinical-grade KLH preparation, two weeks prior to intravesical implantation of tumor cells, followed by intravesical administration of 10 or 100 μg of KLH, resulted in significantly decreased tumor growth (Swerdlow et al., 1994). Prior immunization was required, and no significant histopathological abnormalities were observed. A third model was developed in 1989 that consisted of the induction of a bladder carcinoma in Wistar rats using N-butyl-N-(4-hydroxybutyl) nitrosamine (BBN) (Arentsen et al., 2009). Subcutaneous sensitization with 1 mg of KLH, followed by intravesical and subcutaneous administration twice weekly, led to a decrease of BBN-induced bladder tumors (Recker and Rubben, 1989). A subsequent study demonstrated that subcutaneous administration was more effective than intravesical instillation in terms of tumor growth and rats bearing tumors (Linn et al., 2000).

Finally, more recent studies have evaluated the effect of CCH in the MBT-2 murine model (Becker et al., 2009; Moltedo et al., 2006). Priming with CCH previous subcutaneous implantation of tumor cells, succeeded by subcutaneous immunization with 1 or 0.1 mg of CCH, led to decreases in the incidence and growth of tumors, prolonged survival and the absence of toxic effects (Moltedo et al., 2006). In a subsequent study of the contributions of CCH-A and CCH-B subunits, it was determined that each subunit alone has an anti-tumor effect. However, in terms of tumor incidence and animal survival, CCH-A had the maximum effect (Becker et al., 2009).

4.2. Clinical studies

As a result of complications of complete bladder removal and the possibility of cancer recurrence, some SBCs have been treated with intravesical administration of biological and chemotherapeutic agents in the initial stages of the disease to either treat an established tumor or avoid progression and recurrence after transurethral resection (Perabo and Muller, 2004). The first study in humans was performed in 1974, in which 10 immunocompetent patients subcutaneously primed with 5 mg of KLH and followed with immunization using 200 μg of

KLH had significantly reduced tumor recurrence rates over a period of two years (Olsson et al., 1974). More than 10 years later, a controlled study corroborated that KLH was more effective than mitomycin C (Jurincic et al., 1988). Then, it was determined that the incidence of recurrence in patients with TCC related to urinary schistosomiasis was diminished after KLH treatment (Wishahi et al., 1995). However, studies with patients who were unresponsive to chemotherapeutic agents (Flamm et al., 1990) or who had carcinoma *in situ* (CIS) (Jurincic-Winkler et al., 1995c; Jurincic-Winkler et al., 2000) have not shown any significant effects after KLH treatment.

A Phase III clinical trial was conducted by Intracel Resources (USA) to assess the safety and effectiveness of the KLH BCI-Immune Activator compared to doxorubicin in BCG-intolerant or refractory patients with CIS with or without resected SBC. Nevertheless, although the study was completed, no results have been posted. Recently, Biosyn (USA) evaluated the efficacy and adverse effects of IMMUCOTHEL®, a clinical-grade KLH preparation developed by Biosyn Arzneimittel GmbH (Germany). Their outcomes showed almost no KLH-induced adverse effects, and the efficacy of IMMUCOTHEL® was comparable to mitomycin C.

4.3. Other models

Due to some of the successful results using hemocyanins in SBC therapy, their therapeutic effects have been evaluated in other cancers, such as melanoma, breast, pancreatic, esophageal and prostatic.

4.3.1. In vitro studies

The effectiveness of KLH has been demonstrated in diverse human cancer cell lines, such as estrogen-independent breast (ZR75-1), estrogen-dependent breast (MCF-7), esophagus (SEG-1 and BIC-1), pancreas (PANC-1), melanoma (HTB68 and HTB72) and prostate (DU145), through the inhibition of cellular growth in an apoptotic-dependent or independent manner (McFadden et al., 2003; Riggs et al., 2002; Riggs et al., 2005; Somasundar et al., 2005). In addition, KLH was shown to exert an additive effect with IL-2 and IFN-α in a combined therapy against melanoma, which encourages the use of this type of bivalent therapy as an effective treatment against these types of aggressive disease (McFadden et al., 2007).

4.3.2. In vivo studies

Diverse hemocyanins have been evaluated as a therapy in murine models of melanoma. First, the combined effect of KLH with IL-2 and IFN-α was evaluated in an HTB68 mouse melanoma model. KLH augmented the effect of IFN-α, one of the most common immunotherapeutic agents against melanoma (Rizvi et al., 2007). Then, the effect of diverse glycoconjugates (GCs), which induce NK-cell mediated cytotoxicity *in vitro*, were evaluated with or without KLH in a B16F10 murine melanoma model. However, no synergism was observed, which was attributed to the common epitopes shared between the protein and the GCs (Hulikova et al.). Recently, it was demonstrated that an oxidated-modified CCH, which had enhanced structural stability and immunogenicity, has the same anti-tumor effect in the B16F10 melanoma model as its native counterpart (Arancibia et al., 2012a). In addition, we have recently demonstrated the outstanding immunomodulatory properties of FLH in a B16F10 murine melanoma model. FLH promotes significantly higher antibody titers than CCH and KLH, in addition to exhibiting potent anti-tumor activity that delays the growth of B16F10 melanoma cells and prolongs murine survival (Arancibia et al., 2014).

5. Hemocyanins as carriers/adjuvants in vaccines

Mollusk hemocyanins have been widely used in therapeutic and prophylactic vaccines, enhancing the immune response by building on hemocyanin's carrier properties and adjuvant capacities (Del Campo et al., 2011). In order to generate immunity against antigens, pathogens, TAAs and certain chemical substances, such as commonly abused drugs, it is necessary to chemically couple the compound to the hemocyanin and then immunize the patient. The hemocyanins can also be used as genuine adjuvants to further enhance T cell reactivity to tumors in DC vaccine therapy; in this case, hemocyanins contribute to the reversal of the DC tolerogenic profile in cancer patients toward an immunostimulatory profile (Presicce et al., 2008). Indeed, the generation of an optimal cytotoxic T cell (CTL) immune response requires the presence of T helper lymphocytes (CD4+) and the expression of both helper-and CTL-defined antigen determinants on the same DC (Shimizu et al., 2001; Timmerman and Levy, 2000). Thus, hemocyanins produce a bystander effect, inducing a potent specific memory T cell response associated with the secretion of cytokines that indirectly promote the specific cellular response against the antigen of interest, whether a tumor cell, a pathogen or a deleterious compound.

The following overview offers a brief look at the experimental vaccines that have used hemocyanins in their formulations.

5.1. Vaccines against pathogens

Pathogenic immunodominant peptides or polysaccharides coupled to hemocyanin have been tested in the development of experimental vaccines that are intended to prevent diseases caused by bacteria, viruses and fungi. We next present some examples.

5.1.1. Vaccines against bacteria

For *Pseudomonas aeruginosa,* which causes pulmonary infection, the use of synthetic peptides representing surface-exposed, linear B-cell epitopes of outer membrane protein F (Hughes and Gilleland, 1995) or mucoid exopolysaccharide (MEP) coupled to KLH demonstrated that significantly enhances its immunogenicity and the capacity to elicit opsonic antibodies in mice and rabbits (Theilacker et al., 2003). For *Streptococcus pneumonia,* which causes pneumococcal infection, administration of a DNA plasmid encoding the FLt3 ligand gene as a mucosal adjuvant plus phosphorylcholine (PC) conjugated to KLH demonstrated elicitation of PC-specific immune responses at the mucosal and serum levels (Baatarjav et al., 2011). For *Coxiella burnetii,* which causes acute and chronic Q fever in humans, a lipopolysaccharide (LPS) mimetic peptide was coupled to KLH; immunized mice were able to inhibit *C. burnetii* infection and to develop significant protection against *C. burnetii* challenge (Peng et al., 2012).

5.1.2. Vaccines against viruses

For papillomavirus, peptide fragments were used that mimicked B-cell epitopes of the capsid protein L1 of human papillomavirus (HPV) type 31 coupled to KLH, generating specific anti-peptide antibodies in mice (Andreev et al., 2012). For influenza, a conjugate vaccine consisting of the peptide of the highly conserved M2 membrane protein coupled to KLH was highly immunogenic and able to confer protection against lethal challenge with either H1N1 or H3N1 virus in mice (Fan et al., 2004; Kiraly et al., 2011). For HIV-1, aiming to develop neutralizing antibodies in a caprine model, KLH was coupled with a synthetic peptide representative of the p17 functional epitope (AT20) derived from HIV-1 or with MPR peptide from the gp41 membrane proximal region to prevent transmission of the virus through colostrum. This conjugated vaccine effectively induced specific sIgA and IgG in the colostrum of a lactating species.(Dorosko et al., 2008).

5.1.3. Vaccines against fungi

For *Cryptococcus neoformans,* which causes meningoencephalitis in AIDS patients, one component of the cryptococcal capsular polysaccharide was coupled to KLH, producing antibodies that were protective against the pathogen (May et al., 2003). However, a protective epitope of *Candida albicans* conjugated to KLH induced a Th1-type cytokine expression pattern in C57BL/6J mice (Su et al., 2007).

5.2. Antitumor vaccines

The antitumoral vaccines are intended to treat an existing cancer by strengthening the body's natural defenses against cancer and have emerged as alternatives to anti-proliferative treatments, such as chemo-or radio-therapy. The design of such vaccines is focused on the search for specific epitopes in tumor cells to raise antibodies against them. These epitopes are usually aberrant branches of polysaccharides located on the cell surface. Some of them are glycolipids, such as Globo H, Lewis Y, GM2, GD2, GD3 and fucosyl-GM1, and others are glycoproteins, such as MUC-1, Tn, sialyl-Tn and TF (Galonic and Gin, 2007). The aim of these vaccines is to transform these tumor antigens into immunogens powerful enough to achieve an immune response. Furthermore, hemocyanins are used as immunomodulatory agents in DC vaccines in which these autologous presenting cells are loaded with tumor antigen, whether as tumor lysate, recombinant antigen or transfecting cell tumor RNA, in the presence of hemocyanins (Steinman and Banchereau, 2007). In this case, the patient's responses are measured by DTH tests against hemocyanins or tumor extract (Escobar et al., 2005). In addition to the extensive use of KLH for this purpose, promising results have been obtained with CCH as an adjuvant in a DC vaccine administered to patients with CRPC (Reyes et al., 2013). Next, we review selected antitumor vaccine clinical trials with hemocyanins that have been approved by the US National Institutes of Health (NIH).

5.3. Breast, ovary, fallopian tube and peritoneal cancers

Sialyl-Tn (STn) is the tumor antigen most frequently expressed in breast, ovary, colon, rectal, stomach and pancreas adenocarcinomas. This antigen, conjugated to KLH, has been named Theratope and is capable of generating positive serological results, inducing significant titers of IgM and IgG antibodies against STn (Gilewski et al., 2007). The results of a Phase III multicenter clinical trial, which included 1,028 women with metastatic breast cancer, showed that the sialyl-Tn (STn)-KLH vaccine was well tolerated by the patients, but no overall benefit in time to progression or survival was observed (Miles et al., 2011). However, women who also received endocrine therapy and showed greater antibody response to the STn-KLH vaccine had significantly longer median overall survival than those who had lower antibody responses, demonstrating that this dual treatment may improve clinical outcomes in women with metastatic breast cancer (Miles et al., 2011). Other monovalent vaccines have been developed in which a single carbohydrate antigen, including Globo-H, fucosyl GM1 and Lewis^y (Le^y), were coupled to KLH with saponin fractions (QS21 or OPT-82142) added as adjuvants; these vaccines have exhibited varying degrees of promise in early clinical settings (Ragupathi et al., 2011; Zhu et al., 2009). Additionally, multivalent vaccines have been formulated with GM2, Globo-H, Lewis Y, Tn (c), STn (c), TF (c) and Tn-MUC1, each individually conjugated to KLH. QS21 was added as an adjuvant to this cocktail of conjugates and was evaluated in patients with either epithelial ovarian, fallopian tube or peritoneal cancer in second or greater complete clinical remission, demonstrating that this heptavalent vaccine was safe and induced antibody responses against five of seven antigens (Sabbatini et al., 2007). Currently, more elaborate constructs have been designed in a new vaccine against ovarian cancer, based on clusters of a globotriaosylceramide (Gb3) antigen and incorporating a MUC5AC peptide epitope that mimics the surfaces of targeted tumor cells (Zhu et al., 2009).

5.4. Melanomas

Vaccines were designed with the gangliosides GM2, GD2 and GD3 conjugated to KLH plus the adjuvant QS21. These vaccines produced high titers of IgM and IgG in patients with melanoma compared to vaccines with GM2 and BCG as adjuvants (Ragupathi et al., 2000). Although it was initially postulated that immunotherapy against GM2 was effective in reducing the risk of relapse in post-surgery patients with stage III melanoma, the vaccine was ineffective in a Phase III clinical trial in 1314 patients (Eggermont et al., 2013). Additionally, gangliosides GD2-L and GD3-L have been used as therapeutic targets, generating higher titers of IgM and IgG (Ragupathi et al., 2003).

Regarding cellular vaccines, the first clinical study included patients with advanced melanoma who were treated with DCs loaded with tumor lysate or a mixture of melanoma peptides in the presence of KLH. Patients tolerated the vaccine and did not develop autoimmunity (Nestle et al., 1998). Currently, other antigens, such as MART-1/MelanA, tyrosinase, MAGE-3 and gp100 (Fay et al., 2006; Tittarelli et al.; Tittarelli et al., 2012), in addition to the heat-shocked melanoma lysate named TRIMEL (Aguilera et al., 2011), with KLH as an adjuvant have been loaded on DCs, yielding promising results in terms of the prolongation of overall survival time. Interestingly, in the search for parameters of clinical effectiveness of KLH-containing vaccines and therapies, a quantitative enzyme-linked immunosorbent assay (ELISA) has been developed to measure KLH-specific antibodies as biomarkers in humans, demonstrating that it is possible to monitor the dynamics of both KLH-specific antibody levels and antibody class-switching in individuals who are repeatedly exposed to KLH (Aarntzen et al., 2012).

5.5. Prostate cancer

Numerous tumor antigens coupled to hemocyanins have been tested in monovalent, divalent or polyvalent vaccines (Zhu et al., 2009). To date, there are 10 clinical trials in various stages of development using primarily the antigen MUC-2 with KLH. When comparing preclinical studies between mono-and polyvalent vaccines, the controversy arises over which strategy is best and why, based on the observations that the monovalent vaccines induced high titers of antibodies, whereas the polyvalent vaccines reached a greater range of antibodies (Slovin et al., 2007). Recently, CCH, as an adjuvant in a cancer vaccine based on DCs loaded with prostate cancer cell lysates and TRIMEL, was used for the first time in CRPC patients. This study demonstrated that CCH is safe and is capable of inducing memory T cell responses, as determined *in vivo* by a DTH test (Reyes et al., 2013), thus indicating that CCH can complement or substitute KLH in such therapies.

5.6. Lung cancer

In the eradication of micrometastases in chemotherapy-resistant small cell lung cancer (SCLC), the ganglioside fucosyl-GM1 is used as a therapeutic target. Therefore, in a clinical study, 11 patients with SCLC were vaccinated by injection with this synthetic antigen coupled to KLH. Higher IgM titers against fucosyl-GM1 were detected in eight of the patients, and only one patient developed IgG with a similar titer; these results led to a Phase II study (Krug et al., 2004). Recently, vaccination with N-propionyl polysialic acid-KLH conjugate plus QS-21 in patients with SCLC has demonstrated that this vaccine is safe and results in consistent high-titer antibody responses. These results open up the possibility of incorporating polysialic acid into a polyvalent vaccine against SCLC with four glycolipid antigens that are also widely expressed in SCLC, such as GD2, GD3, fucosylated GM1 and globo H (Krug et al., 2012). In consideration of the fact that tumor angiogenesis is critical for tumor growth, infiltration and metastasis, another promising approach includes the generation of a mimotope of Bevacizumab (Avastin), a monoclonal antibody that reacts directly against vascular endothelial growth factor (VEGF) conjugated to KLH, which induces humoral immunity and results in the induction of anti-angiogenesis responses in mice (Li et al., 2013).

5.7. Lymphomas and myelomas

For the non-Hodgkins lymphomas, the strategy of conjugating the variable regions of the immunoglobulin to the tumorigenic clone with KLH has been used. These variable regions act as tumor antigens. The principle of these vaccines is that the clonal immunoglobulin idiotype displayed on the surface of most malignant B cells is not only tumor-specific; it is also a patient-specific antigen that can be used for therapeutic vaccination (Bendandi, 2006; de Cerio et al., 2007). These idiotype vaccines have shown some degrees of both biological efficacy and improved clinical outcomes in lymphoma (Bendandi, 2009). The effect of this type of vaccine has been enhanced by incorporating granulocyte macrophage colony-stimulating factor (GM-CSF); showing DCs recruiment and activation of CD4+and CD8+T lymphocytes (Bendandi et al., 1999). These encouraging results led to the initiation of Phase III clinical trials to establish the clinical benefits induced by anti-idiotypic vaccines (Neelapu and Kwak, 2007). In addition, DC-based anti-idiotype vaccination using KLH as an adjuvant induces a specific cellular immune response in patients with stage 1 myeloma (Rollig et al., 2011).

5.8. Vaccines against abused drugs

Experimental vaccines have been developed to curb recidivism in the consumption of addictive drugs, including cocaine and nicotine. The aim of these vaccines is to generate antibodies that reduce blood concentrations of the given drug and its effect on the central nervous system by preventing the drug from crossing the blood-brain barrier. The experimental strategies to induce protective and specific antibodies against cocaine included subcutaneous and intranasal immunization (Hrafnkelsdottir et al., 2007). Preclinical studies using KLH as a carrier of these drugs are promising (Moreno and Janda, 2009). However, the only clinical evidence with good results for the effectiveness of these vaccines used cholera toxin as a carrier of the cocaine-B subunit (Martell et al., 2009). Another interesting experimental approach is the generation of two complementary but mechanistically distinct active vaccines (i.e., non-catalytic and catalytic hapten designs) using a cocaine-like hapten, GNE, and a cocaine transition-state analogue, GNT, coupled to KLH. Although GNT-KLH induced higher titers of catalytic antibodies, these titers were not sufficient to provide protection in mice challenged with cocaine (Cai et al., 2013). Additionally, an anti-nicotine vaccine that used nicotine coupled to KLH, which was named Niccine®, was no better than the placebo (Gorelick, 2012).

6. The mechanisms of hemocyanin immunostimulation

6.1. At the innate immunity level

The effects induced by hemocyanins during the early phases of the immune response and the identities of the target cell type(s) have been scarcely studied. Several authors have suggested that the oligosaccharides may play a role in this process. As mentioned, the carbohydrate compositions of hemocyanins are quite diverse; however, the most abundant monosaccharide is mannose, which is often found in high-mannose or hybrid structures of oligosaccharides. The mammalian innate immune system has a variety of cell types that express several receptors on the cell surface. In this context, specialized professional antigen-presenting cells (APCs), such as macrophages and DCs, are key players in immune surveillance. These cells present a broad range of germ-line encoded pattern recognition receptors that recognize conserved pathogen-associated molecular patterns. Among these receptors, the C-type lectin family of receptors recognizes several types of oligosaccharides present on pathogens and foreign molecules (McGreal et al., 2006; van Vliet et al., 2008). The biological role of the high mannose oligosaccharides on mollusk hemocyanins has not been clearly demonstrated. However, it has been reported that KLH promotes the *in vitro* maturation of human DCs through its engagement of the mannose receptor, as assessed by the up-regulation of the cell surface expression of major histocompatibility complex (MHC) class II and co-stimulatory molecules (Presicce et al., 2008). It seems that this phenomenon has been described only for human DCs; in mice, neither KLH nor CCH induce DC maturation *in vitro* through canonical mechanisms (i.e., via up-regulation of MHCII and co-stimulatory molecules) during the early hours of *in vitro* culture (Arancibia et al., 2012a). Moreover, Teitz-Tennenbaum and collaborators (2008) demonstrated that murine DCs pulsed with KLH for 18 h *in vitro* did not undergo DC maturation, a result that is consistent with *in vivo* experiments performed by Moltedo et al. 2009 (Moltedo et al., 2009; Teitz-Tennenbaum et al., 2008). Recently, we observed that mouse DCs internalized this hemocyanin but did not mature within 72 h of culture *in vitro* with CCH. Remarkably, FLH, unlike KLH or CCH, promoted the high secretion of pro-inflammatory cytokines, such as IL-6, IL-12p40, TNF-α and IL-23, from murine DCs *in vitro* (Arancibia et al., 2014). Moreover, the secretion of cytokines was dependent on the presence of oligosaccharides on FLH, indicating a role for lectin-like receptors in the response. These results indicate the complexity of the immune response and demonstrate that different hemocyanins can activate diverse molecular and cellular pathways. In addition, the divergence regarding the role of DCs in hemocyanin recognition highlights the importance of studying those mechanisms in human cells.

Once hemocyanins are internalized by APCs, the proteolytic machinery of the cell degrades them slowly in comparison to classical antigens, thus increasing antigen persistence. This process permits the presence of hemocyanins for longer periods of time, resulting in augmented immunogenicity, as demonstrated for CCH (Arancibia et al., 2012a). In fact, using electron microscopy, we have determined that CCH molecules are internalized by DCs mainly through macropinocytosis and are then localized intact in lysosomes for up to 24 h. Moreover, we compared the antigen-processing kinetics of DCs for CCH and ovalbumin, a widely used antigen model, demonstrating the persistence of a band of approximately 49 kDa in DC cultures with CCH for 72 h; in contrast, in cultures of DCs pulsed with ovalbumin, the antigen was completely degraded by this time.

6.2. At the adaptive immunity level

Hemocyanins are thymus-dependent antigens; therefore, they require the interaction between T and B lymphocytes to initiate antibody production. In fact, it has been established that non-specific immunotherapeutic effects of hemocyanins in superficial bladder cancer rely on adequate priming, emphasizing the importance of the adaptive immune response in this property. Considering that the antitumor effect is induced by hemocyanins themselves without adjuvant, we assume that KLH and CCH have common structural features that promote inflammation and maintain innate immunity, leading to the onset of an antitumor adaptive immune response. These common characteristics of hemocyanins may rely on carbohydrates, which may act as natural adjuvants. A proposed alternative mechanism is that CD4+T lymphocytes reacting to preserved xenogenic peptidic sequences stimulate T lymphocytes to secrete Th1 cytokines that, in turn, break tumor tolerance via a bystander effect, thus braking tolerance to tumor antigens and enhancing the immune response against the tumor. This hypothesis is supported by the high secretion of cytokines, such as IFNγ and IL-2, observed in the regional lymph nodes (Arancibia et al., 2012b) after hemocyanin challenge. Accordingly, mice that were primed with CCH or KLH, challenged with MBT-2 cells and then subjected to immunotherapy with the respective hemocyanin increased natural killer cell activity and exhibited cytokine environment polarization toward a Th1 response (i.e., IFNγ production increased significantly in mouse sera), which correlated with antibodies belonging to the Th1 isotypes (Moltedo et al., 2006). Moreover, in patients with superficial bladder cancer under intravesical KLH therapy, a significant increase of CD4+T lymphocytes in the submucosa and among urothelial cells was observed, in contrast to a slight increase in CD8+T lymphocytes (Jurincic-Winkler et al., 1995a; Jurincic-Winkler et al., 1995b). In addition, KLH-conjugated vaccines against cancer using mucin-like or ganglioside epitopes have induced tumor-specific antibodies of the IgG1 and IgG3 isotypes (Musselli et al., 2001).

7. Future prospects

The information available shows that the mollusk hemocyanins presented herein – including KLH, the traditional and most utilized hemocyanin in biomedicine, and **CCH**, **RtH**, **HtH** and **FLH,** the most recently characterized hemocyanins – differ in their immunogenicity and non-specific immunostimulatory properties, opening basic questions on the structural characteristics responsible for these differences. Moreover, it is important to note that although several subunits of these hemocyanins have been sequenced via cDNA and that the complete amino acid sequences for these subunits are currently available, until now, it has not been possible to express heterologous or synthetic hemocyanins, mainly because of their size, complex structures and glycosylations. Therefore, all of the hemocyanins mentioned in this review can be obtained only as purified biological products from their natural sources, emphasizing the importance of pre-clinically evaluating diverse sources of hemocyanins for biomedical purposes. In this respect, only CCH hemocyanin from *Concholepas,* which has been pre-clinically evaluated in a murine experimental model of superficial bladder cancer (Moltedo et al., 2006) and has been recently used as an adjuvant in DC immunotherapy of patients with prostate cancer, is considered a safe complement or alternative to KLH (Reyes et al., 2013; Salazar-Onfray et a. 2013).

Finally, from a basic science perspective, a detailed molecular understanding of the receptors and signaling pathways involved in hemocyanin-induced immunostimulatory processes in mammals will be required to determine the basis of the qualitative and quantitative differences in the effects of the different hemocyanins on tumor immunology. Undoubtedly, this knowledge will support the development of new and better biomedical applications of these proteins, as hemocyanins exert their effects as immunopotentiators without the unwanted inflammatory side effects of classical adjuvants that drive cell-mediated immune responses.

Acknowledgements

This work was partially supported by research grant from **FONDECYT 1110651** to María Inés Becker.

Author details

María Inés Becker[1,2], Sergio Arancibia[1], Fabián Salazar[1], Miguel Del Campo[1] and Alfredo De Ioannes[2]

1 Fundación Ciencia y Tecnología para el Desarrollo (FUCITED), Santiago, Chile

2 Biosonda Corporation, Santiago, Chile

References

[1] Aarntzen, E.H., I.J. de Vries, J.H. Goertz, M. Beldhuis-Valkis, H.M. Brouwers, M.W. van de Rakt, R.G. van der Molen, C.J. Punt, G.J. Adema, P.J. Tacken, I. Joosten, and J.F. Jacobs. 2012. Humoral anti-KLH responses in cancer patients treated with dendritic cell-based immunotherapy are dictated by different vaccination parameters. *Cancer Immunol Immunother*. 61:2003-2011.

[2] Aguilera, R., C. Saffie, A. Tittarelli, F.E. Gonzalez, M. Ramirez, D. Reyes, C. Pereda, D. Hevia, T. Garcia, L. Salazar, A. Ferreira, M. Hermoso, A. Mendoza-Naranjo, C. Ferrada, P. Garrido, M.N. Lopez, and F. Salazar-Onfray. 2011. Heat-shock induction of tumor-derived danger signals mediates rapid monocyte differentiation into clinically effective dendritic cells. *Clin Cancer Res*. 17:2474-2483.

[3] Altenhein, B., J. Markl, and B. Lieb. 2002. Gene structure and hemocyanin isoform HtH2 from the mollusc Haliotis tuberculata indicate early and late intron hot spots. *Gene*. 301:53-60.

[4] Andreev, S.M., A.V. Giliazova, M.R. Khaitov, and D.G. Kozlov. 2012. [Anti-peptide antibodies specifically recognize the L1 protein of human papilloma virus type 31]. *Bioorg Khim*. 38:667-675.

[5] Arancibia, S., M. Del Campo, E. Nova, F. Salazar, and M.I. Becker. 2012a. Enhanced structural stability of Concholepas hemocyanin increases its immunogenicity and maintains its non-specific immunostimulatory effects. *Eur J Immunol*. 42:688-699.

[6] Arancibia, S., C. Espinoza, F. Salazar, M. Del Campo, R. Tampe, T. Zhong, P. De Ioannes, B. Moltedo, J. Ferreira, E.C. Lavelle, A. Manubens, and M.I. Becker. 2014. A Novel Immunomodulatory Hemocyanin from the Limpet Fissurella latimarginata

Promotes Potent Anti-tumor Activity in Melanoma. *Plos One.* doi:10.1371/journal.pone.0087240

[7] Arancibia, S., F. Salazar, and M.I. Becker. 2012b. Hemocyanins in the Immunotherapy of Superficial Bladder Cancer. *In* Bladder Cancer. Janeza, Croatia: INTECH. pp 221-242.

[8] Arentsen, H.C., K. Hendricksen, E. Oosterwijk, and J.A. Witjes. 2009. Experimental rat bladder urothelial cell carcinoma models. *World J Urol.* 27:313-317.

[9] Atala, A. 2006. This Month in Investigative Urology. *J Urol.* 176:2335-2336.

[10] Baatarjav, T., K. Kataoka, R.S. Gilbert, Y. Terao, M. Fukui, M. Goto, S. Kawabata, M. Yamamoto, K. Fujihashi, and H.O. Ito. 2011. Mucosal immune features to phosphorylcholine by nasal Flt3 ligand cDNA-based vaccination. *Vaccine.* 29:5747-5757.

[11] Becker, M.I., I. Carrasco, C. Beltran, M. Torres, B. Jaureguiberry, and A.E. De Ioannes. 1998. Development of monoclonal antibodies to gizzerosine, a toxic component present in fish meal. *Hybridoma.* 17:373-381.

[12] Becker, M.I., A. Fuentes, M. Del Campo, A. Manubens, E. Nova, H. Oliva, F. Faunes, M.A. Valenzuela, M. Campos-Vallette, A. Aliaga, J. Ferreira, A.E. De Ioannes, P. De Ioannes, and B. Moltedo. 2009. Immunodominant role of CCHA subunit of Concholepas hemocyanin is associated with unique biochemical properties. *Int Immunopharmacol.* 9:330-339.

[13] Bendandi, M. 2006. Clinical benefit of idiotype vaccines: too many trials for a clever demonstration? *Rev Recent Clin Trials.* 1:67-74.

[14] Bendandi, M., C.D. Gocke, C.B. Kobrin, F.A. Benko, L.A. Sternas, R. Pennington, T.M. Watson, C.W. Reynolds, B.L. Gause, P.L. Duffey, E.S. Jaffe, S.P. Creekmore, D.L. Longo, and L.W. Kwak. 1999. Complete molecular remissions induced by patient-specific vaccination plus granulocyte-monocyte colony-stimulating factor against lymphoma. *Nat Med.* 5:1171-1177.

[15] Cai, X., T. Whitfield, M.S. Hixon, Y. Grant, G.F. Koob, and K.D. Janda. 2013. Probing active cocaine vaccination performance through catalytic and noncatalytic hapten design. *J Med Chem.* 56:3701-3709.

[16] Curtis, J.E., E.M. Hersh, W.T. Butler, and R.D. Rossen. 1971. Antigen dose in the human immune response. Dose-relationships in the human immune response to Keyhole limpet hemocyanin. *J Lab Clin Med.* 78:61-69.

[17] Curtis, J.E., E.M. Hersh, J.E. Harris, C. McBride, and E.J. Freireich. 1970. The human primary immune response to keyhole limpet haemocyanin: interrelationships of delayed hypersensitivity, antibody response and in vitro blast transformation. *Clin Exp Immunol.* 6:473-491.

[18] de Cerio, A.L., N. Zabalegui, M. Rodriguez-Calvillo, S. Inoges, and M. Bendandi. 2007. Anti-idiotype antibodies in cancer treatment. *Oncogene*. 26:3594-3602.

[19] De Ioannes, P., B. Moltedo, H. Oliva, R. Pacheco, F. Faunes, A.E. De Ioannes, and M.I. Becker. 2004. Hemocyanin of the molluscan Concholepas concholepas exhibits an unusual heterodecameric array of subunits. *J Biol Chem*. 279:26134-26142.

[20] Decker, H., N. Hellmann, E. Jaenicke, B. Lieb, U. Meissner, and J. Markl. 2007. Minireview: Recent progress in hemocyanin research. *Integr Comp Biol*. 47:631-644.

[21] Del Campo, M., S. Arancibia, E. Nova, F. Salazar, A. Gonzalez, B. Moltedo, P. De Ioannes, J. Ferreira, A. Manubens, and M.I. Becker. 2011. [Hemocyanins as immunostimulants]. *Rev Med Chil*. 139:236-246.

[22] Dorosko, S.M., S.L. Ayres, and R.I. Connor. 2008. Induction of HIV-1 MPR(649-684)-specific IgA and IgG antibodies in caprine colostrum using a peptide-based vaccine. *Vaccine*. 26:5416-5422.

[23] Duvillie, B., M. Attali, V. Aiello, E. Quemeneur, and R. Scharfmann. 2003. Label-retaining cells in the rat pancreas: location and differentiation potential in vitro. *Diabetes*. 52:2035-2042.

[24] Edwards, F.R., and F. Whitwell. 1974. Use of BCG as an immunostimulant in the surgical treatment of carcinoma of the lung. *Thorax*. 29:654-658.

[25] Eggermont, A.M., S. Suciu, P. Rutkowski, J. Marsden, M. Santinami, P. Corrie, S. Aamdal, P.A. Ascierto, P.M. Patel, W.H. Kruit, L. Bastholt, L. Borgognoni, M.G. Bernengo, N. Davidson, L. Polders, M. Praet, and A. Spatz. 2013. Adjuvant ganglioside GM2-KLH/QS-21 vaccination versus observation after resection of primary tumor > 1.5 mm in Patients with stage II melanoma: results of the EORTC 18961 randomized phase III trial. *J Clinical Oncol*. 31:3831-3837.

[26] Escobar, A., M. Lopez, A. Serrano, M. Ramirez, C. Perez, A. Aguirre, R. Gonzalez, J. Alfaro, M. Larrondo, M. Fodor, C. Ferrada, and F. Salazar-Onfray. 2005. Dendritic cell immunizations alone or combined with low doses of interleukin-2 induce specific immune responses in melanoma patients. *Clin Exp Immunol*. 142:555-568.

[27] Fan, J., X. Liang, M.S. Horton, H.C. Perry, M.P. Citron, G.J. Heidecker, T.M. Fu, J. Joyce, C.T. Przysiecki, P.M. Keller, V.M. Garsky, R. Ionescu, Y. Rippeon, L. Shi, M.A. Chastain, J.H. Condra, M.E. Davies, J. Liao, E.A. Emini, and J.W. Shiver. 2004. Preclinical study of influenza virus A M2 peptide conjugate vaccines in mice, ferrets, and rhesus monkeys. *Vaccine*. 22:2993-3003.

[28] Fay, J.W., A.K. Palucka, S. Paczesny, M. Dhodapkar, D.A. Johnston, S. Burkeholder, H. Ueno, and J. Banchereau. 2006. Long-term outcomes in patients with metastatic melanoma vaccinated with melanoma peptide-pulsed CD34(+) progenitor-derived dendritic cells. *Cancer Immunol Immunother*. 55:1209-1218.

[29] Flamm, J., A. Bucher, W. Holtl, and W. Albrecht. 1990. Recurrent superficial transitional cell carcinoma of the bladder: adjuvant topical chemotherapy versus immunotherapy. A prospective randomized trial. *J Urol*. 144:260-263.

[30] Galonic, D.P., and D.Y. Gin. 2007. Chemical glycosylation in the synthesis of glycoconjugate antitumour vaccines. *Nature*. 446:1000-1007.

[31] Gathuru, J.K., F. Koide, G. Ragupathi, J.L. Adams, R.T. Kerns, T.P. Coleman, and P.O. Livingston. 2005. Identification of DHBcAg as a potent carrier protein comparable to KLH for augmenting MUC1 antigenicity. *Vaccine*. 23:4727-4733.

[32] Gatsogiannis, C., and J. Markl. 2009. Keyhole limpet hemocyanin: 9-A CryoEM structure and molecular model of the KLH1 didecamer reveal the interfaces and intricate topology of the 160 functional units. *J Mol Biol*. 385:963-983.

[33] Gebauer, W., J.R. Harris, G. Geisthardt, and J. Markl. 1999a. Keyhole limpet hemocyanin type 2 (KLH2): detection and immunolocalization of a labile functional unit h. *J Struct Biol*. 128:280-286.

[34] Gebauer, W., S. Stoeva, W. Voelter, E. Dainese, B. Salvato, M. Beltramini, and J. Markl. 1999b. Hemocyanin subunit organization of the gastropod Rapana thomasiana. *Arch Biochem Biophys*. 372:128-134.

[35] Genova-Kalou, P., D. Dundarova, K. Idakieva, A. Mohmmed, S. Dundarov, and R. Argirova. 2008. Anti-herpes effect of hemocyanin derived from the mollusk Rapana thomasiana. *Z Naturforsch C*. 63:429-434.

[36] Gesheva, V., K. Idakieva, N. Kerekov, K. Nikolova, N. Mihaylova, L. Doumanova, and A. Tchorbanov. 2011. Marine gastropod hemocyanins as adjuvants of non-conjugated bacterial and viral proteins. *Fish Shellfish Immunol*. 30:135-142.

[37] Geyer, H., M. Wuhrer, A. Resemann, and R. Geyer. 2005. Identification and characterization of keyhole limpet hemocyanin N-glycans mediating cross-reactivity with Schistosoma mansoni. *J Biol Chem*. 280:40731-40748.

[38] Gilewski, T.A., G. Ragupathi, M. Dickler, S. Powell, S. Bhuta, K. Panageas, R.R. Koganty, J. Chin-Eng, C. Hudis, L. Norton, A.N. Houghton, and P.O. Livingston. 2007. Immunization of high-risk breast cancer patients with clustered sTn-KLH conjugate plus the immunologic adjuvant QS-21. *Clin Cancer Res*. 13:2977-2985.

[39] Gorelick, D.A. 2012. Pharmacokinetic strategies for treatment of drug overdose and addiction. *Future Med Chem*. 4:227-243.

[40] Grenegard, M., K. Vretenbrant-Oberg, M. Nylander, S. Desilets, E.G. Lindstrom, A. Larsson, I. Ramstrom, S. Ramstrom, and T.L. Lindahl. 2008. The ATP-gated P2X1 receptor plays a pivotal role in activation of aspirin-treated platelets by thrombin and epinephrine. *J Biol Chem*. 283:18493-18504.

[41] Gunther, J.H., A. Jurczok, T. Wulf, S. Brandau, I. Deinert, D. Jocham, and A. Bohle. 1999. Optimizing syngeneic orthotopic murine bladder cancer (MB49). *Cancer Res.* 59:2834-2837.

[42] Hall, R.L., and E.J. Wood. 1976. The carbohydrate content of gastropod haemocyanins. *Biochem Soc Trans*. 4:307-309.

[43] Harris, J.R., and J. Markl. 1999. Keyhole limpet hemocyanin (KLH): a biomedical review. *Micron*. 30:597-623.

[44] Hrafnkelsdottir, K., J. Valgeirsson, S. Bjarnadottir, S. Olafsdottir, K. Olafsdottir, S.T. Hedinsdottir, E.V. Magnusdottir, and S. Gizurarson. 2007. Immunization prevents DDT buildup in mouse tissues. *Int Immunopharmacol*. 7:1179-1184.

[45] Hughes, E.E., and H.E. Gilleland, Jr. 1995. Ability of synthetic peptides representing epitopes of outer membrane protein F of Pseudomonas aeruginosa to afford protection against P. aeruginosa infection in a murine acute pneumonia model. *Vaccine*. 13:1750-1753.

[46] Hulikova, K., V. Grobarova, R. Krivohlava, and A. Fiserova. Antitumor activity of N-acetyl-D-glucosamine-substituted glycoconjugates and combined therapy with keyhole limpet hemocyanin in B16F10 mouse melanoma model. *Folia Microbiol (Praha)*. 55:528-532.

[47] Idakieva, K., S. Severov, I. Svendsen, N. Genov, S. Stoeva, M. Beltramini, G. Tognon, P. Di Muro, and B. Salvato. 1993. Structural properties of Rapana thomasiana grosse hemocyanin: isolation, characterization and N-terminal amino acid sequence of two different dissociation products. *Comp Biochem Physiol B*. 106:53-59.

[48] Idakieva, K., S. Stoeva, W. Voelter, and C. Gielens. 2004. Glycosylation of Rapana thomasiana hemocyanin. Comparison with other prosobranch (gastropod) hemocyanins. *Comp Biochem Physiol B Biochem Mol Biol*. 138:221-228.

[49] Jurincic-Winkler, C., K.A. Metz, J. Beuth, U. Engelmann, and K.F. Klippel. 1995a. Immunohistological findings in patients with superficial bladder carcinoma after intravesical instillation of keyhole limpet haemocyanin. *Br J Urol*. 76:702-707.

[50] Jurincic-Winkler, C., K.A. Metz, J. Beuth, J. Sippel, and K.F. Klippel. 1995b. Effect of keyhole limpet hemocyanin (KLH) and bacillus Calmette-Guerin (BCG) instillation on carcinoma in situ of the urinary bladder. *Anticancer Res*. 15:2771-2776.

[51] Jurincic-Winkler, C.D., H. Gallati, M. Alvarez-Mon, J. Sippel, J. Carballido, and K.F. Klippel. 1995c. Urinary interleukin-1 alpha levels are increased by intravesical instillation with keyhole limpet hemocyanin in patients with superficial transitional cell carcinoma of the bladder. *Eur Urol*. 28:334-339.

[52] Jurincic-Winkler, C.D., K.A. Metz, J. Beuth, and K.F. Klippel. 2000. Keyhole limpet hemocyanin for carcinoma in situ of the bladder: a long-term follow-up study. *Eur Urol*. 37 Suppl 3:45-49.

[53] Jurincic, C.D., U. Engelmann, J. Gasch, and K.F. Klippel. 1988. Immunotherapy in bladder cancer with keyhole-limpet hemocyanin: a randomized study. *J Urol*. 139:723-726.

[54] Keller, H., B. Lieb, B. Altenhein, D. Gebauer, S. Richter, S. Stricker, and J. Markl. 1999. Abalone (Haliotis tuberculata) hemocyanin type 1 (HtH1). Organization of the approximately 400 kDa subunit, and amino acid sequence of its functional units f, g and h. *Eur J Biochem*. 264:27-38.

[55] Kiraly, J., E. Vareckova, V. Mucha, and F. Kostolansky. 2011. Evaluation of anti-influenza efficiency of polyclonal IgG antibodies specific to the ectodomain of M2 protein of influenza A virus by passive immunization of mice. *Acta Virol*. 55:261-265.

[56] Krug, L.M., G. Ragupathi, C. Hood, C. George, F. Hong, R. Shen, L. Abrey, H.J. Jennings, M.G. Kris, and P.O. Livingston. 2012. Immunization with N-propionyl polysialic acid-KLH conjugate in patients with small cell lung cancer is safe and induces IgM antibodies reactive with SCLC cells and bactericidal against group B meningococci. *Cancer Immunol Immunother*. 61:9-18.

[57] Krug, L.M., G. Ragupathi, K.K. Ng, C. Hood, H.J. Jennings, Z. Guo, M.G. Kris, V. Miller, B. Pizzo, L. Tyson, V. Baez, and P.O. Livingston. 2004. Vaccination of small cell lung cancer patients with polysialic acid or N-propionylated polysialic acid conjugated to keyhole limpet hemocyanin. *Clin Cancer Res*. 10:916-923.

[58] Lamm, D.L. 2003. Intravesical therapy for superficial bladder cancer: slow but steady progress. *J Clin Oncol*. 21:4259-4260.

[59] Lamm, D.L., J.I. DeHaven, D.R. Riggs, C. Delgra, and R. Burrell. 1993a. Keyhole limpet hemocyanin immunotherapy of murine bladder cancer. *Urol Res*. 21:33-37.

[60] Lamm, D.L., J.I. DeHaven, D.R. Riggs, and R.F. Ebert. 1993b. Immunotherapy of murine bladder cancer with keyhole limpet hemocyanin (KLH). *J Urol*. 149:648-652.

[61] Lamm, D.L., J.A. Reyna, and D.F. Reichert. 1981. Keyhole-limpet haemacyanin and immune ribonucleic acid immunotherapy of murine transitional cell carcinoma. *Urol Res*. 9:227-230.

[62] Lamm, D.L., D.E. Thor, V.D. Stogdill, and H.M. Radwin. 1982. Bladder cancer immunotherapy. *J Urol*. 128:931-935.

[63] Lau, B.H., J.L. Woolley, C.L. Marsh, G.R. Barker, D.H. Koobs, and R.R. Torrey. 1986. Superiority of intralesional immunotherapy with Corynebacterium parvum and Allium sativum in control of murine transitional cell carcinoma. *J Urol*. 136:701-705.

[64] Li, W., Y. Ran, M. Li, K. Zhang, X. Qin, X. Xue, C. Zhang, Q. Hao, W. Zhang, and Y. Zhang. 2013. Mimotope vaccination for epitope-specific induction of anti-VEGF antibodies. *BMC Biotechnol*. 13:77.

[65] Lieb, B., B. Altenhein, and J. Markl. 2000. The sequence of a gastropod hemocyanin (HtH1 from Haliotis tuberculata). *J Biol Chem*. 275:5675-5681.

[66] Linn, J.F., P. Black, K. Derksen, H. Rubben, and J.W. Thuroff. 2000. Keyhole limpet haemocyanin in experimental bladder cancer: literature review and own results. *Eur Urol*. 37 Suppl 3:34-40.

[67] Markl, J., B. Lieb, W. Gebauer, B. Altenhein, U. Meissner, and J.R. Harris. 2001. Marine tumor vaccine carriers: structure of the molluscan hemocyanins KLH and htH. *J Cancer Res Clin Oncol*. 127 Suppl 2:R3-9.

[68] Markl, J. 2013. Evolution of molluscan hemocyanin structures. *Biochim Biophys Acta*. 1834:1840-1852.

[69] Marsh, C.L., R.R. Torrey, J.L. Woolley, G.R. Barker, and B.H. Lau. 1987. Superiority of intravesical immunotherapy with Corynebacterium parvum and Allium sativum in control of murine bladder cancer. *J Urol*. 137:359-362.

[70] Martell, B.A., F.M. Orson, J. Poling, E. Mitchell, R.D. Rossen, T. Gardner, and T.R. Kosten. 2009. Cocaine vaccine for the treatment of cocaine dependence in methadone-maintained patients: a randomized, double-blind, placebo-controlled efficacy trial. *Arch Gen Psychiatry*. 66:1116-1123.

[71] Matus, S., P.V. Burgos, M. Bravo-Zehnder, R. Kraft, O.H. Porras, P. Farias, L.F. Barros, F. Torrealba, L. Massardo, S. Jacobelli, and A. Gonzalez. 2007. Antiribosomal-P autoantibodies from psychiatric lupus target a novel neuronal surface protein causing calcium influx and apoptosis. *J Exp Med*. 204:3221-3234.

[72] May, R.J., D.O. Beenhouwer, and M.D. Scharff. 2003. Antibodies to keyhole limpet hemocyanin cross-react with an epitope on the polysaccharide capsule of Cryptococcus neoformans and other carbohydrates: implications for vaccine development. *J Immunol*. 171:4905-4912.

[73] McFadden, D.W., D.R. Riggs, B.J. Jackson, A. Ng, and C. Cunningham. 2007. Keyhole limpet hemocyanin potentiates standard immunotherapy for melanoma. *Am J Surg*. 193:284-287.

[74] McFadden, D.W., D.R. Riggs, B.J. Jackson, and L. Vona-Davis. 2003. Keyhole limpet hemocyanin, a novel immune stimulant with promising anticancer activity in Barrett's esophageal adenocarcinoma. *Am J Surg*. 186:552-555.

[75] McGreal, E.P., M. Rosas, G.D. Brown, S. Zamze, S.Y. Wong, S. Gordon, L. Martinez-Pomares, and P.R. Taylor. 2006. The carbohydrate-recognition domain of Dectin-2 is a C-type lectin with specificity for high mannose. *Glycobiology*. 16:422-430.

[76] Milas, L., and H.R. Withers. 1976. Nonspecific immunotherapy of malignant tumors. *Radiology*. 118:211-218.

[77] Miles, D., H. Roche, M. Martin, T.J. Perren, D.A. Cameron, J. Glaspy, D. Dodwell, J. Parker, J. Mayordomo, A. Tres, J.L. Murray, N.K. Ibrahim, and G. Theratope Study.

2011. Phase III multicenter clinical trial of the sialyl-TN (STn)-keyhole limpet hemocyanin (KLH) vaccine for metastatic breast cancer. *Oncologist*. 16:1092-1100.

[78] Miller, L.A., J.P. Gionfriddo, K.A. Fagerstone, J.C. Rhyan, and G.J. Killian. 2008. The single-shot GnRH immunocontraceptive vaccine (GonaCon) in white-tailed deer: comparison of several GnRH preparations. *Am J Reprod Immunol*. 60:214-223.

[79] Moltedo, B., F. Faunes, D. Haussmann, P. De Ioannes, A.E. De Ioannes, J. Puente, and M.I. Becker. 2006. Immunotherapeutic effect of Concholepas hemocyanin in the murine bladder cancer model: evidence for conserved antitumor properties among hemocyanins. *J Urol*. 176:2690-2695.

[80] Moltedo, B., C.B. Lopez, M. Pazos, M.I. Becker, T. Hermesh, and T.M. Moran. 2009. Cutting edge: stealth influenza virus replication precedes the initiation of adaptive immunity. *J Immunol*. 183:3569-3573.

[81] Morales, A., D. Eidinger, and A.W. Bruce. 1976. Intracavitary Bacillus Calmette-Guerin in the treatment of superficial bladder tumors. *J Urol*. 116:180-183.

[82] Moreno, A.Y., and K.D. Janda. 2009. Immunopharmacotherapy: vaccination strategies as a treatment for drug abuse and dependence. *Pharmacol Biochem Behav*. 92:199-205.

[83] Mura, C.V., M.I. Becker, A. Orellana, and D. Wolff. 2002. Immunopurification of Golgi vesicles by magnetic sorting. *J Immunol Methods*. 260:263-271.

[84] Musselli, C., P.O. Livingston, and G. Ragupathi. 2001. Keyhole limpet hemocyanin conjugate vaccines against cancer: the Memorial Sloan Kettering experience. *J Cancer Res Clin Oncol*. 127 Suppl 2:R20-26.

[85] Neelapu, S.S., and L.W. Kwak. 2007. Vaccine therapy for B-cell lymphomas: next-generation strategies. *Hematology Am Soc Hematol Educ Program*. 2007:243-249.

[86] Nelson, E.L., X. Li, F.J. Hsu, L.W. Kwak, R. Levy, C. Clayberger, and A.M. Krensky. 1996. Tumor-specific, cytotoxic T-lymphocyte response after idiotype vaccination for B-cell, non-Hodgkin's lymphoma. *Blood*. 88:580-589.

[87] Nestle, F.O., S. Alijagic, M. Gilliet, Y. Sun, S. Grabbe, R. Dummer, G. Burg, and D. Schadendorf. 1998. Vaccination of melanoma patients with peptide- or tumor lysate-pulsed dendritic cells. *Nat Med*. 4:328-332.

[88] Nseyo, U.O., and D.L. Lamm. 1997. Immunotherapy of bladder cancer. *Semin Surg Oncol*. 13:342-349.

[89] Olsson, C.A., R. Chute, and C.N. Rao. 1974. Immunologic reduction of bladder cancer recurrence rate. *J Urol*. 111:173-176.

[90] Paccagnella, M., L. Bologna, M. Beccaro, I. Micetic, P. Di Muro, and B. Salvato. 2004. Structural subunit organization of molluscan hemocyanins. *Micron*. 35:21-22.

[91] Peng, Y., Y. Zhang, W.J. Mitchell, and G. Zhang. 2012. Development of a lipopolysaccharide-targeted peptide mimic vaccine against Q fever. *J Immunol*. 189:4909-4920.

[92] Perabo, F.G., and S.C. Muller. 2004. Current and new strategies in immunotherapy for superficial bladder cancer. *Urology*. 64:409-421.

[93] Pilon, J., C. Loiacono, D. Okeson, S. Lund, K. Vercauteren, J. Rhyan, and L. Miller. 2007. Anti-prion activity generated by a novel vaccine formulation. *Neurosci Lett*. 429:161-164.

[94] Presicce, P., A. Taddeo, A. Conti, M.L. Villa, and S. Della Bella. 2008. Keyhole limpet hemocyanin induces the activation and maturation of human dendritic cells through the involvement of mannose receptor. *Mol Immunol*. 45:1136-1145.

[95] Ragupathi, G., J.R. Gardner, P.O. Livingston, and D.Y. Gin. 2011. Natural and synthetic saponin adjuvant QS-21 for vaccines against cancer. *Expert Rev Vaccines*. 10:463-470.

[96] Ragupathi, G., P.O. Livingston, C. Hood, J. Gathuru, S.E. Krown, P.B. Chapman, J.D. Wolchok, L.J. Williams, R.C. Oldfield, and W.J. Hwu. 2003. Consistent antibody response against ganglioside GD2 induced in patients with melanoma by a GD2 lactone-keyhole limpet hemocyanin conjugate vaccine plus immunological adjuvant QS-21. *Clin Cancer Res*. 9:5214-5220.

[97] Ragupathi, G., M. Meyers, S. Adluri, L. Howard, C. Musselli, and P.O. Livingston. 2000. Induction of antibodies against GD3 ganglioside in melanoma patients by vaccination with GD3-lactone-KLH conjugate plus immunological adjuvant QS-21. *Int J Cancer*. 85:659-666.

[98] Recker, F., and H. Rubben. 1989. Variation of the immunosystem by ciclosporin and keyhole-limpet hemocyanin--are there effects on chemically induced bladder carcinoma? *Urol Int*. 44:77-80.

[99] Reyes, D., L. Salazar, E. Espinoza, C. Pereda, E. Castellon, R. Valdevenito, C. Huidobro, M. Ines Becker, A. Lladser, M.N. Lopez, and F. Salazar-Onfray. 2013. Tumour cell lysate-loaded dendritic cell vaccine induces biochemical and memory immune response in castration-resistant prostate cancer patients. *Br J Cancer*. 109:1488-1497.

[100] Riggs, D.R., B. Jackson, L. Vona-Davis, and D. McFadden. 2002. In vitro anticancer effects of a novel immunostimulant: keyhole limpet hemocyanin. *J Surg Res*. 108:279-284.

[101] Riggs, D.R., B.J. Jackson, L. Vona-Davis, A. Nigam, and D.W. McFadden. 2005. In vitro effects of keyhole limpet hemocyanin in breast and pancreatic cancer in regards to cell growth, cytokine production, and apoptosis. *Am J Surg*. 189:680-684.

[102] Riggs, D.R., W.F. Tarry, J.I. DeHaven, J. Sosnowski, and D.L. Lamm. 1992. Immunotherapy of murine transitional cell carcinoma of the bladder using alpha and gamma interferon in combination with other forms of immunotherapy. *J Urol*. 147:212-214.

[103] Rizvi, I., D.R. Riggs, B.J. Jackson, and D.W. McFadden. 2007. Keyhole limpet hemocyanin: an effective adjunct against melanoma in vivo. *Am J Surg*. 194:628-632.

[104] Rollig, C., C. Schmidt, M. Bornhauser, G. Ehninger, M. Schmitz, and S. Auffermann-Gretzinger. 2011. Induction of cellular immune responses in patients with stage-I multiple myeloma after vaccination with autologous idiotype-pulsed dendritic cells. *J Immunother*. 34:100-106.

[105] Sabbatini, P.J., G. Ragupathi, C. Hood, C.A. Aghajanian, M. Juretzka, A. Iasonos, M.L. Hensley, M.K. Spassova, O. Ouerfelli, D.R. Spriggs, W.P. Tew, J. Konner, H. Clausen, N. Abu Rustum, S.J. Dansihefsky, and P.O. Livingston. 2007. Pilot study of a heptavalent vaccine-keyhole limpet hemocyanin conjugate plus QS21 in patients with epithelial ovarian, fallopian tube, or peritoneal cancer. *Clin Cancer Res*. 13:4170-4177.

[106] Salazar-Onfray, F., Pereda, C., Reyes, D, and M.N, López. 2013. TAPCells, the Chilean dendritic cell vaccine against melanoma and prostate cancer. Biol Res. ; 46:431-440.

[107] Schenkman, E., and D.L. Lamm. 2004. Superficial bladder cancer therapy. *ScientificWorldJournal*. 4 Suppl 1:387-399.

[108] Shimizu, K., E.K. Thomas, M. Giedlin, and J.J. Mule. 2001. Enhancement of tumor lysate- and peptide-pulsed dendritic cell-based vaccines by the addition of foreign helper protein. *Cancer Res*. 61:2618-2624.

[109] Slovin, S.F., G. Ragupathi, C. Fernandez, M. Diani, M.P. Jefferson, A. Wilton, W.K. Kelly, M. Morris, D. Solit, H. Clausen, P. Livingston, and H.I. Scher. 2007. A polyvalent vaccine for high-risk prostate patients: "are more antigens better?". *Cancer Immunol Immunother*. 56:1921-1930.

[110] Somasundar, P., D.R. Riggs, B.J. Jackson, and D.W. McFadden. 2005. Inhibition of melanoma growth by hemocyanin occurs via early apoptotic pathways. *Am J Surg*. 190:713-716.

[111] Steinman, R.M., and J. Banchereau. 2007. Taking dendritic cells into medicine. *Nature*. 449:419-426.

[112] Su, Q.P., D.Z. Wen, Q. Yang, Y.H. Zhang, C. Liu, and L. Wang. 2007. Comparison of phage pVIII and KLH as vector in inducing the production of cytokines in C57BL/6J mice. *Vaccine*. 25:970-975.

[113] Swerdlow, R.D., R.F. Ebert, P. Lee, C. Bonaventura, and K.I. Miller. 1996. Keyhole limpet hemocyanin: structural and functional characterization of two different subunits and multimers. *Comp Biochem Physiol B Biochem Mol Biol*. 113:537-548.

[114] Swerdlow, R.D., T.L. Ratliff, M. La Regina, J.K. Ritchey, and R.F. Ebert. 1994. Immunotherapy with keyhole limpet hemocyanin: efficacy and safety in the MB-49 intravesical murine bladder tumor model. *J Urol*. 151:1718-1722.

[115] Tchorbanov, A., K. Idakieva, N. Mihaylova, and L. Doumanova. 2008. Modulation of the immune response using Rapana thomasiana hemocyanin. *Int Immunopharmacol.* 8:1033-1038.

[116] Teitz-Tennenbaum, S., Q. Li, M.A. Davis, and A.E. Chang. 2008. Dendritic cells pulsed with keyhole limpet hemocyanin and cryopreserved maintain anti-tumor activity in a murine melanoma model. *Clin Immunol.* 129:482-491.

[117] Theilacker, C., F.T. Coleman, S. Mueschenborn, N. Llosa, M. Grout, and G.B. Pier. 2003. Construction and characterization of a Pseudomonas aeruginosa mucoid exopolysaccharide-alginate conjugate vaccine. *Infect Immun.* 71:3875-3884.

[118] Timmerman, J.M., and R. Levy. 2000. Linkage of foreign carrier protein to a self-tumor antigen enhances the immunogenicity of a pulsed dendritic cell vaccine. *J Immunol.* 164:4797-4803.

[119] Tittarelli, A., F.E. Gonzalez, C. Pereda, G. Mora, L. Munoz, C. Saffie, T. Garcia, D. Diaz, C. Falcon, M. Hermoso, M.N. Lopez, and F. Salazar-Onfray. Toll-like receptor 4 gene polymorphism influences dendritic cell in vitro function and clinical outcomes in vaccinated melanoma patients. *Cancer Immunol Immunother.* 61:2067-2077.

[120] Tittarelli, A., F.E. Gonzalez, C. Pereda, G. Mora, L. Munoz, C. Saffie, T. Garcia, D. Diaz, C. Falcon, M. Hermoso, M.N. Lopez, and F. Salazar-Onfray. 2012. Toll-like receptor 4 gene polymorphism influences dendritic cell in vitro function and clinical outcomes in vaccinated melanoma patients. *Cancer Immunol Immunother.* 61:2067-2077.

[121] Torres, M., H. Manosalva, I. Carrasco, A.E. De Ioannes, and M.I. Becker. 1999. Procedure for radiolabeling gizzerosine and basis for a radioimmunoassay. *J Agric Food Chem.* 47:4231-4236.

[122] van Holde, K.E., and K.I. Miller. 1995. Hemocyanins. *Adv Protein Chem.* 47:1-81.

[123] van Vliet, S.J., J.J. Garcia-Vallejo, and Y. van Kooyk. 2008. Dendritic cells and C-type lectin receptors: coupling innate to adaptive immune responses. *Immunol Cell Biol.* 86:580-587.

[124] Velkova, L., P. Dolashka, B. Lieb, A. Dolashki, W. Voelter, J. Van Beeumen, and B. Devreese. Glycan structures of the structural subunit (HtH1) of Haliotis tuberculata hemocyanin. *Glycoconj J.* 28:385-395.

[125] Walsh, W.G., P. Tomashefsky, C.A. Olsson, and R. deVere White. 1983. Keyhole-limpet haemocyanin (KLH) immunotherapy of murine transitional cell carcinoma. *Urol Res.* 11:263-265.

[126] Wishahi, M.M., I.M. Ismail, H. Ruebben, and T. Otto. 1995. Keyhole-limpet hemocyanin immunotherapy in the bilharzial bladder: a new treatment modality? Phase II trial: superficial bladder cancer. *J Urol.* 153:926-928.

[127] Zanjani, N.T., F. Sairi, G. Marshall, M.M. Saksena, P. Valtchev, V.G. Gomes, A.L. Cunningham, and F. Dehghani. 2013. Formulation of abalone hemocyanin with high antiviral activity and stability. *Eur J Pharm Sci*. 53:77-85.

[128] Zhu, J., Q. Wan, D. Lee, G. Yang, M.K. Spassova, O. Ouerfelli, G. Ragupathi, P. Damani, P.O. Livingston, and S.J. Danishefsky. 2009. From synthesis to biologics: preclinical data on a chemistry derived anticancer vaccine. *J Am Chem Soc*. 131:9298-9303.

Section 2

Immunomodulation

Chapter 3

Manipulating Immune Regulatory Pathways to Enhance T Cell Stimulation

Joeri J. Pen, Joeri. L. Aerts, Thérèse Liechtenstein,
David Escors and Karine Breckpot

Additional information is available at the end of the chapter

http://dx.doi.org/10.5772/57539

1. Introduction

Cancer immunotherapy aspires to treat malignant disease by activating cancer specific immune responses. It is generally accepted that the latter can only be achieved by an approach in which tumor specific T cells are educated to recognize and kill tumor cells, whilst they are furthermore empowered to overcome immunosuppressive mechanisms present both at peripheral sites and in the tumor environment. Dendritic cells (DCs) have been extensively explored as a cellular vaccine for the stimulation of tumor specific T cells. Several strategies have been devised to manipulate these cells to become strongly activated tumor associated antigen (TAA) presenting cells. Our growing knowledge on the biology of DCs and the co-stimulatory as well as inhibitory molecules expressed by them, provides us with opportunities to generate DCs that are capable of hyper-activating cytotoxic T lymphocytes (CTLs) whilst they impact on regulatory T cells (T_{reg}), which are now well established to be an important contributor to failure of cancer vaccines. In this chapter, we will focus on the cross talk between DCs and T cells mediated by the CD70/CD27 and PD-L1/PD-1 axis as these have been identified as critical pathways in the regulation of immunity versus tolerance.

2. Cancer — A therapeutic challenge

Cancer is a disease in which cells divide abnormally and acquire the ability to invade other tissues. Given the fact that virtually any tissue in the body can become transformed from normal cells towards cancer cells, a large degree of heterogeneity exists. This implies that cancer is an overall name covering a group of over 100 different diseases, which have in common the occurrence of abnormal cells, which grow out of control and can be present within different parts of the body. Therefore, it is not surprising that cancer is a frequently occurring disease, affecting about one in three people during their lifetime in developed countries [1].

Despite the enormous amount of research and rapid developments in prevention, diagnosis and treatment, cancer remains one of the most difficult diseases to cure. Today, the first line treatment for most solid cancer types is surgical resection or radiotherapy to remove or necrose the primary tumor. Since these strategies do not tackle residual tumor cells or metastases, a commonly encountered problem is disease relapse. Therefore, the aforementioned treatment strategies are often combined with chemotherapy, a systemic but aggressive and non-selective approach to eradicate tumor cells. Despite major improvements in these conventional treatment strategies, the requirement to develop alternative treatment modalities that are tumor cell specific and provide better long-term protection to avoid recurrence of tumor cells remains high [2].

A very promising new approach that fulfills these criteria is immunotherapy. The main premise of cancer immunotherapy is to harness the patients' immune system to specifically recognize and kill tumor cells. This is based on the knowledge that our immune system can discriminate healthy cells from cancer cells as the latter express TAAs [3]. Several strategies have been developed to achieve destruction of TAA expressing cancer cells. These are extensively reviewed in [4]. Of these the exploitation of dendritic cells (DCs), the professional antigen presenting cells of our immune system, to present TAAs to $CD4^+$T helper 1 (T_H1) cells and $CD8^+$cytotoxic T lymphocytes (CTLs) is considered to be very promising. Of note, in 2010 the FDA approved a first DC-vaccine, Sipuleucel-T (Provenge®), which was shown to be effective in metastatic, asymptomatic, hormone refractory prostate cancer [5, 6]. Thus, cancer immunotherapy could be a powerful new treatment strategy that oncologists can offer to patients.

It needs to be clarified that cancer development is a complex progressive process that involves a sequence of interactions between cancer cells and immune cells. As mentioned above, the immune system can specifically identify and eliminate cancer cells based on the expression of TAAs. This process was first described by Burnet and Thomas and is generally referred to as tumor immunosurveillance [7]. It occurs physiologically to protect the body from tumor formation. Nevertheless, this process is not perfect and tumors can develop despite tumor immunosurveillance. In fact, the manifestation of malignancy means that the disease has eventually prevailed over immunity. The latter can be explained by the more recently described notion of "tumor immunoediting", a process that comprises three phases [8]. The first phase is the elimination phase in which most immunogenic tumor cells are eliminated by CTLs and natural killer (NK) cells. This phase is followed by an equilibrium phase in which tumor cells that show a reduced immunogenicity are selected for. These tumor cell variants enable the third phase, the escape phase, as they are no longer sensitive to the host immune system. Nonetheless, T cells recognizing these tumor cell variants are often isolated from blood and tumor of cancer patients. Thus the question arises why these cells are unable to eradicate tumor cells?

One of the major hurdles in the fight against cancer is the presence of regulatory T cells (T_{reg}) in the tumor environment as well as in the periphery [9, 10]. Recruitment, expansion and *de novo* generation of T_{reg} is a common theme in cancer (Figure 1). For instance, melanoma cells can secrete transforming growth factor-β (TGF-β) and interleukin-10 (IL-10), factors that are linked to expansion of natural T_{reg} and differentiation of naive $CD4^{+}$T cells to inducible T_{reg} [11]. Another well-described mechanism is the expression of the enzyme indoleamine 2,3-dioxygenase (IDO) by tumor cells and tumor associated antigen presenting cells, which mediates conversion of $CD4^{+}$T cells to T_{reg} [12]. The expression of IDO is only one out of many mechanisms that are exploited by DCs to drive $CD4^{+}$T cell differentiation towards T_{reg} [13]. Nonetheless, it highlights that not only tumor cells drive the stimulation of T_{reg} but that DCs, in particular immature DCs, trapped within the tumor environment, also have an important role in this process. Furthermore, it is well known that T_{reg} prevent full maturation of DCs and as such are at the basis of a vicious circle [14]. The suppressive activity of T_{reg} is mediated by various mechanisms [13]. As mentioned, they hamper full DC maturation [14]. Moreover, T_{reg} can hijack the co-stimulatory molecules CD80 and CD86 from the membrane of DCs through transendocytosis via interactions with cytotoxic T lymphocyte antigen-4 (CTLA-4 or CD152). As such they deprive effector T (T_{eff}) cells from co-stimulatory signals [15]. It has furthermore been shown that T_{reg} influence the character of T cell differentiation by selectively dampening T_H1 responses and CTLs [16, 17]. Importantly, T_{reg} not only hamper DCs in their ability to induce CTL mediated anti-tumor immune responses, they furthermore hamper the functionality of T_{eff} cells or can cause T_{eff} cell death through exocytosis of granzymes and perforin [18]. It has also been described that T_{reg}, which express high levels of the IL-2 receptor CD25, are capable of scavenging IL-2, thus depriving T_{eff} from this cytokine [19]. Finally, T_{reg} can disrupt metabolic pathways through tryptophan conversion [20] or adenosine secretion [21], which leads to the production of suppressive metabolites. In this way, T_{reg} are able to control the induction and/or presence of CTLs as well as their functionality.

Taken together, therapeutic vaccination against tumors takes place in the presence of a milieu that counteracts tumor specific T-cell responses. Therefore, the method of vaccination, *e.g.* DC-based vaccination, should fulfill several requirements. It should result in strong activation of tumor specific CTLs that are able to migrate to the tumor site, recognize and kill tumor cells. Furthermore, the activated CTLs should be refractory to the immunosuppressive mechanisms exerted for instance by T_{reg}. Linked herewith, the vaccination strategy should avoid expansion of T_{reg} or even drive the TGF-β characterized T_{reg} signature into a more favorable IFN-γ signature [22-24].

3. The rationale behind therapeutic anti-cancer vaccination: tumor antigens

Active therapeutic vaccination builds on the power and specificity of the patient's immune system to eradicate cancer cells. The latter is based on the ability of immune cells to discriminate healthy cells from tumor cells, mainly based on the expression of distinct antigens, the so called TAAs. It has to be noted that in contrast to environmentally induced or virus-related tumors (e.g. HPV induced cervix carcinoma, causing genomic mutations

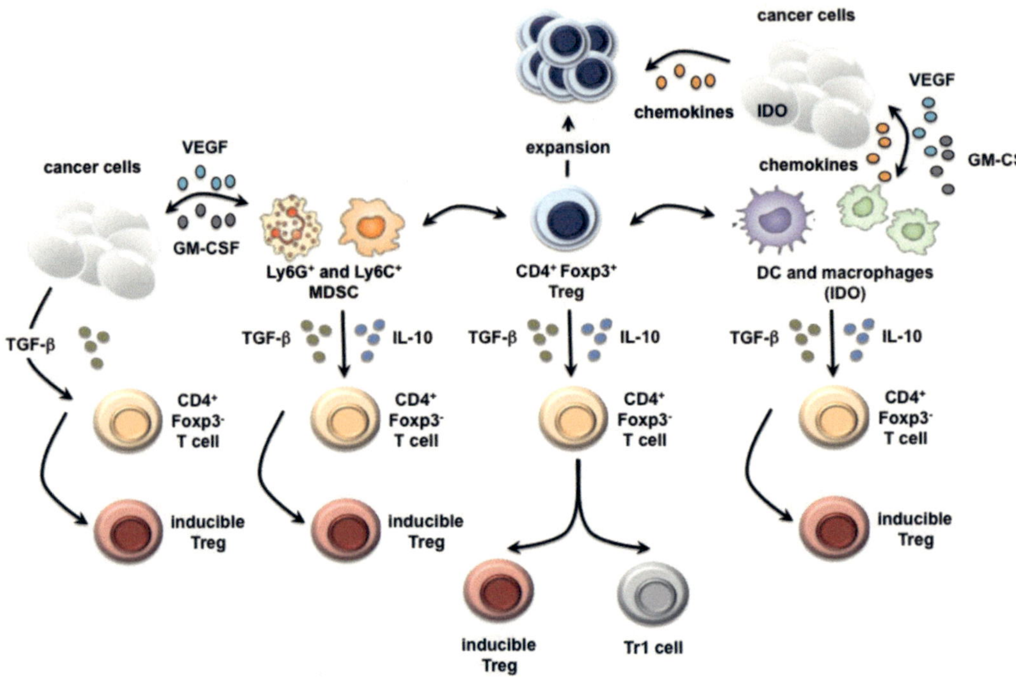

Figure 1. T_{reg} are a major hurdle in cancer. It is well known T_{reg} can be found at elevated numbers in cancers. Three main mechanisms are at the basis of this phenomenon. Firstly, $CD4^+CD25^+Foxp3^+T_{reg}$ or so-called naturally occurring T_{reg} infiltrate the tumor. The latter is driven by the expression of the chemokine receptor CCR4 on the T_{reg} and the expression of its ligand CCL22 in the tumor environment. Secondly, several immune cells found in the tumor environment, including MDSCs, DCs, macrophages and natural T_{reg}, as well as tumor cells themselves drive the differentiation of $CD4^+Foxp3^-$cells into so-called inducible T_{reg} ($Foxp3^+$) and/or IL-10 producing Tr1 cells ($CD4^+IL\text{-}10^+Foxp3^-$) through the secretion of TGF-β and/or IL-10. Thirdly, it is well known that dysfunctional myeloid cells within the tumor environment further stimulate T_{reg} expansion. Importantly, there is an extensive cross talk between the different immune cells found within the tumor as well as between these immune cells and the tumor cells themselves. This cross talk ensures that the tumor environment remains a sanctuary for immunosuppresive cells, such as the T_{reg}.

resulting in strongly immogenic antigens), for most tumors the etiology is unclear and that they are not particularly immunogenic. Nonetheless, several TAAs have been identified as immunological targets. TAAs can be classified in different classes, dependent on their expression pattern. The most important classes are the cancer-testis antigens (e.g. MAGE-family), differentiation antigens (e.g. MART-1/Melan-A, CEA), mutated antigens (e.g. BRAF), antigens that are overexpressed in tumors (e.g. hTERT, WT-1). Examples hereof are carcinoembryonic antigen in colorectal carcinoma [25], α-fetoprotein in hepatocellular carcinoma [26] and members of the melanoma antigen gene (MAGE) family in melanoma [27].

The immune cells that are responsible for the specific recognition of TAAs are T cells. Peptides derived from a TAA can be presented in major histocompatibility class (MHC) molecules to the T-cell receptor (TCR) of T cells offering the opportunity to induce specific and long lasting immune reactivity against TAAs [28, 29]. As mentioned above, CTLs are critical in the immunological control of cancer cells [30]. Initiation of CTL mediated immune responses requires antigen presentation in MHC I molecules that are present on antigen presenting cells, to the TCR of CD8⁺T lymphocytes. In particular, DCs are equipped with specialized machinery that promote effective display of antigenic peptide/MHC I complexes. Importantly, DCs also present peptides in the context of MHC II molecules to CD4⁺T cells, which through delicate interactions with DCs and CD8⁺T cells help in the induction, expansion and maintenance of CTLs [31]. Although antigen presentation is a first prerequisite for stimulation of CTLs, additional signals, co-stimulation by surface expressed stimulatory molecules and an inflammatory environment provided by the secretion of a plethora of cytokines, are required. Both can be delivered by DCs when these are appropriately activated [32].

Over a hundred TAAs that are recognized by T cells have been identified to date [33]. The question which TAAs has the most potential as a target for therapeutic vaccination was recently addressed in a pilot study in which 75 TAAs were ranked according to predefined and weighted objective criteria, including its therapeutic function, immunogenicity and specificity. This study brought the Wilms' Tumor 1 (WT-1) antigen forward as an excellent, nearly universal TAA [34].

Over the years, several strategies have been developed to introduce TAAs to DCs. Generally these approaches are divided into viral and non-viral strategies. Examples hereof are lentiviral modification and mRNA electroporation of DCs, respectively [35-41]. Both strategies have been shown to be efficient for delivery of TAAs to DCs [42]. Of note, these approaches have later on been fine tuned to furthermore provide immune modulating signals to the DCs [32, 43-46]. A thorough review of the use of lentiviral vectors and mRNA for modification of DCs is provided in references [47, 48] and [49, 50] respectively.

3.1. Dendritic cells guide CD8⁺T cell activation

Dendritic cells, the most potent antigen presenting cells of our immune system, are at the centre of our immune system. They bridge the innate and adaptive immune system, and orchestrate amongst others T-cell mediated immune responses. Therefore, it is not surprising that DCs are frequently targeted to generate therapeutic immunity against cancer cells [51].

Immature DCs have the intrinsic capacity to scan peripheral tissues for antigens (both self-antigens and foreign antigens) and capture these antigens using several complementary mechanisms [52]. Intrinsically, DCs have a poor T-cell activating capacity as they express low levels of MHC and co-stimulatory molecules. In order to potently stimulate antigen-specific T-cell responses, DCs need to be fully matured, which will be described below. It is however important to note that immature DCs are not immunologically quiescent as they induce T-cell tolerance against self-antigens through several mechanisms such as depletion of T cells, induction of T-cell anergy, T_{reg} amplification or differentiation [53-55]. When immature DCs capture an antigen under pro-inflammatory circumstances, in the presence of pathogen associated molecular patterns or danger associated molecular patterns they undergo a maturation process [56]. This process is characterized by a decreased capacity for phagocytosis and an increased expression of MHC and co-stimulatory molecules, such as CD80 and CD86. In addition, the chemokine receptor CCR7 is up-regulated, allowing DCs to migrate to lymphoid organs. While DCs migrate to lymph nodes, they process the captured antigens into peptides that primarily bind to MHC II molecules for presentation to $CD4^+$T cells. Importantly, exogenous antigens can enter the MHC I presentation pathway for presentation to $CD8^+$T cells through a process called cross-presentation. Although the mechanisms allowing exogenous antigens to enter the MHC I pathway are not fully understood, two main pathways have been described, leakage of antigens from phagosomes/endosomes to the cytosol and loading of peptides generated by lysosomal degradation onto MHC I molecules that are recycled [57]. The ability to cross-present exogenous antigens, such as TAAs, acquired from for instance dying tumor cells is of utmost importance in cancer immunosurveillance [58].

In the lymph nodes, fully mature, antigen presenting DCs can activate naive $CD4^+$and $CD8^+$T cells. While naive $CD8^+$T cells can differentiate into CTLs, naive $CD4^+$T cells can differentiate into different T_H cell types, of which T_H1 cells are critical in the induction of potent anti-tumor immune responses. In this context, it is important to note that both $CD4^+$and $CD8^+$T cells require a minimum level of MHC/peptide-TCR interactions for proper activation. Too few MHC/peptide-TCR interactions can result in T-cell ignorance or tolerance while persistent interactions can lead to induction of T-cell anergy or deletion [59]. Although recognition of antigen, presented on DCs as peptide/MHC complexes is considered the first signal required for T-cell activation, it is not sufficient. Adequate activation of T cells at least requires co-stimulation, the so-called second signal, delivered by surface expressed molecules. Co-stimulation can promote more efficient engagement of TCR molecules in order to enhance the immunological synapse or can provide additional signals to promote cell proliferation, augment cell survival or induce effector functions such as cytokine secretion or cytotoxicity [60]. Signaling via the TCR and additional co-stimulatory receptors initiates clonal expansion and acquisition of effector functions by primed T cells [61]. The requirement for a third signal, delivered as inflammatory cytokines such as IL-12, to stimulate antigen dependent proliferation is variable. When antigen levels are low, the third signal is critical to induce maximal T-cell proliferation. However, at high antigen levels extensive proliferation can occur in its absence. Importantly, in the absence of a third signal proliferating T cells often fail to develop full effector functions. Thus, proliferation and development of cytolytic function can be fully uncoupled and the absence of the third signal can render T cells functionally tolerant, in the sense that subsequent re-stimulation with a potent stimulus results in limited clonal expansion, impaired IFN-γ production and no cytolytic function. Thus, the presence or absence of the third signal appears to be a critical variable in determining whether antigenic challenge results in tolerance *versus* development of effector function and establishment of a responsive memory population [62]. It is important to note that activated $CD8^+$CTLs disseminate to the periphery (*e.g.* tumor site) and mediate efficient and rapid killing of target cells by various mechanisms, including secretion of cytokines such as tumor necrosis factor-α (TNF-α), exocytosis of lytic granules containing granzymes and perforin, or by ligation of death receptors such as Fas on target cells [63].

3.2. Co-signaling by dendritic cells

Mature DCs express a plethora of diverse co-signaling molecules. These bind to their partnering receptor on T cells and as such deliver various signals that contribute in their own way to the quality of the T cell response. Co-signaling molecules can act on particular aspects of T cell activation, such as survival, cell cycle progression and differentiation to either T_{eff} cell or memory T cells [64]. It is furthermore important to note that intracellular signals may be transduced through both the co-signaling ligand and its receptor, a concept known as bidirectional signaling [65-68]. Consequently, co-signaling can affect both the antigen presenting cell and T cells [69].

The function of a particular co-signaling molecule is strongly related to the timing of its action, as early co-signaling molecules are functionally distinct from those that act late during the T-cell response. It is for this reason that the expression of each co-signaling molecule and/or its receptor is tightly regulated and depends on the activation status of the cell [70].

Another important issue is that the outcome of the signaling is not necessarily stimulatory hence co-signaling molecules can be categorized as being co-stimulatory or co-inhibitory based on the outcome of their signals. Linked herewith, it is worthwhile noting that co-signaling molecules are as essential in determining the expansion and function of T_{eff} cells as they are for the development and function of T_{reg} (defined as $CD4^{+}CD25^{+}Foxp3^{+}$cells) [71].

3.3. Co-stimulation: focus on the CD70/CD27 pathway

There is a growing list of co-stimulatory molecules, of which most belong to either the B7 or the TNF receptor superfamily, and are expressed on DCs and other antigen presenting cells [60, 72, 73]. Some co-stimulatory molecules however, exemplified by CD83 and the CD300 family, which is also expressed on mature DCs, cannot be classified in either of these groups [74, 75].

The co-stimulatory function of B7.1 (CD80) and B7.2 (CD86), which are the founding members of the B7 family and which themselves belong to the immunoglobulin superfamily, have been studied most extensively. These co-stimulatory molecules and their receptor CD28 were extensively discussed in [76] and are therefore not addressed in this chapter. It needs to be highlighted that the B7 family now encompasses several other members, which were more recently described. These include inducible co-stimulator ligand (ICOS-L), programmed death 1 receptor-ligand 1 (PD-L1 or B7-H1), PD-L2 (B7-DC), B7-H3 and B7-H4. The corresponding ligands that are inducibly expressed on T cells are ICOS, programmed death 1 receptor (PD-1), and B and T Lymphocyte Attenuator (BTLA). Although their function in T-cell activation is not yet fully understood, it is clear that these B7 members are not innocent bystanders [77]. In this regard, we will discuss the PD-L1/PD-1 axis in more detail in the section "Co-inhibition: focus on the PD-L1/PD-1 pathway".

The second group of co-stimulatory receptors expressed on T cells consists of the TNF receptor type family and includes CD27, OX40 (CD134), glucocorticoid induced TNF receptor family related protein (GITR, TNFRSF18; CD357) and 4-1BB (CD137). Their corresponding ligands CD70, OX40L (CD252), GITRL (TNFSF18) and 4-1BBL (TNFSF9) are expressed on DCs [73]. A common theme for the members of this family is their coordinated expression at the interface between T cells and DCs, and their ability to shape the environment that sets the stage for the cross talk between T cells and DCs. In the remainder of this section we will focus on the CD70/CD27 pathway as this pathway has been identified as a critical regulator of immunity *versus* tolerance.

Similar to the B7 receptor CD28, the receptor CD27 is expressed on naive T cells [78]. Although initially up-regulated upon T cell activation, its expression decreases to undetectable levels after T cells undergo several rounds of division [79]. However, CD27 expression has been reported on central memory T cells [80]. The expression of its ligand CD70 is highly restricted and activation dependent, as it is only transiently expressed on activated T and B cells as well as DCs [81-83]. Studies using CD27 deficient mice have provided insights into the role of CD27 in the generation of T cell immunity. It was indicated that CD27 is of importance in the stimulation of both primary and memory T-cell responses [84]. Although, CD27 seemingly was not required to induce T-cell proliferation, it was shown that CD27 enhances T-cell survival upon successive rounds of cell division [85]. Nonetheless, a role for CD27 in $CD8^{+}$T cell proliferation was shown in the absence of IL-2, although no functional differentiation was detected [86]. In this regard, CD27 has been linked to the induction of IL-2 and IFN-γ secretion by $CD4^{+}$T cells, as such instructing the latter to support $CD8^{+}$T-cell activation [87]. These findings were confirmed in mouse studies using blocking anti-CD70 antibodies [88, 89]. An observation that pinpointed the CD27/CD70 pathway as one of the most important co-stimulatory pathways known today, is the observation that due to their CD70 expression, $DEC205^{+}$spleen DCs are able to prime $CD4^{+}$T cells in the absence of a third signal, *e.g.* IL-12 [90]. Moreover, it was demonstrated in mice that stimulation of T cells by DCs that constitutively express CD70 is effective in the absence of signal 3, suggesting that TCR triggering and CD27/CD70 interaction-at least in mice-is sufficient to promote CTL responses [91]. Many of these studies were performed in the context of infectious diseases. Also in cancer, the CD27/CD70 interaction has been described to help immune cell survival and induction of potent CTL responses [92-95]. Importantly, our group has developed a potent DC-based anti-cancer vaccine based on the use of mRNA to introduce CD70 in addition to two DC activating stimuli CD40 ligand and a constitutive active form of toll-like receptor 4, collectively referred to as TriMix (Figure 2) [43]. It has been demonstrated that these DCs are able to strongly activate allogeneic naive $CD4^{+}CD45RA^{+}$T cells and when loaded with TAA derived peptides are able to hyper-activate $CD8^{+}$T cells (>500-fold increase in Melan A-specific $CD8^{+}$T cells was observed when compared with immature DCs, and a >200-fold increase when compared with DCs activated with a classical cytokine cocktail). Simultaneous introduction of TAA and TriMix mRNA was shown to be feasible [96]. These data formed the basis for clinical evaluation of these so-called TriMix-DCs as a cellular vaccine for immunization of advanced stage melanoma patients [97]. Extensive immunomonitoring of delayed type hypersensitivity reactions [98] and/or blood samples [99] obtained from these vaccinated patients, demonstrated priming of $CD4^{+}$and $CD8^{+}$T cell responses against multiple epitopes of the TAAs present within the DC-vaccine. More importantly, in a small-scale (15 patients) phase IB clinical trial in advanced melanoma, it was shown that combined intradermal/intravenous vaccination with TriMix-DCs induces anti-tumor activity with durable disease control in a number of patients [100].

http://dx.doi.org/10.5772/57539

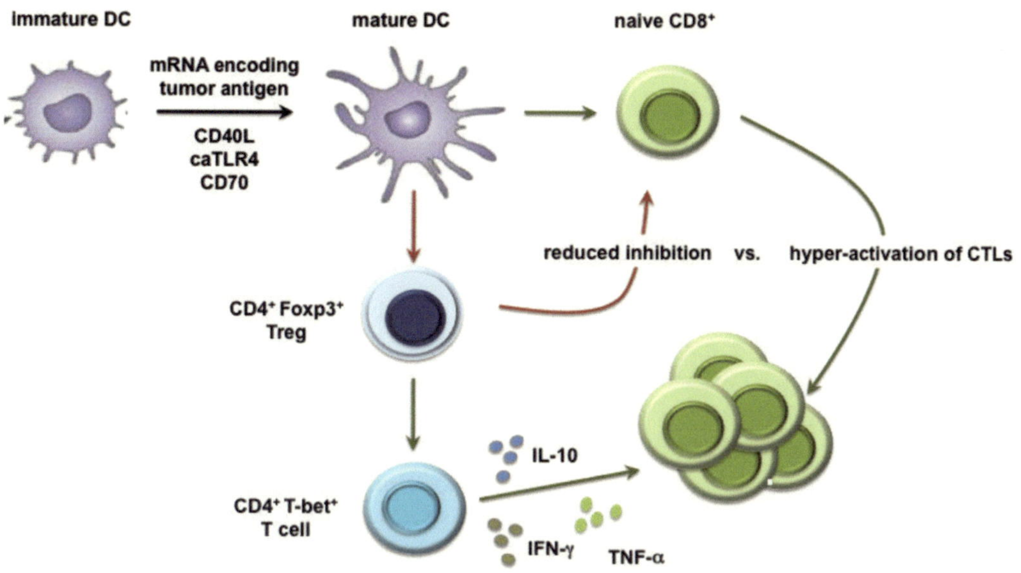

Figure 2. TriMix-DCs hyper-activate CTLs that are partially protected from T_{reg} suppression and drive T_{reg} towards a T_H1 phenotype. Immature DCs can be artificially maturated using genetic modification. To obtain strong T-cell responses, DCs can be electroporated with a cocktail of mRNA molecules encoding constitutive active toll like receptor 4, CD40 ligand and CD70, not only maturing the DCs but also providing them with a powerful co-stimulatory molecule. These DCs are able to stimulate both naive $CD4^+$and $CD8^+$T cells. $CD8^+$T cells will become activated to CTLs, while $CD4^+T_H1$ cells will facilitate this process. Moreover, it has recently been shown that these DCs are also able to thwart the function of T_{reg}, whereby their suppressive effect on DCs, $CD4^+$and $CD8^+$T cells is largely incapacitated. As a consequence, the stimulatory potential of these DCs is enhanced because they do not only provide co-stimulation, but also counter immune inhibition.

As mentioned co-stimulatory molecules can also affect T_{reg}. For instance, it was described that triggering OX40 (human and mouse), GITR (mouse) or 4-1BB leads to a reduced Treg suppression [45, 101-106].

Given its important role in T-cell stimulation as described above, it is worthwhile discussing the role of the co-stimulatory CD70/CD27 pathway in the context of T_{reg} suppression. Although it is well described that T_{reg} express high levels of CD27, the effect of CD27/CD70 signaling on the function of T_{reg} has not been studied in detail in the context of cancer [107-109]. Importantly, it is worthwhile to note that different effects of CD70/CD27 signaling on T_{reg} have been described and that these effects seem to be dependent on the context of the CD70 expression. For instance, Claus and colleagues demonstrated that CD70/CD27 interaction in the chronically inflamed tumor environment increased the frequency of T_{reg}, resulting in reduced tumor specific T cell responses and the promotion of tumor growth. The latter was shown to be due to an enhanced survival of T_{reg}, which was linked to the stimulation of $CD4^+T_{eff}$ cells to produce IL-2 a well-known survival factor for T_{reg} [107, 110]. It has been suggested by Moser and colleagues that in a pro-inflammatory environment, such as secondary lymphoid organs, priming of T_H1 cells (a necessary component for efficient priming of CTLs) is driven by IL-12 or CD70/CD27 signaling, depending on the function of T_{reg}. They observed that enhanced T_H1

priming in the absence of T_{reg} is CD70 dependent, whereas IL-12 is required for T_H1 development when T_{reg} are at place. The fact that CD70 can exert its co-stimulatory function for T_H1 cells in the absence of T_{reg}, might be explained by their observation that the expression of CD70 on DCs was abrogated by T_{reg} *in vitro* [16]. More recently, we extensively investigated the influence of CD70 expressing TriMix-DCs on T_{reg} (Figure 2). We demonstrated that these DCs do not induce T_{reg} starting from $CD4^+CD25^-$T cells. More importantly, the stimulation of $CD8^+$T cells by TriMix-DCs was only marginally influenced by the presence of T_{reg}. In addition, we showed that $CD8^+$T cells that were cultured with TriMix-DCs were partially protected from subsequent T_{reg} suppression. Besides desensitization of $CD8^+$T cells to T_{reg}, we further showed that T_{reg} co-cultured in the presence of TriMix-DCs partially lost their suppressive capacity, a phenomenon that was accompanied by a decrease in CD27 and CD25 expression on these T_{reg}, as well as an increase in the expression of the transcription factor T-bet and secretion of cytokines linked to a T_H1 phenotype. Although the assays were performed *in vitro* and their outcome cannot solely be attributed to CD70, these data further underline the notion that the effect of CD70/CD27 signaling on T_{reg} might depend on its context. Importantly, these data suggest that the potency of CD70 expressing TriMix-DCs is linked to their ability to hyper-activate CTLs that are refractory to T_{reg} as well as on their ability to suppress the function of T_{reg}, even reprogram them to T_H1 cells under certain circumstances [108].

3.4. Co-inhibition: focus on the PD-L1/PD-1 pathway

Over the years, two negative stimulatory (co-inhibitory) receptors on T cells have been extensively studied in the context of cancer. These are CTLA-4 and PD-1, which are both members of the B7 receptor family. Moreover, they are both considered to be critical immune checkpoints that can be exploited to enhance anti-tumor T-cell responses.

The role of CTLA-4 in dampening T cell mediated immune responses has been extensively reviewed in [111, 112]. Briefly, CTLA-4 is up-regulated on activated T cells. At that time CTLA-4 interacts with the same B7 molecules as the CD28 receptor but outcompetes the CD28 receptor due to its higher affinity for these B7 molecules. The net effect of this B7.1 or B7.2/ CTLA-4 signaling is a decrease in T-cell activity hence dampening of the immune response. Several mechanisms have been described by which CTLA-4 inhibits effector T-cell functions, including induction of reduced contact period between antigen presenting cells and T cells [113] and by transendocytosis of CD80/CD86, thus compromising the T-cell stimulatory capacity of antigen presenting cells [15]. Furthermore, CTLA-4 is constitutively expressed on T_{reg} and has been shown to be essential for their suppressive function [14]. Today, it is evidenced that unleashing this immunological break through delivery of blocking anti-CTLA-4 antibodies (*e.g.* ipilimumab) is therapeutically beneficial in the fight against cancer [114].

One of the more recently identified B7 receptor family members PD-1 is a distant homologue of CTLA-4, which was originally identified as a gene that was highly expressed by cells undergoing programmed cell death hence its name programmed death 1 receptor [115]. Similar to CTLA-4, PD-1 is up-regulated upon stimulation of T cells, although it has been shown on human T cells that PD-1 can be up-regulated in the absence of TCR triggering through the addition of cytokines [116]. Importantly, its expression is not limited to activated T cells, as it is also expressed on activated B cells and myeloid cells [117, 118]. Although PD-1 is not present on the surface of freshly isolated T_{reg}, it can be found at high levels intracellularly. Here it is stored for export to the cell surface upon TCR stimulation [119].

The ligands for PD-1 are B7-H1 (PD-L1) and B7-DC (PD-L2). These show a distinct expression pattern. Whereas expression of B7-H1 can be induced on several different cell types, including monocytes, DCs, mast cells, T and B cells, epithelial, endothelial and muscle cells, the expression of B7-DC is more restricted to DCs, macrophages and mast cells [120-122]. Importantly, B7-H1 expression was also found on several human and mouse tumors [123, 124]. Of note, to emphasize that both B7-H1 and B7-DC bind PD-1, they were renamed as PD-L1 and PD-L2, respectively. However, PD-L1 is polyamorous, it can bind to PD-1 as well as B7.1. Therefore, this nomenclature does not reflect the complexity of the signaling pathways that involve PD-L1 [125, 126]. For instance, it was shown that B7.1 (CD80) expressed on T cells transduces an inhibitory signal to T cells following its ligation with B7-H1 *in vitro* [125, 127]. Conversely, B7-H1 expressed on T cells transduced an inhibitory signal to T cells after its interaction with B7.1 (CD80) [125]. So far, it has not been demonstrated that similar T cell-T cell interactions occur *in vivo*. Moreover, it remains to be clarified whether interaction of B7.1 (CD80) expressed on myeloid cells, *e.g.* DCs and myeloid derived suppressor cells (MDSCs), with B7-H1 on T cells would result in a similar inhibitory signal.

The role of the receptor PD-1 is predominantly described as being inhibitory for immune responses (Figure 3), a notion that is supported by the phenotype of PD-1 deficient mice [128]. There is little doubt that PD-L1 is the main partner in this inhibitory function as experiments utilizing strategies to either interfere with PD-1 or PD-L1 (*e.g.* antibodies, genetic down-regulation, *etc.*) often have a similar outcome [70]. Of note, whereas PD-1 deficient mice develop severe autoimmunity, this is not the case in PD-L1 deficient mice [129]. In addition, it needs to be mentioned that contradictory results have been obtained *in vitro* showing both negative and positive signaling of B7-H1 on T cell proliferation and cytokine production. These observations caution us to conclude that PD-L1 is exclusively suppressive.

With regard to suppression of immune responses, it has been described that PD-1 plays a critical role in maintaining peripheral tolerance. In this regard, it has been shown that the co-inhibitory PD-1 receptor plays a role in the conversion of naive $CD4^{+}T$ cells to induced $Foxp3^{+}T_{reg}$ [130]. Moreover, PD-1 is up-regulated on T_{reg} upon TCR stimulation and has been suggested to enhance their proliferation [131]. It is furthermore thought that the interaction of PD-L1 with PD-1 is responsible for the lack of T-cell responsiveness in settings of persistent antigen stimulation such as those encountered in cancer and chronic infectious diseases [132-135]. Several modes of action that result in the corruption of the T_{eff} cell functionality have been described, including inhibition of kinases involved in T cell activation [118], induction of cell death [115] and modulation of the duration of T cell-DC or T cell-target cell contact by down-regulation of the TCR [136-138]. The physiological importance of TCR down-regulation is yet unclear [139], however most of the experimental evidence points out that TCR down-regulation seems to act at different levels to prevent autoimmunity during the onset of immune responses [140].

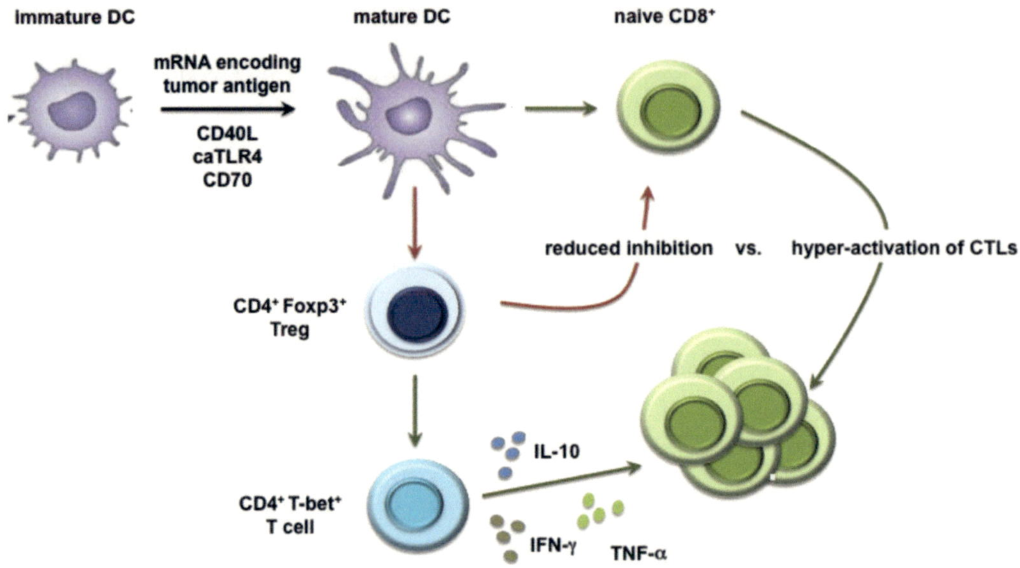

Figure 3. The PD-1/PD-L1 interaction has an inhibitory effect on T cells, while it simultaneously provides survival signals to cancer cells. DCs can be manipulated to stimulate both naive CD4⁺and CD8⁺T cells. Immune stimulation of these T cells leads to up-regulation of the receptor PD-1, interacting with PD-L1 on DCs, to terminate the immune response before causing harm to the host. In the tumor environment, however, PD-1 up-regulation will incapacitate T cells before they are able to tackle tumor cells. Moreover, the tumor itself, can up-regulate PD-L1 to avoid T-cell mediated killing. T_{reg} can be induced from naive CD4⁺T cells. The role of PD-1 in T_{reg} is less documented. Nonetheless it is supposed that T_{reg} are able to express PD-1 and can expand upon PD-1 triggering.

Most studies that have demonstrated negative co-signaling through interaction of PD-1 with PD-L1 during antigen presentation by DCs, have predominantly focused on expansion of T cells and secretion of single cytokines [141]. However, there is a growing appreciation that poly-functional T cells might reflect the effectiveness of the T cells to mediate tumor cell eradication, as was described in the eradication of virally infected cells [142]. In this regard, several studies have found enhanced numbers of tumor-specific poly-functional T cells in patients responding favorably to various forms of immunotherapy, including anti-CTLA-4 antibody therapy [143] and tumor vaccines [144]. In addition, the studies performed by Imai and colleagues [145] suggest that poly-functionality of adoptively transferred CD8⁺T cells is a sensitive immune correlate for successful immunotherapy against malignancy. Therefore, we recently evaluated whether interference of the PD-1/PD-L1 pathway during antigen presentation by DCs impacted on the ability of CD4⁺and CD8⁺T cells to perform multiple functions at the same time [146]. To that end, we genetically engineered monocyte-derived DCs to secrete soluble PD-1 or soluble PD-L1. The latter approach was based on the observation that patients with chronic lymphocytic leukemia that have a splice variants of PD-1, which gives rise to a soluble form of PD-1, have a prolonged survival [147]. Interestingly, we observed that modification of DCs with soluble PD-1 or soluble PD-L1 mRNA resulted in increased levels of the co-stimulatory molecule CD80 and a distinct cytokine profile, characterized by the secretion of IL-10 and TNF-α, respectively. Importantly, these DCs stimulated a significantly higher number of multifunctional T cells that showed increased cytokine secretion, while it did not induce T_{reg}.

Besides antigen presenting cells, tumor cells use the PD-1/PD-L1 pathway to control anti-tumor immunity. Many human cancers have been shown to aberrantly express B7-H1. Up-regulation of B7-H1 is associated to local inflammation (predominantly the presence of IFN-γ) [148]. Importantly, expression of B7-H1 is a poor prognostic factor in several cancer types, including ovarian cancer [149], renal cancer [150, 151], pancreatic cancer [152] and breast cancer [153]. The latter can be explained by three different mechanisms. First, it has been described that binding of PD-1 (T cells) to B7-H1 on cancer cells provides anti-apoptotic stimuli to these cancer cells [65]. Secondly, it was shown in experiments in which cancer cells were modified to express B7-H1, that these cells become refractory to CTL mediated killing [154, 155]. In another model it was shown that this phenomenon was reversible, when the binding of B7-H1 was prevented by blocking antibodies [156]. Thirdly, tumor associated antigen presenting cells utilize the PD-1/PD-L1 (B7-H1) pathway to control anti-tumor T cell responses using the mechanisms that were described above. This results in the stimulation of T_{eff} cells that show high expression of PD-1, are impaired in their function and resemble the exhausted antigen specific T cells that can be found during chronic viral infection. Interaction between PD-L1 expressed on tumor cells and PD-1 expressed on effector T cells was also shown to directly induce apoptosis of T cells [157].

The knowledge that blockade of PD-1/PD-L1 signaling aids the priming of multifunctional T_{eff} cells, avoids expansion of T_{reg} and facilitates anti-tumor immune responses at the tumor site, has instigated research in which stimulation of T cell responses in tumor bearing mice was combined with the administration of anti-PD-1 or anti-PD-L1 blocking antibodies, demonstrating a synergistic effect of both strategies [152, 154, 156, 158, 159]. Of note, treatment of mice with blocking antibodies without other treatment modalities only had marginal effects. So far, four humanized antibodies have been generated and tested in clinical trials to block the PD-1/PD-L1 pathway. Three of them are blocking anti-PD-1 antibodies, CT-011 [160, 161], MDX-1106 [162] and BMS-936558 [163, 164], whereas the fourth antibody is a blocking anti-PD-L1 antibody called BMS-936559 [165]. The antibody CT-011 was used in a phase I clinical trial in 17 patients with advanced hematological malignancies, demonstrating clinical benefit in about 33% of patients of which one complete response. There was no development of autoimmunity reported [160]. The antibody MDX-1106 was tested in 39 patients with advanced solid cancer, including patients with colorectal cancer, melanoma, prostate cancer, non small cell lung carcinoma and renal cell carcinoma. Manageable toxicity, such as anemia, lymphopenia, colitis and arthritis was reported. Clinical benefit was demonstrate in about 10% of patients of which one complete response, two partial responses and two mixed responses [162]. The same team conducted a large-scale study in a similar patient population (over 260 patients) using the anti-PD-1 antibody, BMS-936558. Objective responses were described in approximately one in four to one in five patients with non-small-cell lung cancer, melanoma or renal cell cancer. Again, the adverse event profile did not appear to preclude the use of the tested antibody. Moreover, a relationship between PD-L1 expression on tumor cells and objective response was suggested in this trial [163, 164]. Also the anti-PD-L1 antibody,

BMS-936559, was evaluated by this group in a phase I trial including over 200 patients suffering from the aforementioned cancers. From this study, it was concluded that antibody mediated blockade of PD-L1 induced durable tumor regression (objective response rate of 6 to 17%) and prolonged stabilization of disease (rates of 12 to 41% at 24 weeks) in patients with advanced cancers, including non–small cell lung cancer, melanoma and renal cell cancer [165].

In conclusion, experimental and early clinical results indicate that manipulation of the B7-H1 (PD-L1)/PD-1 pathway provides novel opportunities in anti-tumor therapy. In particular the combination of PD-L1/PD-1 blockade with vaccination strategies might synergize to initially enhance the stimulation of T_{eff} cells, whilst enabling these T_{eff} cells to exert their function in the tumor environment.

4. Discussion

Progress in our understanding on how immune cells interact with each other and how they are affected by cancer cells has led to the development of immunotherapeutic strategies that aim to harness the potential of CTLs in order to improve the outcome for cancer patients. Although CTLs are critical to fight cancer cells, there is a general consensus that stimulation of CTLs will only be successful when they are able to overcome the immunosuppression exerted by cancer cells and cancer associated immune cells, such as T_{reg}. To achieve the latter, research has focused on two approaches. One approach is designing DCs that are able to stimulate CTLs that are no longer sensitive to immunosuppression and to use these DCs as a cellular vaccine. Another approach is to develop strategies to modulate immunosuppressive mechanisms and use these either alone or in combination with vaccination. Our growing knowledge on the expression pattern and function of individual co-signaling molecules and how these educate T cells to respond or not, has been invaluable for the development of both approaches.

Co-signaling molecules start a signal cascade in T cells, which in turn allows them to sense environmental conditions and consequently respond accordingly. There is a growing list of co-signaling molecules that can either transduce stimulatory or inhibitory signals and therefore are often categorized as such. However, whether co-signaling will be stimulatory or inhibitory is dependent on the level and timing of expression of these molecules hence in reality (when multiple co-signaling molecules are expressed on the antigen presenting cell, be it DCs or cancer cells) the situation is much more complex. Nonetheless, major discoveries on new signaling molecules, their interactions and multilevel functionality have had a tremendous impact on cancer immunotherapy over the years. In this regard, important milestones have been the description of the CD70/CD27 and PD-L1/PD-1 pathways. Although it's early days in their clinical exploitation, the pre-clinical and clinical results described in this chapter demonstrate that manipulation of these pathways is promising. In particular, clinical results such as those obtained with improved DC vaccines, e.g. TriMix-DCs or blocking anti-PD-1 or PD-L1 antibodies, re-fuel the enthusiasm that immunotherapy strategies will find their place as an effective fourth treatment modality for cancer.

Author details

Joeri J. Pen[1], Joeri. L. Aerts[1], Thérèse Liechtenstein[2], David Escors[2,3] and Karine Breckpot[1]

*Address all correspondence to: kbreckpo@vub.ac.be

1 Laboratory of Molecular and Cellular Therapy, Vrije Universiteit Brussel (VUB), Brussels, Belgium

2 Division of Infection and Immunity, University College London (UCL), London, UK

3 Biomedical Research Centre Navarrabiomed-Fundacion Miguel Servet, National Health Service of Navarre, Pamplona, Navarre, Spain

References

[1] Bruno, T.C., French, J.D., Jordan, K.R., Ramirez, O., Sippel, T.R., Borges, V.F., Haugen, B.R., McCarter, M.D., Waziri, A., Slansky, J.E. (2013) Influence of human immune cells on cancer: studies at the University of Colorado. *Immunol Res* 55, 22-33.

[2] Jemal, A., Bray, F., Center, M.M., Ferlay, J., Ward, E., Forman, D. (2011) Global cancer statistics. *CA Cancer J Clin* 61, 69-90.

[3] Boon, T., Coulie, P.G., Van den Eynde, B.J., van der Bruggen, P. (2006) Human T cell responses against melanoma. *Annu Rev Immunol* 24, 175-208.

[4] Lizee, G., Overwijk, W.W., Radvanyi, L., Gao, J., Sharma, P., Hwu, P. (2013) Harnessing the power of the immune system to target cancer. *Annu Rev Med* 64, 71-90.

[5] Gardner, T.A., Elzey, B.D., Hahn, N.M. (2012) Sipuleucel-T (Provenge) autologous vaccine approved for treatment of men with asymptomatic or minimally symptomatic castrate-resistant metastatic prostate cancer. *Hum Vaccin Immunother* 8, 534-9.

[6] Kantoff, P.W., Higano, C.S., Small, E.J., Whitmore, J.B., Frohlich, M.W., Schellhammer, P.F. (2012) Re: interdisciplinary critique of sipuleucel-T as immunotherapy in castration-resistant prostate cancer. *J Natl Cancer Inst* 104, 1107-9; author reply 1109-12.

[7] Burnet, F.M. (1970) The concept of immunological surveillance. *Prog Exp Tumor Res* 13, 1-27.

[8] Urosevic, M., Dummer, R. (2008) Human leukocyte antigen-G and cancer immunoediting. *Cancer Res* 68, 627-30.

[9] Jacobs, J.F., Nierkens, S., Figdor, C.G., de Vries, I.J., Adema, G.J. (2012) Regulatory T cells in melanoma: the final hurdle towards effective immunotherapy? *Lancet Oncol* 13, e32-42.

[10] Nishikawa, H., Sakaguchi, S. (2010) Regulatory T cells in tumor immunity. *Int J Cancer* 127, 759-67.

[11] Nizar, S., Meyer, B., Galustian, C., Kumar, D., Dalgleish, A. (2010) T regulatory cells, the evolution of targeted immunotherapy. *Biochim Biophys Acta* 1806, 7-17.

[12] Munn, D.H., Mellor, A.L. (2007) Indoleamine 2,3-dioxygenase and tumor-induced tolerance. *J Clin Invest* 117, 1147-54.

[13] Emeagi, P.U., Goyvaerts, C., Maenhout, S., Pen, J., Thielemans, K., Breckpot, K. (2013) Lentiviral vectors: a versatile tool to fight cancer. *Curr Mol Med* 13, 602-25.

[14] Wing, K., Onishi, Y., Prieto-Martin, P., Yamaguchi, T., Miyara, M., Fehervari, Z., Nomura, T., Sakaguchi, S. (2008) CTLA-4 control over Foxp3+regulatory T cell function. *Science* 322, 271-5.

[15] Qureshi, O.S., Zheng, Y., Nakamura, K., Attridge, K., Manzotti, C., Schmidt, E.M., Baker, J., Jeffery, L.E., Kaur, S., Briggs, Z., Hou, T.Z., Futter, C.E., Anderson, G., Walker, L.S., Sansom, D.M. (2011) Trans-endocytosis of CD80 and CD86: a molecular basis for the cell-extrinsic function of CTLA-4. *Science* 332, 600-3.

[16] Denoeud, J., Moser, M. (2011) Role of CD27/CD70 pathway of activation in immunity and tolerance. *J Leukoc Biol* 89, 195-203.

[17] Oldenhove, G., de Heusch, M., Urbain-Vansanten, G., Urbain, J., Maliszewski, C., Leo, O., Moser, M. (2003) CD4+CD25+regulatory T cells control T helper cell type 1 responses to foreign antigens induced by mature dendritic cells in vivo. *J Exp Med* 198, 259-66.

[18] Cao, X., Cai, S.F., Fehniger, T.A., Song, J., Collins, L.I., Piwnica-Worms, D.R., Ley, T.J. (2007) Granzyme B and perforin are important for regulatory T cell-mediated suppression of tumor clearance. *Immunity* 27, 635-46.

[19] Barthlott, T., Moncrieffe, H., Veldhoen, M., Atkins, C.J., Christensen, J., O'Garra, A., Stockinger, B. (2005) CD25+CD4+T cells compete with naive CD4+T cells for IL-2 and exploit it for the induction of IL-10 production. *Int Immunol* 17, 279-88.

[20] Fallarino, F., Grohmann, U., Hwang, K.W., Orabona, C., Vacca, C., Bianchi, R., Belladonna, M.L., Fioretti, M.C., Alegre, M.L., Puccetti, P. (2003) Modulation of tryptophan catabolism by regulatory T cells. *Nat Immunol* 4, 1206-12.

[21] Kobie, J.J., Shah, P.R., Yang, L., Rebhahn, J.A., Fowell, D.J., Mosmann, T.R. (2006) T regulatory and primed uncommitted CD4 T cells express CD73, which suppresses effector CD4 T cells by converting 5'-adenosine monophosphate to adenosine. *J Immunol* 177, 6780-6.

[22] McClymont, S.A., Putnam, A.L., Lee, M.R., Esensten, J.H., Liu, W., Hulme, M.A., Hoffmuller, U., Baron, U., Olek, S., Bluestone, J.A., Brusko, T.M. (2011) Plasticity of human regulatory T cells in healthy subjects and patients with type 1 diabetes. *J Immunol* 186, 3918-26.

[23] Oldenhove, G., Bouladoux, N., Wohlfert, E.A., Hall, J.A., Chou, D., Dos Santos, L., O'Brien, S., Blank, R., Lamb, E., Natarajan, S., Kastenmayer, R., Hunter, C., Grigg, M.E., Belkaid, Y. (2009) Decrease of Foxp3+Treg cell number and acquisition of effector cell phenotype during lethal infection. *Immunity* 31, 772-86.

[24] Wei, G., Wei, L., Zhu, J., Zang, C., Hu-Li, J., Yao, Z., Cui, K., Kanno, Y., Roh, T.Y., Watford, W.T., Schones, D.E., Peng, W., Sun, H.W., Paul, W.E., O'Shea, J.J., Zhao, K. (2009) Global mapping of H3K4me3 and H3K27me3 reveals specificity and plasticity in lineage fate determination of differentiating CD4+T cells. *Immunity* 30, 155-67.

[25] Gold, P., Freedman, S.O. (1965) Demonstration of Tumor-Specific Antigens in Human Colonic Carcinomata by Immunological Tolerance and Absorption Techniques. *J Exp Med* 121, 439-62.

[26] Abelev, G.I., Tsvetkov, V.S., Biriulina, T.I., El'gort, D.A., Olovnikov, A.M. (1971) [Evaluation of the use of highly sensitive methods of determining alpha-fetoprotein for the diagnosis of hepatocellular cancer and teratoblastoma]. *Biull Eksp Biol Med* 71, 75-81.

[27] Knuth, A., Wolfel, T., Klehmann, E., Boon, T., Meyer zum Buschenfelde, K.H. (1989) Cytolytic T-cell clones against an autologous human melanoma: specificity study and definition of three antigens by immunoselection. *Proc Natl Acad Sci U S A* 86, 2804-8.

[28] Boon, T., van der Bruggen, P. (1996) Human tumor antigens recognized by T lymphocytes. *J Exp Med* 183, 725-9.

[29] Van den Eynde, B.J., Boon, T. (1997) Tumor antigens recognized by T lymphocytes. *Int J Clin Lab Res* 27, 81-6.

[30] Foged, C., Hansen, J., Agger, E.M. (2012) License to kill: Formulation requirements for optimal priming of CD8(+) CTL responses with particulate vaccine delivery systems. *Eur J Pharm Sci* 45, 482-91.

[31] Bonehill, A., Heirman, C., Thielemans, K. (2005) Genetic approaches for the induction of a CD4+T cell response in cancer immunotherapy. *J Gene Med* 7, 686-95.

[32] Breckpot, K., Escors, D. (2009) Dendritic cells for active anti-cancer immunotherapy: targeting activation pathways through genetic modification. *Endocr Metab Immune Disord Drug Targets* 9, 328-43.

[33] Novellino, L., Castelli, C., Parmiani, G. (2005) A listing of human tumor antigens recognized by T cells: March 2004 update. *Cancer Immunol Immunother* 54, 187-207.

[34] Cheever, M.A., Allison, J.P., Ferris, A.S., Finn, O.J., Hastings, B.M., Hecht, T.T., Mellman, I., Prindiville, S.A., Viner, J.L., Weiner, L.M., Matrisian, L.M. (2009) The prioriti-

zation of cancer antigens: a national cancer institute pilot project for the acceleration of translational research. *Clin Cancer Res* 15, 5323-37.

[35] Breckpot, K., Dullaers, M., Bonehill, A., van Meirvenne, S., Heirman, C., de Greef, C., van der Bruggen, P., Thielemans, K. (2003) Lentivirally transduced dendritic cells as a tool for cancer immunotherapy. *J Gene Med* 5, 654-67.

[36] Dyall, J., Latouche, J.B., Schnell, S., Sadelain, M. (2001) Lentivirus-transduced human monocyte-derived dendritic cells efficiently stimulate antigen-specific cytotoxic T lymphocytes. *Blood* 97, 114-21.

[37] Michiels, A., Tuyaerts, S., Bonehill, A., Heirman, C., Corthals, J., Thielemans, K. (2008) Delivery of tumor-antigen-encoding mRNA into dendritic cells for vaccination. *Methods Mol Biol* 423, 155-63.

[38] Ponsaerts, P., Van den Bosch, G., Cools, N., Van Driessche, A., Nijs, G., Lenjou, M., Lardon, F., Van Broeckhoven, C., Van Bockstaele, D.R., Berneman, Z.N., Van Tendeloo, V.F. (2002) Messenger RNA electroporation of human monocytes, followed by rapid in vitro differentiation, leads to highly stimulatory antigen-loaded mature dendritic cells. *J Immunol* 169, 1669-75.

[39] Schroers, R., Sinha, I., Segall, H., Schmidt-Wolf, I.G., Rooney, C.M., Brenner, M.K., Sutton, R.E., Chen, S.Y. (2000) Transduction of human PBMC-derived dendritic cells and macrophages by an HIV-1-based lentiviral vector system. *Mol Ther* 1, 171-9.

[40] Tuyaerts, S., Noppe, S.M., Corthals, J., Breckpot, K., Heirman, C., De Greef, C., Van Riet, I., Thielemans, K. (2002) Generation of large numbers of dendritic cells in a closed system using Cell Factories. *J Immunol Methods* 264, 135-51.

[41] Van Tendeloo, V.F., Ponsaerts, P., Lardon, F., Nijs, G., Lenjou, M., Van Broeckhoven, C., Van Bockstaele, D.R., Berneman, Z.N. (2001) Highly efficient gene delivery by mRNA electroporation in human hematopoietic cells: superiority to lipofection and passive pulsing of mRNA and to electroporation of plasmid cDNA for tumor antigen loading of dendritic cells. *Blood* 98, 49-56.

[42] Dullaers, M., Breckpot, K., Van Meirvenne, S., Bonehill, A., Tuyaerts, S., Michiels, A., Straetman, L., Heirman, C., De Greef, C., Van Der Bruggen, P., Thielemans, K. (2004) Side-by-side comparison of lentivirally transduced and mRNA-electroporated dendritic cells: implications for cancer immunotherapy protocols. *Mol Ther* 10, 768-79.

[43] Bonehill, A., Tuyaerts, S., Van Nuffel, A.M., Heirman, C., Bos, T.J., Fostier, K., Neyns, B., Thielemans, K. (2008) Enhancing the T-cell stimulatory capacity of human dendritic cells by co-electroporation with CD40L, CD70 and constitutively active TLR4 encoding mRNA. *Mol Ther* 16, 1170-80.

[44] Breckpot, K., Heirman, C., Neyns, B., Thielemans, K. (2004) Exploiting dendritic cells for cancer immunotherapy: genetic modification of dendritic cells. *J Gene Med* 6, 1175-88.

[45] De Keersmaecker, B., Heirman, C., Corthals, J., Empsen, C., van Grunsven, L.A., Allard, S.D., Pen, J., Lacor, P., Thielemans, K., Aerts, J.L. (2011) The combination of 4-1BBL and CD40L strongly enhances the capacity of dendritic cells to stimulate HIV-specific T cell responses. *J Leukoc Biol* 89, 989-99.

[46] Escors, D., Breckpot, K. (2010) Lentiviral vectors in gene therapy: their current status and future potential. *Arch Immunol Ther Exp (Warsz)* 58, 107-19.

[47] Breckpot, K., Aerts, J.L., Thielemans, K. (2007) Lentiviral vectors for cancer immunotherapy: transforming infectious particles into therapeutics. *Gene Ther* 14, 847-62.

[48] Breckpot, K., Emeagi, P.U., Thielemans, K. (2008) Lentiviral vectors for anti-tumor immunotherapy. *Curr Gene Ther* 8, 438-48.

[49] Boudreau, J.E., Bonehill, A., Thielemans, K., Wan, Y. (2011) Engineering dendritic cells to enhance cancer immunotherapy. *Mol Ther* 19, 841-53.

[50] Van Lint, S., Heirman, C., Thielemans, K., Breckpot, K. (2013) mRNA: From a chemical blueprint for protein production to an off-the-shelf therapeutic. *Hum Vaccin Immunother* 9.

[51] Steinman, R.M. (2007) Dendritic cells: understanding immunogenicity. *Eur J Immunol* 37 Suppl 1, S53-60.

[52] Trombetta, E.S., Mellman, I. (2005) Cell biology of antigen processing in vitro and in vivo. *Annu Rev Immunol* 23, 975-1028.

[53] Cools, N., Ponsaerts, P., Van Tendeloo, V.F., Berneman, Z.N. (2007) Balancing between immunity and tolerance: an interplay between dendritic cells, regulatory T cells, and effector T cells. *J Leukoc Biol* 82, 1365-74.

[54] Mahnke, K., Schmitt, E., Bonifaz, L., Enk, A.H., Jonuleit, H. (2002) Immature, but not inactive: the tolerogenic function of immature dendritic cells. *Immunol Cell Biol* 80, 477-83.

[55] Yamazaki, S., Inaba, K., Tarbell, K.V., Steinman, R.M. (2006) Dendritic cells expand antigen-specific Foxp3+CD25+CD4+regulatory T cells including suppressors of alloreactivity. *Immunol Rev* 212, 314-29.

[56] Steinman, R.M. (2003) Some interfaces of dendritic cell biology. *Apmis* 111, 675-97.

[57] Lin, H.H., Ray, S., Tongchusak, S., Reinherz, E.L., Brusic, V. (2008) Evaluation of MHC class I peptide binding prediction servers: applications for vaccine research. *BMC Immunol* 9, 8.

[58] Kurts, C., Wagner, H. (2011) Grand challenges in molecular antigen-presenting cellbiology. *Front Immunol* 2, 8.

[59] Nierkens, S., den Brok, M.H., Garcia, Z., Togher, S., Wagenaars, J., Wassink, M., Boon, L., Ruers, T.J., Figdor, C.G., Schoenberger, S.P., Adema, G.J., Janssen, E.M. (2011) Immune adjuvant efficacy of CpG oligonucleotide in cancer treatment is

founded specifically upon TLR9 function in plasmacytoid dendritic cells. *Cancer Res* 71, 6428-37.

[60] Croft, M. (2003) Co-stimulatory members of the TNFR family: keys to effective T-cell immunity? *Nat Rev Immunol* 3, 609-20.

[61] Villadangos, J.A., Schnorrer, P. (2007) Intrinsic and cooperative antigen-presenting functions of dendritic-cell subsets in vivo. *Nat Rev Immunol* 7, 543-55.

[62] Curtsinger, J.M., Lins, D.C., Mescher, M.F. (2003) Signal 3 determines tolerance versus full activation of naive CD8 T cells: dissociating proliferation and development of effector function. *J Exp Med* 197, 1141-51.

[63] Griffiths, G.M. (1995) The cell biology of CTL killing. *Curr Opin Immunol* 7, 343-8.

[64] Nolte, M.A., van Olffen, R.W., van Gisbergen, K.P., van Lier, R.A. (2009) Timing and tuning of CD27-CD70 interactions: the impact of signal strength in setting the balance between adaptive responses and immunopathology. *Immunol Rev* 229, 216-31.

[65] Azuma, T., Yao, S., Zhu, G., Flies, A.S., Flies, S.J., Chen, L. (2008) B7-H1 is a ubiquitous antiapoptotic receptor on cancer cells. *Blood* 111, 3635-43.

[66] Grohmann, U., Volpi, C., Fallarino, F., Bozza, S., Bianchi, R., Vacca, C., Orabona, C., Belladonna, M.L., Ayroldi, E., Nocentini, G., Boon, L., Bistoni, F., Fioretti, M.C., Romani, L., Riccardi, C., Puccetti, P. (2007) Reverse signaling through GITR ligand enables dexamethasone to activate IDO in allergy. *Nat Med* 13, 579-86.

[67] Orabona, C., Grohmann, U., Belladonna, M.L., Fallarino, F., Vacca, C., Bianchi, R., Bozza, S., Volpi, C., Salomon, B.L., Fioretti, M.C., Romani, L., Puccetti, P. (2004) CD28 induces immunostimulatory signals in dendritic cells via CD80 and CD86. *Nat Immunol* 5, 1134-42.

[68] Zhao, F., Cannons, J.L., Dutta, M., Griffiths, G.M., Schwartzberg, P.L. (2009) Positive and negative signaling through SLAM receptors regulate synapse organization and thresholds of cytolysis. *Immunity* 36, 1003-16.

[69] Aerts-Toegaert, C., Heirman, C., Tuyaerts, S., Corthals, J., Aerts, J.L., Bonehill, A., Thielemans, K., Breckpot, K. (2007) CD83 expression on dendritic cells and T cells: correlation with effective immune responses. *Eur J Immunol* 37, 686-95.

[70] Chen, L., Flies, D.B. (2013) Molecular mechanisms of T cell co-stimulation and co-inhibition. *Nat Rev Immunol* 13, 227-42.

[71] Bour-Jordan, H., Bluestone, J.A. (2009) Regulating the regulators: costimulatory signals control the homeostasis and function of regulatory T cells. *Immunol Rev* 229, 41-66.

[72] Carreno, B.M., Collins, M. (2002) The B7 family of ligands and its receptors: new pathways for costimulation and inhibition of immune responses. *Annu Rev Immunol* 20, 29-53.

[73] Watts, T.H. (2005) TNF/TNFR family members in costimulation of T cell responses. *Annu Rev Immunol* 23, 23-68.

[74] Ju, X., Zenke, M., Hart, D.N., Clark, G.J. (2008) CD300a/c regulate type I interferon and TNF-alpha secretion by human plasmacytoid dendritic cells stimulated with TLR7 and TLR9 ligands. *Blood* 112, 1184-94.

[75] Lechmann, M., Berchtold, S., Hauber, J., Steinkasserer, A. (2002) CD83 on dendritic cells: more than just a marker for maturation. *Trends Immunol* 23, 273-5.

[76] Sharpe, A.H., Freeman, G.J. (2002) The B7-CD28 superfamily. *Nat Rev Immunol* 2, 116-26.

[77] Wang, S., Chen, L. (2004) Co-signaling molecules of the B7-CD28 family in positive and negative regulation of T lymphocyte responses. *Microbes Infect* 6, 759-66.

[78] de Jong, D.M., Pate, J.L., Kirkland, T.N., Taylor, C.E., Baker, P.J., Takayama, K. (1991) Lipopolysaccharidelike immunological properties of cell wall glycoproteins isolated from Cytophaga johnsonae. *Infect Immun* 59, 2631-7.

[79] Baars, P.A., Sierro, S., Arens, R., Tesselaar, K., Hooibrink, B., Klenerman, P., van Lier, R.A. (2005) Properties of murine (CD8+)CD27-T cells. *Eur J Immunol* 35, 3131-41.

[80] Wherry, E.J., Teichgraber, V., Becker, T.C., Masopust, D., Kaech, S.M., Antia, R., von Andrian, U.H., Ahmed, R. (2003) Lineage relationship and protective immunity of memory CD8 T cell subsets. *Nat Immunol* 4, 225-34.

[81] Bowman, M.R., Crimmins, M.A., Yetz-Aldape, J., Kriz, R., Kelleher, K., Herrmann, S. (1994) The cloning of CD70 and its identification as the ligand for CD27. *J Immunol* 152, 1756-61.

[82] Hintzen, R.Q., Lens, S.M., Beckmann, M.P., Goodwin, R.G., Lynch, D., van Lier, R.A. (1994) Characterization of the human CD27 ligand, a novel member of the TNF gene family. *J Immunol* 152, 1762-73.

[83] Tesselaar, K., Gravestein, L.A., van Schijndel, G.M., Borst, J., van Lier, R.A. (1997) Characterization of murine CD70, the ligand of the TNF receptor family member CD27. *J Immunol* 159, 4959-65.

[84] Hendriks, J., Gravestein, L.A., Tesselaar, K., van Lier, R.A., Schumacher, T.N., Borst, J. (2000) CD27 is required for generation and long-term maintenance of T cell immunity. *Nat Immunol* 1, 433-40.

[85] Hendriks, J., Xiao, Y., Borst, J. (2003) CD27 promotes survival of activated T cells and complements CD28 in generation and establishment of the effector T cell pool. *J Exp Med* 198, 1369-80.

[86] Carr, J.M., Carrasco, M.J., Thaventhiran, J.E., Bambrough, P.J., Kraman, M., Edwards, A.D., Al-Shamkhani, A., Fearon, D.T. (2006) CD27 mediates interleukin-2-independ-

ent clonal expansion of the CD8+T cell without effector differentiation. *Proc Natl Acad Sci U S A* 103, 19454-9.

[87] Xiao, Y., Peperzak, V., Keller, A.M., Borst, J. (2008) CD27 instructs CD4+T cells to provide help for the memory CD8+T cell response after protein immunization. *J Immunol* 181, 1071-82.

[88] Dolfi, D.V., Boesteanu, A.C., Petrovas, C., Xia, D., Butz, E.A., Katsikis, P.D. (2008) Late signals from CD27 prevent Fas-dependent apoptosis of primary CD8+T cells. *J Immunol* 180, 2912-21.

[89] Taraban, V.Y., Rowley, T.F., Tough, D.F., Al-Shamkhani, A. (2006) Requirement for CD70 in CD4+Th cell-dependent and innate receptor-mediated CD8+T cell priming. *J Immunol* 177, 2969-75.

[90] Soares, H., Waechter, H., Glaichenhaus, N., Mougneau, E., Yagita, H., Mizenina, O., Dudziak, D., Nussenzweig, M.C., Steinman, R.M. (2007) A subset of dendritic cells induces CD4+T cells to produce IFN-gamma by an IL-12-independent but CD70-dependent mechanism in vivo. *J Exp Med* 204, 1095-106.

[91] Keller, A.M., Schildknecht, A., Xiao, Y., van den Broek, M., Borst, J. (2008) Expression of costimulatory ligand CD70 on steady-state dendritic cells breaks CD8+T cell tolerance and permits effective immunity. *Immunity* 29, 934-46.

[92] Arens, R., Schepers, K., Nolte, M.A., van Oosterwijk, M.F., van Lier, R.A., Schumacher, T.N., van Oers, M.H. (2004) Tumor rejection induced by CD70-mediated quantitative and qualitative effects on effector CD8+T cell formation. *J Exp Med* 199, 1595-605.

[93] Aulwurm, S., Wischhusen, J., Friese, M., Borst, J., Weller, M. (2006) Immune stimulatory effects of CD70 override CD70-mediated immune cell apoptosis in rodent glioma models and confer long-lasting antiglioma immunity in vivo. *Int J Cancer* 118, 1728-35.

[94] French, R.R., Taraban, V.Y., Crowther, G.R., Rowley, T.F., Gray, J.C., Johnson, P.W., Tutt, A.L., Al-Shamkhani, A., Glennie, M.J. (2007) Eradication of lymphoma by CD8 T cells following anti-CD40 monoclonal antibody therapy is critically dependent on CD27 costimulation. *Blood* 109, 4810-5.

[95] Roberts, D.J., Franklin, N.A., Kingeter, L.M., Yagita, H., Tutt, A.L., Glennie, M.J., Bullock, T.N. (2010) Control of established melanoma by CD27 stimulation is associated with enhanced effector function and persistence, and reduced PD-1 expression of tumor infiltrating CD8(+) T cells. *J Immunother* 33, 769-79.

[96] Bonehill, A., Van Nuffel, A.M., Corthals, J., Tuyaerts, S., Heirman, C., Francois, V., Colau, D., van der Bruggen, P., Neyns, B., Thielemans, K. (2009) Single-step antigen loading and activation of dendritic cells by mRNA electroporation for the purpose of therapeutic vaccination in melanoma patients. *Clin Cancer Res* 15, 3366-75.

[97] Wilgenhof, S., Van Nuffel, A.M., Corthals, J., Heirman, C., Tuyaerts, S., Benteyn, D., De Coninck, A., Van Riet, I., Verfaillie, G., Vandeloo, J., Bonehill, A., Thielemans, K.,

Neyns, B. (2011) Therapeutic vaccination with an autologous mRNA electroporated dendritic cell vaccine in patients with advanced melanoma. *J Immunother* 34, 448-56.

[98] Van Nuffel, A.M., Tuyaerts, S., Benteyn, D., Wilgenhof, S., Corthals, J., Heirman, C., Neyns, B., Thielemans, K., Bonehill, A. (2012) Epitope and HLA-type independent monitoring of antigen-specific T-cells after treatment with dendritic cells presenting full-length tumor antigens. *J Immunol Methods* 377, 23-36.

[99] Benteyn, D., Van Nuffel, A.M., Wilgenhof, S., Corthals, J., Heirman, C., Neyns, B., Thielemans, K., Bonehill, A. (2013) Characterization of CD8+T-cell responses in the peripheral blood and skin injection sites of melanoma patients treated with mRNA electroporated autologous dendritic cells (TriMixDC-MEL). *Biomed Res Int* 2013, 976383.

[100] Wilgenhof, S., Van Nuffel, A.M., Benteyn, D., Corthals, J., Aerts, C., Heirman, C., Van Riet, I., Bonehill, A., Thielemans, K., Neyns, B. (2013) A phase IB study on intravenous synthetic mRNA electroporated dendritic cell immunotherapy in pretreated advanced melanoma patients. *Ann Oncol.*

[101] Valzasina, B., Guiducci, C., Dislich, H., Killeen, N., Weinberg, A.D., Colombo, M.P. (2005) Triggering of OX40 (CD134) on CD4(+)CD25+T cells blocks their inhibitory activity: a novel regulatory role for OX40 and its comparison with GITR. *Blood* 105, 2845-51.

[102] Piconese, S., Valzasina, B., Colombo, M.P. (2008) OX40 triggering blocks suppression by regulatory T cells and facilitates tumor rejection. *J Exp Med* 205, 825-39.

[103] Shimizu, J., Yamazaki, S., Takahashi, T., Ishida, Y., Sakaguchi, S. (2002) Stimulation of CD25(+)CD4(+) regulatory T cells through GITR breaks immunological self-tolerance. *Nat Immunol* 3, 135-42.

[104] Jame, D.W., West, J.M., Dooley, P.C., Stephenson, D.G. (2004) Differential effects of arginine, glutamate and phosphoarginine on Ca(2+)-activation properties of muscle fibres from crayfish and rat. *J Muscle Res Cell Motil* 25, 497-508.

[105] Stephens, G.L., McHugh, R.S., Whitters, M.J., Young, D.A., Luxenberg, D., Carreno, B.M., Collins, M., Shevach, E.M. (2004) Engagement of glucocorticoid-induced TNFR family-related receptor on effector T cells by its ligand mediates resistance to suppression by CD4+CD25+T cells. *J Immunol* 173, 5008-20.

[106] Choi, B.K., Bae, J.S., Choi, E.M., Kang, W.J., Sakaguchi, S., Vinay, D.S., Kwon, B.S. (2004) 4-1BB-dependent inhibition of immunosuppression by activated CD4+CD25+T cells. *J Leukoc Biol* 75, 785-91.

[107] Claus, C., Riether, C., Schurch, C., Matter, M.S., Hilmenyuk, T., Ochsenbein, A.F. (2012) CD27 signaling increases the frequency of regulatory T cells and promotes tumor growth. *Cancer Res* 72, 3664-76.

[108] Pen, J.J., De Keersmaecker, B., Maenhout, S.K., Van Nuffel, A.M., Heirman, C., Corthals, J., Escors, D., Bonehill, A., Thielemans, K., Breckpot, K., Aerts, J.L. (2013) Mod-

ulation of Regulatory T Cell Function by Monocyte-Derived Dendritic Cells Matured through Electroporation with mRNA Encoding CD40 Ligand, Constitutively Active TLR4, and CD70. *J Immunol* 191, 1976-83.

[109] Pepe, C.A., Ricci, R., Cortelazzi, C., Mori, G., Zambito, F., Campanini, N., Aimi, F., Santoro, S., Lombardi, M., Santini, M., de Panfilis, G. (2011) The vast majority of lymphocytes infiltrating primary cutaneous melanoma express the CD27 costimulatory receptor: implications for melanoma progression. *Eur J Dermatol* 21, 178-83.

[110] Riether, C., Schurch, C., Ochsenbein, A.F. (2012) Modulating CD27 signaling to treat cancer. *Oncoimmunology* 1, 1604-1606.

[111] Keilholz, U. (2008) CTLA-4: negative regulator of the immune response and a target for cancer therapy. *J Immunother* 31, 431-9.

[112] Pentcheva-Hoang, T., Corse, E., Allison, J.P. (2009) Negative regulators of T-cell activation: potential targets for therapeutic intervention in cancer, autoimmune disease, and persistent infections. *Immunol Rev* 229, 67-87.

[113] Schneider, H., Downey, J., Smith, A., Zinselmeyer, B.H., Rush, C., Brewer, J.M., Wei, B., Hogg, N., Garside, P., Rudd, C.E. (2006) Reversal of the TCR stop signal by CTLA-4. *Science* 313, 1972-5.

[114] Dequen, P., Lorigan, P., Jansen, J.P., van Baardewijk, M., Ouwens, M.J., Kotapati, S. (2012) Systematic review and network meta-analysis of overall survival comparing 3 mg/kg ipilimumab with alternative therapies in the management of pretreated patients with unresectable stage III or IV melanoma. *Oncologist* 17, 1376-85.

[115] Ishida, Y., Agata, Y., Shibahara, K., Honjo, T. (1992) Induced expression of PD-1, a novel member of the immunoglobulin gene superfamily, upon programmed cell death. *Embo J* 11, 3887-95.

[116] Kinter, A.L., Godbout, E.J., McNally, J.P., Sereti, I., Roby, G.A., O'Shea, M.A., Fauci, A.S. (2008) The common gamma-chain cytokines IL-2, IL-7, IL-15, and IL-21 induce the expression of programmed death-1 and its ligands. *J Immunol* 181, 6738-46.

[117] Agata, Y., Kawasaki, A., Nishimura, H., Ishida, Y., Tsubata, T., Yagita, H., Honjo, T. (1996) Expression of the PD-1 antigen on the surface of stimulated mouse T and B lymphocytes. *Int Immunol* 8, 765-72.

[118] Freeman, G.J., Long, A.J., Iwai, Y., Bourque, K., Chernova, T., Nishimura, H., Fitz, L.J., Malenkovich, N., Okazaki, T., Byrne, M.C., Horton, H.F., Fouser, L., Carter, L., Ling, V., Bowman, M.R., Carreno, B.M., Collins, M., Wood, C.R., Honjo, T. (2000) Engagement of the PD-1 immunoinhibitory receptor by a novel B7 family member leads to negative regulation of lymphocyte activation. *J Exp Med* 192, 1027-34.

[119] Raimondi, G., Shufesky, W.J., Tokita, D., Morelli, A.E., Thomson, A.W. (2006) Regulated compartmentalization of programmed cell death-1 discriminates CD4+CD25+resting regulatory T cells from activated T cells. *J Immunol* 176, 2808-16.

[120] Dong, H., Zhu, G., Tamada, K., Chen, L. (1999) B7-H1, a third member of the B7 family, co-stimulates T-cell proliferation and interleukin-10 secretion. *Nat Med* 5, 1365-9.

[121] Tamura, H., Dong, H., Zhu, G., Sica, G.L., Flies, D.B., Tamada, K., Chen, L. (2001) B7-H1 costimulation preferentially enhances CD28-independent T-helper cell function. *Blood* 97, 1809-16.

[122] Tseng, S.Y., Otsuji, M., Gorski, K., Huang, X., Slansky, J.E., Pai, S.I., Shalabi, A., Shin, T., Pardoll, D.M., Tsuchiya, H. (2001) B7-DC, a new dendritic cell molecule with potent costimulatory properties for T cells. *J Exp Med* 193, 839-46.

[123] Blank, C., Gajewski, T.F., Mackensen, A. (2005) Interaction of PD-L1 on tumor cells with PD-1 on tumor-specific T cells as a mechanism of immune evasion: implications for tumor immunotherapy. *Cancer Immunol Immunother* 54, 307-14.

[124] Blank, C., Kuball, J., Voelkl, S., Wiendl, H., Becker, B., Walter, B., Majdic, O., Gajewski, T.F., Theobald, M., Andreesen, R., Mackensen, A. (2006) Blockade of PD-L1 (B7-H1) augments human tumor-specific T cell responses in vitro. *Int J Cancer* 119, 317-27.

[125] Butte, M.J., Keir, M.E., Phamduy, T.B., Sharpe, A.H., Freeman, G.J. (2007) Programmed death-1 ligand 1 interacts specifically with the B7-1 costimulatory molecule to inhibit T cell responses. *Immunity* 27, 111-22.

[126] Butte, M.J., Pena-Cruz, V., Kim, M.J., Freeman, G.J., Sharpe, A.H. (2008) Interaction of human PD-L1 and B7-1. *Mol Immunol* 45, 3567-72.

[127] Park, J.J., Omiya, R., Matsumura, Y., Sakoda, Y., Kuramasu, A., Augustine, M.M., Yao, S., Tsushima, F., Narazaki, H., Anand, S., Liu, Y., Strome, S.E., Chen, L., Tamada, K. (2010) B7-H1/CD80 interaction is required for the induction and maintenance of peripheral T-cell tolerance. *Blood* 116, 1291-8.

[128] Okazaki, T., Honjo, T. (2006) The PD-1-PD-L pathway in immunological tolerance. *Trends Immunol* 27, 195-201.

[129] Dong, H., Zhu, G., Tamada, K., Flies, D.B., van Deursen, J.M., Chen, L. (2004) B7-H1 determines accumulation and deletion of intrahepatic CD8(+) T lymphocytes. *Immunity* 20, 327-36.

[130] Wang, L., Pino-Lagos, K., de Vries, V.C., Guleria, I., Sayegh, M.H., Noelle, R.J. (2008) Programmed death 1 ligand signaling regulates the generation of adaptive Foxp3+CD4+regulatory T cells. *Proc Natl Acad Sci U S A* 105, 9331-6.

[131] Francisco, L.M., Salinas, V.H., Brown, K.E., Vanguri, V.K., Freeman, G.J., Kuchroo, V.K., Sharpe, A.H. (2009) PD-L1 regulates the development, maintenance, and function of induced regulatory T cells. *J Exp Med* 206, 3015-29.

[132] Ahmadzadeh, M., Johnson, L.A., Heemskerk, B., Wunderlich, J.R., Dudley, M.E., White, D.E., Rosenberg, S.A. (2009) Tumor antigen-specific CD8 T cells infiltrating

the tumor express high levels of PD-1 and are functionally impaired. *Blood* 114, 1537-44.

[133] Francisco, L.M., Sage, P.T., Sharpe, A.H. (2010) The PD-1 pathway in tolerance and autoimmunity. *Immunol Rev* 236, 219-42.

[134] Radziewicz, H., Ibegbu, C.C., Fernandez, M.L., Workowski, K.A., Obideen, K., Wehbi, M., Hanson, H.L., Steinberg, J.P., Masopust, D., Wherry, E.J., Altman, J.D., Rouse, B.T., Freeman, G.J., Ahmed, R., Grakoui, A. (2007) Liver-infiltrating lymphocytes in chronic human hepatitis C virus infection display an exhausted phenotype with high levels of PD-1 and low levels of CD127 expression. *J Virol* 81, 2545-53.

[135] Rutebemberwa, A., Ray, S.C., Astemborski, J., Levine, J., Liu, L., Dowd, K.A., Clute, S., Wang, C., Korman, A., Sette, A., Sidney, J., Pardoll, D.M., Cox, A.L. (2008) High-programmed death-1 levels on hepatitis C virus-specific T cells during acute infection are associated with viral persistence and require preservation of cognate antigen during chronic infection. *J Immunol* 181, 8215-25.

[136] Fife, B.T., Pauken, K.E., Eagar, T.N., Obu, T., Wu, J., Tang, Q., Azuma, M., Krummel, M.F., Bluestone, J.A. (2009) Interactions between PD-1 and PD-L1 promote tolerance by blocking the TCR-induced stop signal. *Nat Immunol* 10, 1185-92.

[137] Karwacz, K., Arce, F., Bricogne, C., Kochan, G., Escors, D. (2012) PD-L1 co-stimulation, ligand-induced TCR down-modulation and anti-tumor immunotherapy. *Oncoimmunology* 1, 86-88.

[138] Karwacz, K., Bricogne, C., MacDonald, D., Arce, F., Bennett, C.L., Collins, M., Escors, D. (2011) PD-L1 co-stimulation contributes to ligand-induced T cell receptor down-modulation on CD8+T cells. *EMBO Mol Med* 3, 581-92.

[139] Cai, Z., Kishimoto, H., Brunmark, A., Jackson, M.R., Peterson, P.A., Sprent, J. (1997) Requirements for peptide-induced T cell receptor downregulation on naive CD8+T cells. *J Exp Med* 185, 641-51.

[140] Escors, D., Bricogne, C., Arce, F., Kochan, G., Karwacz, K. (2011) On the Mechanism of T cell receptor down-modulation and its physiological significance. *J Biosci Med* 1.

[141] Liechtenstein, T., Dufait, I., Bricogne, C., Lanna, A., Pen, J., Breckpot, K., Escors, D. (2012) PD-L1/PD-1 Co-Stimulation, a Brake for T cell Activation and a T cell Differentiation Signal. *J Clin Cell Immunol* S12.

[142] Seder, R.A., Darrah, P.A., Roederer, M. (2008) T-cell quality in memory and protection: implications for vaccine design. *Nat Rev Immunol* 8, 247-58.

[143] Yuan, J., Gnjatic, S., Li, H., Powel, S., Gallardo, H.F., Ritter, E., Ku, G.Y., Jungbluth, A.A., Segal, N.H., Rasalan, T.S., Manukian, G., Xu, Y., Roman, R.A., Terzulli, S.L., Heywood, M., Pogoriler, E., Ritter, G., Old, L.J., Allison, J.P., Wolchok, J.D. (2008) CTLA-4 blockade enhances polyfunctional NY-ESO-1 specific T cell responses in

metastatic melanoma patients with clinical benefit. *Proc Natl Acad Sci U S A* 105, 20410-5.

[144] Perales, M.A., Yuan, J., Powel, S., Gallardo, H.F., Rasalan, T.S., Gonzalez, C., Manukian, G., Wang, J., Zhang, Y., Chapman, P.B., Krown, S.E., Livingston, P.O., Ejadi, S., Panageas, K.S., Engelhorn, M.E., Terzulli, S.L., Houghton, A.N., Wolchok, J.D. (2008) Phase I/II study of GM-CSF DNA as an adjuvant for a multipeptide cancer vaccine in patients with advanced melanoma. *Mol Ther* 16, 2022-9.

[145] Imai, N., Ikeda, H., Tawara, I., Shiku, H. (2009) Tumor progression inhibits the induction of multifunctionality in adoptively transferred tumor-specific CD8+T cells. *Eur J Immunol* 39, 241-53.

[146] Pen, J. J., B. D. Keersmaecker, C. Heirman, J. Corthals, T. Liechtenstein, D. Escors, K. Thielemans, and K. Breckpot. 2014. Interference with PD-L1/PD-1 co-stimulation during antigen presentation enhances the multifunctionality of antigen-specific T cells. *Gene Ther* 21:262-271.

[147] Grzywnowicz, M., Zaleska, J., Mertens, D., Tomczak, W., Wlasiuk, P., Kosior, K., Piechnik, A., Bojarska-Junak, A., Dmoszynska, A., Giannopoulos, K. (2012) Programmed death-1 and its ligand are novel immunotolerant molecules expressed on leukemic B cells in chronic lymphocytic leukemia. *PLoS One* 7, e35178.

[148] Keir, M.E., Butte, M.J., Freeman, G.J., Sharpe, A.H. (2008) PD-1 and its ligands in tolerance and immunity. *Annu Rev Immunol* 26, 677-704.

[149] Hamanishi, J., Mandai, M., Iwasaki, M., Okazaki, T., Tanaka, Y., Yamaguchi, K., Higuchi, T., Yagi, H., Takakura, K., Minato, N., Honjo, T., Fujii, S. (2007) Programmed cell death 1 ligand 1 and tumor-infiltrating CD8+T lymphocytes are prognostic factors of human ovarian cancer. *Proc Natl Acad Sci U S A* 104, 3360-5.

[150] Thompson, R.H., Gillett, M.D., Cheville, J.C., Lohse, C.M., Dong, H., Webster, W.S., Krejci, K.G., Lobo, J.R., Sengupta, S., Chen, L., Zincke, H., Blute, M.L., Strome, S.E., Leibovich, B.C., Kwon, E.D. (2004) Costimulatory B7-H1 in renal cell carcinoma patients: Indicator of tumor aggressiveness and potential therapeutic target. *Proc Natl Acad Sci U S A* 101, 17174-9.

[151] Thompson, R.H., Kuntz, S.M., Leibovich, B.C., Dong, H., Lohse, C.M., Webster, W.S., Sengupta, S., Frank, I., Parker, A.S., Zincke, H., Blute, M.L., Sebo, T.J., Cheville, J.C., Kwon, E.D. (2006) Tumor B7-H1 is associated with poor prognosis in renal cell carcinoma patients with long-term follow-up. *Cancer Res* 66, 3381-5.

[152] Nomi, T., Sho, M., Akahori, T., Hamada, K., Kubo, A., Kanehiro, H., Nakamura, S., Enomoto, K., Yagita, H., Azuma, M., Nakajima, Y. (2007) Clinical significance and therapeutic potential of the programmed death-1 ligand/programmed death-1 pathway in human pancreatic cancer. *Clin Cancer Res* 13, 2151-7.

[153] Ghebeh, H., Mohammed, S., Al-Omair, A., Qattan, A., Lehe, C., Al-Qudaihi, G., Elkum, N., Alshabanah, M., Bin Amer, S., Tulbah, A., Ajarim, D., Al-Tweigeri, T., Der-

mime, S. (2006) The B7-H1 (PD-L1) T lymphocyte-inhibitory molecule is expressed in breast cancer patients with infiltrating ductal carcinoma: correlation with important high-risk prognostic factors. *Neoplasia* 8, 190-8.

[154] Hirano, F., Kaneko, K., Tamura, H., Dong, H., Wang, S., Ichikawa, M., Rietz, C., Flies, D.B., Lau, J.S., Zhu, G., Tamada, K., Chen, L. (2005) Blockade of B7-H1 and PD-1 by monoclonal antibodies potentiates cancer therapeutic immunity. *Cancer Res* 65, 1089-96.

[155] Iwai, Y., Ishida, M., Tanaka, Y., Okazaki, T., Honjo, T., Minato, N. (2002) Involvement of PD-L1 on tumor cells in the escape from host immune system and tumor immunotherapy by PD-L1 blockade. *Proc Natl Acad Sci U S A* 99, 12293-7.

[156] Strome, S.E., Dong, H., Tamura, H., Voss, S.G., Flies, D.B., Tamada, K., Salomao, D., Cheville, J., Hirano, F., Lin, W., Kasperbauer, J.L., Ballman, K.V., Chen, L. (2003) B7-H1 blockade augments adoptive T-cell immunotherapy for squamous cell carcinoma. *Cancer Res* 63, 6501-5.

[157] Dong, H., Strome, S.E., Salomao, D.R., Tamura, H., Hirano, F., Flies, D.B., Roche, P.C., Lu, J., Zhu, G., Tamada, K., Lennon, V.A., Celis, E., Chen, L. (2002) Tumor-associated B7-H1 promotes T-cell apoptosis: a potential mechanism of immune evasion. *Nat Med* 8, 793-800.

[158] Curiel, T.J., Wei, S., Dong, H., Alvarez, X., Cheng, P., Mottram, P., Krzysiek, R., Knutson, K.L., Daniel, B., Zimmermann, M.C., David, O., Burow, M., Gordon, A., Dhurandhar, N., Myers, L., Berggren, R., Hemminki, A., Alvarez, R.D., Emilie, D., Curiel, D.T., Chen, L., Zou, W. (2003) Blockade of B7-H1 improves myeloid dendritic cell-mediated antitumor immunity. *Nat Med* 9, 562-7.

[159] Webster, W.S., Thompson, R.H., Harris, K.J., Frigola, X., Kuntz, S., Inman, B.A., Dong, H. (2007) Targeting molecular and cellular inhibitory mechanisms for improvement of antitumor memory responses reactivated by tumor cell vaccine. *J Immunol* 179, 2860-9.

[160] Berger, R., Rotem-Yehudar, R., Slama, G., Landes, S., Kneller, A., Leiba, M., Koren-Michowitz, M., Shimoni, A., Nagler, A. (2008) Phase I safety and pharmacokinetic study of CT-011, a humanized antibody interacting with PD-1, in patients with advanced hematologic malignancies. *Clin Cancer Res* 14, 3044-51.

[161] Wong, R.M., Scotland, R.R., Lau, R.L., Wang, C., Korman, A.J., Kast, W.M., Weber, J.S. (2007) Programmed death-1 blockade enhances expansion and functional capacity of human melanoma antigen-specific CTLs. *Int Immunol* 19, 1223-34.

[162] Brahmer, J.R., Drake, C.G., Wollner, I., Powderly, J.D., Picus, J., Sharfman, W.H., Stankevich, E., Pons, A., Salay, T.M., McMiller, T.L., Gilson, M.M., Wang, C., Selby, M., Taube, J.M., Anders, R., Chen, L., Korman, A.J., Pardoll, D.M., Lowy, I., Topalian, S.L. (2010) Phase I study of single-agent anti-programmed death-1 (MDX-1106) in re-

fractory solid tumors: safety, clinical activity, pharmacodynamics, and immunologic correlates. *J Clin Oncol* 28, 3167-75.

[163] Lipson, E.J., Sharfman, W.H., Drake, C.G., Wollner, I., Taube, J.M., Anders, R.A., Xu, H., Yao, S., Pons, A., Chen, L., Pardoll, D.M., Brahmer, J.R., Topalian, S.L. (2013) Durable cancer regression off-treatment and effective reinduction therapy with an anti-PD-1 antibody. *Clin Cancer Res* 19, 462-8.

[164] Topalian, S.L., Hodi, F.S., Brahmer, J.R., Gettinger, S.N., Smith, D.C., McDermott, D.F., Powderly, J.D., Carvajal, R.D., Sosman, J.A., Atkins, M.B., Leming, P.D., Spigel, D.R., Antonia, S.J., Horn, L., Drake, C.G., Pardoll, D.M., Chen, L., Sharfman, W.H., Anders, R.A., Taube, J.M., McMiller, T.L., Xu, H., Korman, A.J., Jure-Kunkel, M., Agrawal, S., McDonald, D., Kollia, G.D., Gupta, A., Wigginton, J.M., Sznol, M. (2012) Safety, activity, and immune correlates of anti-PD-1 antibody in cancer. *N Engl J Med* 366, 2443-54.

[165] Brahmer, J.R., Tykodi, S.S., Chow, L.Q., Hwu, W.J., Topalian, S.L., Hwu, P., Drake, C.G., Camacho, L.H., Kauh, J., Odunsi, K., Pitot, H.C., Hamid, O., Bhatia, S., Martins, R., Eaton, K., Chen, S., Salay, T.M., Alaparthy, S., Grosso, J.F., Korman, A.J., Parker, S.M., Agrawal, S., Goldberg, S.M., Pardoll, D.M., Gupta, A., Wigginton, J.M. (2012) Safety and activity of anti-PD-L1 antibody in patients with advanced cancer. N Engl J Med 366, 2455-65.

Chapter 4

Negative Immunomodulators – Blunting Immunostimulation and Facilitating Infection

Jeddidiah Griffin, Marie Moulton,
Rabab Elmezayen and Jonathan Moorman

Additional information is available at the end of the chapter

http://dx.doi.org/10.5772/57540

1. Introduction

The human immune system requires a delicate balance of positive and negative regulators to provide appropriate responses to different stimuli. It is important to control the extent of the response and limit the response at the conclusion of an immune event. The immune system has many negative immunomodulators that assist in this function, including such recently described molecules as PD-1, KLRG1, SOCS1, and Tim-3. These immunomodulators, amongst others, are under direct or indirect control of a group of small non-coding RNAs called microRNAs (miRNAs) that regulate gene expression via degradation or translational repression of their target mRNAs. While these modulators perform a vital function during normal immune responses, they have also been implicated in the pathology of chronic infections, including hepatitis C virus (HCV), herpes simplex virus (HSV) and human immunodeficiency virus (HIV) (Table 1). It is believed that these viruses alter the expression of negative immunomodulators to blunt appropriate immune responses, facilitating persistent viral infection. Because of the role of these modulators and the involved miRNAs, they are being investigated as possible treatments for chronic infections. This review is not exhaustive but highlights several lines of research in regard to negative immunomodulators in innate and adaptive immune responses to stimulation.

Molecule	Ligand	Expression
PD-1	PD-L1/PD-L2	B cells, T cells, DC, NK T cells, Treg, monocytes
Tim-3	Gal-9	T cells, Treg, monocytes, macrophages, DC
KLRG1	E-cadherin	NK cells, T cells
SOCS1	JAK 2, cytokine receptors	Multiple somatic cells

Table 1. Negative Immunomodulators implicated in Chronic Infection

2. Negative immunomodulators — The players

2.1. PD-1

The gene for Programmed Death-1 (PD-1) was first discovered in 1992 during experimentation with T cell hybridomas [1]; PD-1 was found to be upregulated in cells undergoing apoptosis, and is a type 1transmembrane protein 288 amino acids long [2]. It contains an intracellular domain, a transmembrane domain, a stalk approximately 20 aa in length, and an immunoglobulin superfamily domain that contains an immunoreceptor tyrosine-based switch motif (ITSM) and an immunoreceptor tyrosine-based inhibitory motif (ITIM). PD-1 is expressed on T cells, B cells, dendritic cells (DC), natural killer T cells (NKT cells), and monocytes that have been activated, and two ligands, PD-L1 and PD-L2, have been described. PD-1 expression leads to inhibition of cytokine production, including TNF-α, IFN-γ, IL-2, and possibly the cell survival factor Bcl-xL [2, 3]. PD-1 signals have an inverse relationship with TCR stimulation; at lower levels of TCR stimulation, PD-1 signals are stronger; CD28 signaling, however, can overpower the inhibitory effects of PD-1 [4].When PD-1 binds to its ligand, TCR signaling is decreased, highlighting a function of PD-1 in adaptive immunity. On the cell surface, PD-1 activation induces the phosphorylation of cytoplasmic tyrosines [5, 6]. SHP-2 associates with the PD-1 ITSM, dephosphorylating signals via the P13K pathway and Akt and ultimately decreasing the expression of cytokines such as IL-2, TNF-α, and IFN-γ [2, 5]. Decreases in IL-2 have been associated with cell death, revealing a possible mechanism of function of PD-1 in apoptosis.

2.2. Tim-3

Tim-3 (T cell immunoglobulin and mucin domain 3) was initially found to be expressed on Th1 cells but has since been identified on monocytes, DC, mast cells, and microglia [7-10]. Tim-3 has an IgV domain, a mucin domain, a transmembrane domain, and a cytoplasmic tail [11]. Studies indicate that only the IgV domain binds to the ligand [10]. The most studied ligand of Tim-3 is galectin-9 (Gal-9) [12]. Tim-3 is thought to play a role in both innate and adaptive immune responses. In inactive immune cells, Tim-3 is expressed on DC and functions through Toll-like receptors (TLRs) to facilitate inflammation [13]. However, when Th1 cells are stimulated, Tim-3 expression on those cells is increased and, in the presence of Gal-9, impedes their responses. Tim-3 has also been shown to decrease macrophage activity [13]. Downregulating Tim-3 is associated with an upregulation of the proinflammatory cytokine IL-12, but also IL-10, an anti-inflammatory cytokine, and PD-1 has been inversely correlated with Tim-3 expression. Due to the complexity of Tim-3 interactions, research into the extent and mechanism of the functions of Tim-3 is still ongoing. However, current data suggest Tim-3 is a key regulator in both innate and adaptive immune responses.

2.3. KLRG1

Killer cell lectin like receptor G1 (KLRG1) is found on NK cells and activated T cells [14, 15]. As cells mature and differentiate, they express KLRG1 in higher numbers. KLRG1 also has an ITIM domain, suggesting an inhibitory activity. When bound with its ligand, E-cadherin, KLRG1 has been shown to inhibit degranulation and IFN-γ secretion by NK cells. Furthermore, KLRG1 also inhibits CD4 T cell activity by decreasing CD95 mediated lysis [14, 15]. Henson *et al.* [14, 15] have shown in CD8 T cells that blocking KLRG1 upregulates cyclin D and E and downregulates cyclin inhibitor p27. To prevent T cell activation, both KLRG1 and CD3/TLR need to be stimulated proximally [16], suggesting that both cell signals need to be provided by the same target cell. The KLRG1 ITIM recruits SHIP-1 and SHP-2 phosphatases, facilitating the conversion of PIP3 to PIP2 [17] and thus blocking the actions of PI3K and downstream phosphorylation of Akt [18]. When Akt is not phosphorylated, proliferation is decreased, perhaps by a lack of cyclin D and E and cyclin inhibitor p27 remaining at levels sufficient for inhibition [15].

2.4. SOCS1

SOCS1 is a member of a family called suppressors of cytokine signaling [19]. SOCS members display a wide spectrum of negative cytokine regulation and have a part in preventing harmful cytokine effects in certain organs [20]. SOCS1 is a negative immunomodulator for both cytokine and TLR receptor mediated signaling, and the members of the SOCS family have two key motifs: a SOCS box and a SH2 domain [19]. In addition, SOCS 1 also possesses a kinase-inhibitory region (KIR). The SH2 domain allows SOCS to associate with cytokine receptors and tyrosine kinases, inhibiting cytokine signaling by dampening kinases or making adaptor molecules for receptor sites unavailable [19]. The SOCS box recruits proteins that perform such functions as regulating degradation of proteins bound with SOCS [21]. SOCS1 prefers to use its SH2 domain to bind JAK kinases [20]. SOCS1's inhibitory function comes from reducing JAK kinase activity through the KIR domain and using the SOCS box to degrade JAK kinases. Cytokines such as IL-4, TNF-γ, and some TLR ligands can cause the upregulation of SOCS1 expression [22]. SOCS1 also directly inhibits TLR signaling [21, 22]. The mechanism has not been conclusively demonstrated, but several proposals exist [23, 24].

3. Negative immunomodulators in viral infection — Hepatitis C

Over 180 million people throughout world are infected with Hepatitis C Virus [25]. Of those with an acute HCV infection, 85% become chronic [26]. HCV has developed ways to evade the host immune system, allowing the virus to persist for prolonged periods of time. HCV is a single-stranded RNA virus with a genome of approximately 9.5 kb. A member of the *Flavivirus* family, this virus's genome codes for a single polyprotein precursor that is cleaved into the proteins necessary for viral propagation. The HCV core protein is of particular interest to researchers, as it is implicated in playing a major role in evading host immune responses [27].

Virus-specific cytotoxic T lymphocytes (CTL) are critical for the elimination of the virus-infected cells. Strong viral specific CTL responses have been demonstrated in those individuals who spontaneously resolve HCV infection [28-30]. In chronically HCV-infected patients, however, virus-specific CTL responses are significantly diminished both in the liver and peripheral blood [31, 32]. Numerous additional studies have reported that impaired virus-specific $CD4^+$and $CD8^+$T cell functions are associated with chronic HCV infection [33-36]. This downregulation of cell-mediated T cell responses may contribute to chronic infection; Th $CD4^+$ T cell activation and differentiation may be impaired by HCV [42]. It has been reported that $CD4^+$and $CD8^+$T cell responses, including virus-specific interferon gamma (IFN-γ) production, are severely suppressed in chronically HCV-infected patients through the PD-1 inhibitory pathway [37-39]. Several other investigators have supported these studies, including data suggesting PD-1 blockade can restore T cell functions [40, 41] and that HCV core protein may induce PD-1 upregulation and T cell dysfunction [36].

Additional data on the role of PD-1 in HCV infection has focused on innate immune responses. PD-1 appears to be upregulated in monocytes derived from HCV-infected individuals, and these monocytes are functionally impaired in terms of their ability to express IL-12 [42, 43]. Additionally, both "successful HCV treatment with pegylated interferon/ribavirin as well as blocking PD-1/PDL-1 engagement *ex vivo* were associated with reduced PD-1 expression and improved IL-12 production by monocytes". Studies have also demonstrated that monocyte/macrophages isolated from both healthy and HCV-infected individuals and treated with HCV core protein displayed increased PD-1 expression and decreased IL-12 expression [42, 43].

SOCS1 seems to play an interesting role in chronic HCV infection. Miyoshi *et al.* [44] reported that HCV core protein inhibited SOCS1 expression and Yoshida *et al.* [45] reported SOCS1 gene methylation in hepatitis C patients. These experiments were however performed with hepatocellular carcinomas (HCCs). SOCS1 has been demonstrated to suppress liver cell proliferation [46, 47] and has been implicated as a tumor suppressor, consistent with findings that SOCS1 is downregulated in HCCs [19]. Frazier *et al.* [25] have performed experiments with healthy T cells and found SOCS1 to be upregulated in the presence of HCV core protein. These results suggest HCV core protein increases expression of SOCS1 in T cell populations, decreasing immune responses through the pathways described above; moreover, SOCS1 appears to be downregulated in HCCs in the presence of HCV core protein, altering its role in tumor suppression and liver cell regeneration and further contributing to liver pathology during infection. In innate immune responses, Monocytes isolated from both healthy and HCV-infected individuals and treated with HCV core protein displayed increased SOCS-1 expression and decreased IL-12 expression [43]. PD-1 and SOCS-1 were found to associate by co-immunoprecipitation studies, and either blocking PD-1 or silencing SOCS-1 in $M/M_{\emptyset}$ led to activation of STAT-1 during TLR-stimulated IL-12 production. Silencing SOCS-1 expression

http://dx.doi.org/10.5772/57540

using siRNAs increased IL-12 expression and inhibited PD-1 up-regulation, suggesting crosstalk between the immunomodulators [43].

KLRG1 has been shown to be upregulated in acute hepatitis C infection in T cells but has a relatively low expression in chronic HCV patients [48]. These investigators suggested that, as the number of TCR-triggering events increases, so does the probability that a T cell will express KLRG1. This implies that TCRs are more frequently stimulated in acute HCV infections than chronic infections. Recent studies in NK cells demonstrated that individuals with chronic HCV infection display a reduction in NK cell number and function concomitant with a significant increase in KLRG1 expression. KLRG1 expression was associated with increased NK cell apoptosis and a diminished capacity to undergo cell activation and produce IFNγ, phenomenon; this could be reversed by KLRG1 blockade [49].

Tim-3 has been studied in individuals with HCV infection and found to have a role in both innate and adaptive immune responses. Patients who have a high level of Tim-3 early in infection are more likely to become chronically infected than those with normal levels of Tim-3. The individuals exhibit a higher percentage of CTLs that express both Tim-3 and PD-1 [50]. Tim-3 blockade restores proliferation, cytotoxicity, and killing of HCV-expressing hepatocytes, and blocking PD-1 in the same cells has an even greater effect in most subjects [50].

Tim-3 expression is also up-regulated on Foxp3$^+$Tregulatory cells (Tregs), which could be induced *in vitro* by incubating purified healthy CD4$^+$T cells with HCV-expressing hepatocytes. HCV-infected hepatocytes expressed higher levels of Gal-9 and TGF-β, and drove conventional CD4$^+$T cells into CD25$^+$Foxp3$^+$Tregs that express TGF-β and IL-10 [51, 52]. Additionally, recombinant Gal-9 protein transformed TCR-activated CD4$^+$T cells into Foxp3$^+$Tregs in a dose-dependent manner and blocking Tim-3/Gal-9 ligations abrogated HCV-mediated Treg induction [52].

In innate immune responses, Tim-3 expression was up-regulated on monocytes in HCV-infected individuals and this expression was inversely correlated with IL-12 expression [13, 53]. Tim-3 blockade significantly improved HCV-mediated IL-12 suppression, reduced HCV core-mediated expression of the negative immunoinhibitors PD-1 and SOCS-1, and increased STAT-1 phosphorylation in monocyte macrophages in these studies. Figure 1 represents a potential model for the interplay between the negative immunomodulators during HCV infection.

4. Negative immunomodulators in viral infection— Human Immunodeficiency Virus (HIV)

HIV is a retrovirus with an envelope and is a single-stranded RNA virus. Three enzymes, reverse transcriptase, protease, and integrase, are present in the core of the virus. These proteins are the target of many antiretroviral drugs used for HIV therapy. The HIV pandemic has spurred much of the research into negative immunomodulators, which appear to be involved in many aspects of HIV-mediated immune dysregulation.

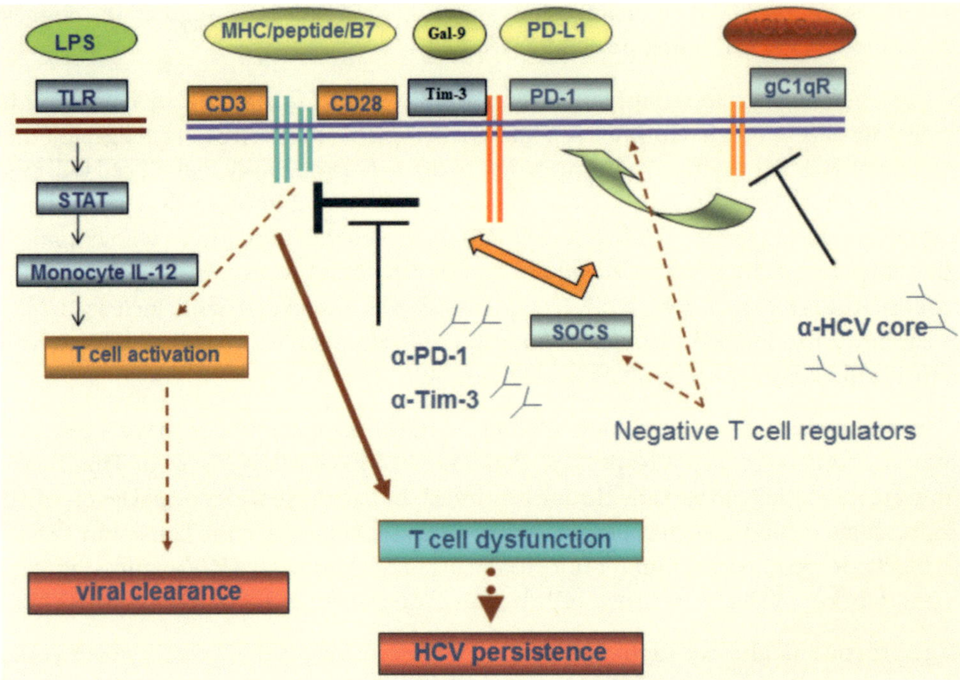

Figure 1. Model for the role of negative immunomodulators during chronic HCV infection.

KLRG1 has been shown by Ibegbu *et al.* [54] to be upregulated on $CD8^+$cells in HIV positive patients. KLRG1 and its ligand, E-cadhedrin, decreased the cytotoxicity of HIV^+CD8^+cells [55]. As noted previously, KLRG1 has also been shown to be co-expressed with other inhibitory molecules such as PD1 in chronic infections such as in HCV infected cells [55]. Chronic latent infections such as Epstein-Barr virus and cytomegalovirus also increase KLRG1 expression, while acute viral infections such as influenza do not [30]. This suggests the persistent antigen stimulation in chronic infections may lead to immune senescence through molecules such as KLRG1, making this cell signal a potential target for therapeutic treatments.

SOCS1 expression is increased in HIV infected cells [56]. SOCS1 may aid in HIV particle maturation and infectivity by interacting with the HIV-1 p55 Gag protein. Viral protease cleaves Gag into domains key to viral replication; SOCS1 promotes the stability of Gag, and the SH2 domain may be of key importance in HIV-1 Gag binding [56]. Other SOCS proteins such as SOCS3 do not increase viral replication, suggesting the role of SOCS1 is unique amongst the proteins with a SOCS box domain.

HIV exposures causes increased expression of PD-1 [57], and PD-1 expression on HIV specific $CD8^+$cells correlates with HIV viral load [58], implying antigen signal strength leads to expression of PD-1 and exhaustion [59]. An HIV protein, Nef, was shown to use a MAPK-dependent pathway to increase the expression of PD-1 [60]. PD-1 has been demonstrated to impair the function of cytotoxic T lymphocytes [59], contributing to the decreased immune response characteristic of HIV infection. However, controlling the viral load through traditional treatment leads to a decrease in PD-1 expression [61]. Blocking the binding of PD-L1 to PD-1 in CTLs has led to an increase in CTLs, which may contribute to a stronger adaptive immune response. These data suggest PD-1 could be a potent target for therapies for HIV. However, PD-1 may protect the vascular system from severe immunological responses during acute infections, with potential difficulties with blocking PD-1 pathways *in vivo* [62, 63].

In HIV-infected patients, Tim-3 expression is increased on T cells [64-66]. The binding of Gal-9 to Tim-3 has been demonstrated to render them less susceptible to HIV-1 infection and replication. The Gal-9/Tim-3 interaction on activated CD4 T cells leads to down-regulation of HIV-1 coreceptors and up-regulation of the cyclin-dependent kinase inhibitor p21 [67]. During the chronic stage of HIV, this interaction can lead to T_H1 and T_C1 cell exhaustion [68]. Thus, T cells expressing Tim-3 during chronic infection have an impaired ability to function properly and to increase in number [64]. $CD8^+$cells that are Tim-3 negative have been shown to have a better ability to degranulate than $Tim\text{-}3^+CD8^+$cells. Blocking Tim-3 pathways in $Tim\text{-}3^+$cells has been shown to increase perforin release, increasing cytotoxic ability and the acquired immune response [68]. These data suggest blocking Tim-3 may prove to be a potent therapeutic technique in the treatment of chronic HIV infection.

5. Negative immunomodulators in viral infection — Herpes simplex virus

The viral family *Herpesviridae* contains linear dsDNA, and HSV is a member of the subfamily *Alphaherpesvirinae*. These viruses lyse infected cells and grow rapidly; frequently, herpes viruses establish chronic subclinical infections in nerve ganglia that can develop into recurrent acute infections. Chronic infection by HSV leads to up-regulation of negative immunomodulators in a manner similar to HCV and HIV chronic infections. Maheller *et al.* [69] noted that SOCS1 is up-regulated during infection by HSV used in gene therapy experimentation, and this up-regulation of SOCS1 aided in viral replication. Because of the role SOCS1 plays in the JAK/STAT pathway, inhibition of this pathway may be what facilitates viral replication. It has also been demonstrated that SOCS3 is required for efficient viral replication of some strains of HSV [70]. This evidence suggests SOCS family cytokines have an important role in viral replication and they warrant further research.

During chronic HSV infections, PD-1 levels are elevated on $CD8^+$T cells [71], perhaps due to frequent antigen stimulation leading to exhaustion. Murine $CD8^+$T cells infected with HSV and expressing increased levels of PD-1 have been shown to produce less cytokines, such as IL-2, INF-γ, and TNF-α, than T cells that express less PD-1. After murine HSV infection, PD-1's ligand, PD-L1, has been found to be upregulated on dendritic cells [71]. It is thought PD-L1 on DCs interacts with PD-1 on $CD8^+$T cells to decrease the immune response in chronic viral infections. Some studies support the possibility of blocking PD-1/PD-L1 interactions to increase immune responses to latent HSV infection [71]. Bryant-Hudson and Carr [72], however, reported an increase in viral load in ganglia and murine cases of keratitis when PD-1/PD-L1 interactions were blocked during acute infections. The pathology associated with keratitis may result from innate immune responses, such as inflammation due to cytokines such as IF-γ [73, 74]. Bryant-Hudson and Carr also hypothesized that PD-L1 may disrupt proper antigen presentation through the down-regulation of costimulatory molecules such as CD80/CD86. The different findings in acute versus latent infections highlight the complex role of many immunomodulators and the difficulties faced in manipulating these molecules in therapeutic settings.

Gal-9 is up-regulated in the presence of both latent and acute HSV infection [75], and the majority of $CD8^{+}$T cells in neural ganglia infected by HSV express Tim-3. This suggests a role for Tim-3 expression in HSV infection. Predictably, it has been demonstrated that Gal-9/Tim-3 interactions decrease the efficiency of $CD8^{+}$T cells in HSV infected neural ganglia [76]. Furthermore, Gal-9:/Tim-3 interaction on $CD8^{+}$T cells increases their apoptosis [77]. Reddy *et al.* [75] have supporting evidence that Tim-3 up-regulation facilitates HSV latency. However, in murine HSV keratitis, the immunoinflammatory-mediated pathology of the cornea is increased when Gal-9 is blocked with mAb [76]. In these studies, at least 50% of T cells associated with murine keratitis express Tim-3. Interestingly, additional Gal-9 decreases the severity of ocular lesions, presumably through decreasing the inflammatory response.

6. MicroRNAs in negative immune regulation

Micro RNAs (miRNAs) have been under extensive research as molecular regulators of negative immunomodulation, with well-described roles in hematopoiesis, inflammation, cancer and many other pathological processes [78, 79]. MicroRNAs are a relatively newly discovered class of non-coding RNAs that function as regulators of gene expression, either by transcriptional inhibition or mRNA degradation. They demonstrate effects either through their loss of function or overexpression, leading to pathologic responses that affect diverse cellular processes including cell differentiation, proliferation, and apoptosis. The effective recognition of viral infection and subsequent triggering of antiviral innate immune responses is controlled by multiple regulators, including miRNAs. A panel of miRNAs has been identified, including miR-124, miR-125, miR-223, miR-155, and miR-146, amongst others, and the role of individual miRNAs has been described in relation to specific pathologic process.

6.1. miRNAs in chronic viral infection — Hepatitis C (HCV)

miR-146a was initially identified during efforts to find miRNAs that are important in the innate immune response to microbial infection. These initial studies confirmed miR-146a as a transcriptional target of NF-kB, and it was thought to have a role as a feedback inhibitor of NF-kB activation. It is highly expressed in mature immune cells, including DC, peritoneal macrophages, granulocytes and splenic B and T cells [80]. Recent studies revealed that Tim-3 expression on T cells is regulated by the Th1 lineage determining transcription factor T-bet (Anderson et al., 2010), which is translationally regulated by miR-146a. Several studies link dysregulation of expression of several miRNAs to HCV and/or its related immunologic phenomenon [81-86].

6.2. miRNA in chronic viral infection — Human Immunodeficiency Virus (HIV)

There are two functional miRNAs, miR-TAR-5p and miR-TAR-3p, which form the transactivating response (TAR) element of human immunodeficiency virus type 1 (HIV-1). Ouellet et al. [87] reported recently that TAR miRNAs derived from HIV-1 can incorporate into host effector Argonaute protein complexes, which is required if these miRNAs are to regulate host mRNA expression. Bioinformatic predictions and reporter gene activity assays identified regulatory elements complementary and responsive to miRTAR-5p and miR-TAR-3p in the 3′ untranslated region (UTR) of several candidate genes involved in apoptosis and cell survival. These include Caspase 8, Aiolos, Ikaros and Nucleophosmin (NPM)/B23. Analyses of Jurkat cells that stably expressed HIV-1 TAR or contained a full-length latent HIV provirus suggested that HIV-1 TAR miRNAs could regulate the expression of genes in T cells that affect the balance between apoptosis and cell survival.

6.3. miRNA in chronic viral infection — Herpes Simplex Virus (HSV)

One of the characteristics of Herpesviruses is their ability to maintain life-long latent infections in their hosts. As reported by Umbach et al. [88], herpes simplex virus 1 (HSV-1) establishes latency in neurons of sensory ganglia, where the only abundant viral gene product is a non-coding RNA. HSV-1 expresses at least two primary miRNA precursors in latently infected neurons that may facilitate the establishment and maintenance of viral latency by post-transcriptionally regulating viral gene expression. These include the latency associated transcript (LAT) [89, 90], which functions as a primary miRNA precursor that encodes four distinct miRNAs in HSV-1 infected cells. One of these miRNAs, miR-H2 3p, is transcribed antisense to ICP0, a viral immediate-early transcriptional activator thought to play a key role in productive HSV-1 replication and reactivation from latency [91].

7. Conclusions

The negative immunomodulators described herein are the targets of researchers attempting to find treatments for chronic diseases. However, the multi-faceted role of many of these molecules makes it difficult to assign specific functions and these immunomodulators likely function in a complex and often interconnected molecular system. The delicate balance of "on" signals and "off" signals within the immune response leads to challenges for this area of research, but the recent strides made in negative immunomodulation are promising.

Acknowledgements

This work was supported by NIH NIAID and an NIH NIDDK grants to JPM. This publication is the result of work supported with resources and the use of facilities at the James H. Quillen Veterans Affairs Medical Center. The contents in this publication do not represent the views of the Department of Veterans Affairs or the United States Government. The authors declare no competing financial interests.

Author details

Jeddidiah Griffin, Marie Moulton[1], Rabab Elmezayen[1] and Jonathan Moorman[1,2*]

*Address all correspondence to: moorman@etsu.edu

1 Department of Internal Medicine, USA

2 James H. Quillen College of Medicine, East Tennessee State University, Johnson City, TN, USA

References

[1] Ishida, Y., et al., *Induced expression of PD-1, a novel member of the immunoglobulin gene superfamily, upon programmed cell death.* EMBO J, 1992. 11(11): p. 3887-95.

[2] Keir, M.E., et al., *PD-1 and its ligands in tolerance and immunity.* Annu Rev Immunol, 2008. 26: p. 677-704.

[3] Chemnitz, J.M., et al., *SHP-1 and SHP-2 associate with immunoreceptor tyrosine-based switch motif of programmed death 1 upon primary human T cell stimulation, but only receptor ligation prevents T cell activation.* J Immunol, 2004. 173(2): p. 945-54.

[4] Freeman, G.J., et al., *Engagement of the PD-1 immunoinhibitory receptor by a novel B7 family member leads to negative regulation of lymphocyte activation.* J Exp Med, 2000. 192(7): p. 1027-34.

[5] Okazaki, T., et al., *PD-1 immunoreceptor inhibits B cell receptor-mediated signaling by recruiting src homology 2-domain-containing tyrosine phosphatase 2 to phosphotyrosine.* Proc Natl Acad Sci U S A, 2001. 98(24): p. 13866-71.

[6] Sheppard, K.A., et al., *PD-1 inhibits T-cell receptor induced phosphorylation of the ZAP70/ CD3zeta signalosome and downstream signaling to PKCtheta.* FEBS Lett, 2004. 574(1-3): p. 37-41.

[7] Anderson AC, Lord GM, Dardalhon V, Lee DH, Sabatos-Peyton CA, Glimcher LH, Kuchroo VK. *T-bet, a Th1 transcription factor regulates the expression of Tim-3.* Eur J Immunol. 2010 Mar;40(3):859-66. doi: 10.1002/eji.200939842.

[8] Monney, L., et al., *Th1-specific cell surface protein Tim-3 regulates macrophage activation and severity of an autoimmune disease.* Nature, 2002. 415(6871): p. 536-41.

[9] Nakae, S., et al., *TIM-1 and TIM-3 enhancement of Th2 cytokine production by mast cells.* Blood, 2007. 110(7): p. 2565-8.

[10] Cao, E., et al., *T cell immunoglobulin mucin-3 crystal structure reveals a galectin-9-independent ligand-binding surface.* Immunity, 2007. 26(3): p. 311-21.

[11] Su, E.W., J.Y. Lin, and L.P. Kane, *TIM-1 and TIM-3 proteins in immune regulation.* Cytokine, 2008. 44(1): p. 9-13.

[12] Zhu, C., et al., *The Tim-3 ligand galectin-9 negatively regulates T helper type 1 immunity.* Nat Immunol, 2005. 6(12): p. 1245-52.

[13] Zhang, Y., et al., *Tim-3 regulates pro-and anti-inflammatory cytokine expression in human CD14+monocytes.* J Leukoc Biol, 2012. 91(2): p. 189-96.

[14] Henson, S.M. and A.N. Akbar, *KLRG1--more than a marker for T cell senescence.* Age (Dordr), 2009. 31(4): p. 285-91.

[15] Henson, S.M., et al., *KLRG1 signaling induces defective Akt (ser473) phosphorylation and proliferative dysfunction of highly differentiated CD8+T cells.* Blood, 2009. 113(26): p. 6619-28.

[16] Rosshart, S., et al., *Interaction of KLRG1 with E-cadherin: new functional and structural insights.* Eur J Immunol, 2008. 38(12): p. 3354-64.

[17] Tessmer, M.S., et al., *KLRG1 binds cadherins and preferentially associates with SHIP-1.* Int Immunol, 2007. 19(4): p. 391-400.

[18] Donahue, A.C. and D.A. Fruman, *PI3K signaling controls cell fate at many points in B lymphocyte development and activation.* Semin Cell Dev Biol, 2004. 15(2): p. 183-97.

[19] Fujimoto, M. and T. Naka, *SOCS1, a Negative Regulator of Cytokine Signals and TLR Responses, in Human Liver Diseases.* Gastroenterol Res Pract, 2010. 2010.

[20] Yoshimura, A., T. Naka, and M. Kubo, *SOCS proteins, cytokine signalling and immune regulation.* Nat Rev Immunol, 2007. 7(6): p. 454-65.

[21] Cassel, S.L. and P.B. Rothman, *Chapter 3: Role of SOCS in allergic and innate immune responses.* Adv Immunol, 2009. 103: p. 49-76.

[22] Naka, T., et al., *Negative regulation of cytokine and TLR signalings by SOCS and others.* Adv Immunol, 2005. 87: p. 61-122.

[23] Gingras, S., et al., *Re-examination of the role of suppressor of cytokine signaling 1 (SOCS1) in the regulation of toll-like receptor signaling.* J Biol Chem, 2004. 279(52): p. 54702-7.

[24] Prele, C.M., et al., *SOCS1 regulates the IFN but not NFkappaB pathway in TLR-stimulated human monocytes and macrophages.* J Immunol, 2008. 181(11): p. 8018-26.

[25] Frazier, A.D., et al., *Programmed death-1 affects suppressor of cytokine signaling-1 expression in T cells during hepatitis C infection.* Viral Immunol, 2010. 23(5): p. 487-95.

[26] Alter, H.J., *HCV natural history: the retrospective and prospective in perspective.* J Hepatol, 2005. 43(4): p. 550-2.

[27] Moorman, J.P., M. Joo, and Y.S. Hahn, *Evasion of host immune surveillance by hepatitis C virus: potential roles in viral persistence.* Arch Immunol Ther Exp (Warsz), 2001. 49(3): p. 189-94.

[28] Cooper, S., et al., *Analysis of a successful immune response against hepatitis C virus.* Immunity, 1999. 10(4): p. 439-49.

[29] Lechner, F., et al., *Analysis of successful immune responses in persons infected with hepatitis C virus.* J Exp Med, 2000. 191(9): p. 1499-512.

[30] Thimme, R., et al., *Increased expression of the NK cell receptor KLRG1 by virus-specific CD8 T cells during persistent antigen stimulation.* J Virol, 2005. 79(18): p. 12112-6.

[31] Lechmann, M., et al., *Decreased frequency of HCV core-specific peripheral blood mononuclear cells with type 1 cytokine secretion in chronic hepatitis C.* J Hepatol, 1999. 31(6): p. 971-8.

[32] Rehermann, B., et al., *Quantitative analysis of the peripheral blood cytotoxic T lymphocyte response in patients with chronic hepatitis C virus infection.* J Clin Invest, 1996. 98(6): p. 1432-40.

[33] King, E., et al., *Hepatitis C: the complications of immune dysfunction.* Expert Rev Clin Immunol, 2007. 3(2): p. 145-57.

[34] Yao, Z.Q., et al., *HCV core/gC1qR interaction arrests T cell cycle progression through stabilization of the cell cycle inhibitor p27Kip1.* Virology, 2003. 314(1): p. 271-82.

[35] Yao, Z.Q., et al., *Direct binding of hepatitis C virus core to gC1qR on CD4+and CD8+T cells leads to impaired activation of Lck and Akt.* J Virol, 2004. 78(12): p. 6409-19.

[36] Yao, Z.Q., et al., *T cell dysfunction by hepatitis C virus core protein involves PD-1/PDL-1 signaling.* Viral Immunol, 2007. 20(2): p. 276-87.

[37] Golden-Mason, L., et al., *Upregulation of PD-1 expression on circulating and intrahepatic hepatitis C virus-specific CD8+T cells associated with reversible immune dysfunction.* J Virol, 2007. 81(17): p. 9249-58.

[38] Nakamoto, N., et al., *Synergistic reversal of intrahepatic HCV-specific CD8 T cell exhaustion by combined PD-1/CTLA-4 blockade.* PLoS Pathog, 2009. 5(2): p. e1000313.

[39] Urbani, S., et al., *PD-1 expression in acute hepatitis C virus (HCV) infection is associated with HCV-specific CD8 exhaustion.* J Virol, 2006. 80(22): p. 11398-403.

[40] Urbani, S., et al., *Restoration of HCV-specific T cell functions by PD-1/PD-L1 blockade in HCV infection: effect of viremia levels and antiviral treatment.* J Hepatol, 2008. 48(4): p. 548-58.

[41] Nakamoto, N., et al., *Functional restoration of HCV-specific CD8 T cells by PD-1 blockade is defined by PD-1 expression and compartmentalization.* Gastroenterology, 2008. 134(7): p. 1927-37, 1937 e1-2.

[42] Ma, C.J., et al., *PD-1 negatively regulates interleukin-12 expression by limiting STAT-1 phosphorylation in monocytes/macrophages during chronic hepatitis C virus infection.* Immunology, 2011. 132(3): p. 421-31.

[43] Zhang, Y., et al., *Cross-talk between programmed death-1 and suppressor of cytokine signaling-1 in inhibition of IL-12 production by monocytes/macrophages in hepatitis C virus infection.* J Immunol, 2011. 186(5): p. 3093-103.

[44] Miyoshi, H., et al., *Hepatitis C virus core protein exerts an inhibitory effect on suppressor of cytokine signaling (SOCS)-1 gene expression.* J Hepatol, 2005. 43(5): p. 757-63.

[45] Yoshida, T., et al., *SOCS1 is a suppressor of liver fibrosis and hepatitis-induced carcinogenesis.* J Exp Med, 2004. 199(12): p. 1701-7.

[46] Brand, S., et al., *IL-22-mediated liver cell regeneration is abrogated by SOCS-1/3 overexpression in vitro.* Am J Physiol Gastrointest Liver Physiol, 2007. 292(4): p. G1019-28.

[47] Seki, E., et al., *Demonstration of cooperative contribution of MET-and EGFR-mediated STAT3 phosphorylation to liver regeneration by exogenous suppressor of cytokine signalings.* J Hepatol, 2008. 48(2): p. 237-45.

[48] Bengsch, B., et al., *Analysis of CD127 and KLRG1 expression on hepatitis C virus-specific CD8+T cells reveals the existence of different memory T-cell subsets in the peripheral blood and liver.* J Virol, 2007. 81(2): p. 945-53.

[49] Wang, J.M., et al., *KLRG1 negatively regulates natural killer (NK) cell functions through Akt pathway in individuals with chronic hepatitis* C. J Virol, 2013.

[50] McMahan, R.H., et al., *Tim-3 expression on PD-1+HCV-specific human CTLs is associated with viral persistence, and its blockade restores hepatocyte-directed in vitro cytotoxicity.* J Clin Invest, 2010. 120(12): p. 4546-57.

[51] Moorman, J.P., et al., *Tim-3 pathway controls regulatory and effector T cell balance during hepatitis C virus infection.* J Immunol, 2012. 189(2): p. 755-66.

[52] Ji, X.J., et al., *HCV-infected hepatocytes drive CD4+CD25+Foxp3+regulatory T-cell development through the Tim-3/Gal-9 pathway.* Eur J Immunol, 2013. 43(2): p. 458-67.

[53] Zhang, Y., et al., *Tim-3 negatively regulates IL-12 expression by monocytes in HCV infection.* PLoS One, 2011. 6(5): p. e19664.

[54] Ibegbu, C.C., et al., *Expression of killer cell lectin-like receptor G1 on antigen-specific human CD8+T lymphocytes during active, latent, and resolved infection and its relation with CD57.* J Immunol, 2005. 174(10): p. 6088-94.

[55] Bengsch, B., et al., *Coexpression of PD-1, 2B4, CD160 and KLRG1 on exhausted HCV-specific CD8+T cells is linked to antigen recognition and T cell differentiation.* PLoS Pathog, 2010. 6(6): p. e1000947.

[56] Ryo, A., et al., *SOCS1 is an inducible host factor during HIV-1 infection and regulates the intracellular trafficking and stability of HIV-1 Gag.* Proc Natl Acad Sci U S A, 2008. 105(1): p. 294-9.

[57] Wang, X., et al., *B7-H1 up-regulation impairs myeloid DC and correlates with disease progression in chronic HIV-1 infection.* Eur J Immunol, 2008. 38(11): p. 3226-36.

[58] Day, C.L., et al., *PD-1 expression on HIV-specific T cells is associated with T-cell exhaustion and disease progression.* Nature, 2006. 443(7109): p. 350-4.

[59] Trautmann, L., et al., *Upregulation of PD-1 expression on HIV-specific CD8+T cells leads to reversible immune dysfunction.* Nat Med, 2006. 12(10): p. 1198-202.

[60] Muthumani, K., et al., *Human immunodeficiency virus type 1 Nef induces programmed death 1 expression through a p38 mitogen-activated protein kinase-dependent mechanism.* J Virol, 2008. 82(23): p. 11536-44.

[61] Kaufmann, D.E. and B.D. Walker, *PD-1 and CTLA-4 inhibitory cosignaling pathways in HIV infection and the potential for therapeutic intervention.* J Immunol, 2009. 182(10): p. 5891-7.

[62] Freeman, G.J., et al., *Reinvigorating exhausted HIV-specific T cells via PD-1-PD-1 ligand blockade.* J Exp Med, 2006. 203(10): p. 2223-7.

[63] Okazaki, T. and T. Honjo, *The PD-1-PD-L pathway in immunological tolerance.* Trends Immunol, 2006. 27(4): p. 195-201.

[64] Jones, R.B., et al., *Tim-3 expression defines a novel population of dysfunctional T cells with highly elevated frequencies in progressive HIV-1 infection.* J Exp Med, 2008. 205(12): p. 2763-79.

[65] Sakhdari, A., et al., *Tim-3 negatively regulates cytotoxicity in exhausted CD8+T cells in HIV infection.* PLoS One, 2012. 7(7): p. e40146.

[66] Vali, B., et al., *HCV-specific T cells in HCV/HIV co-infection show elevated frequencies of dual Tim-3/PD-1 expression that correlate with liver disease progression.* Eur J Immunol, 2010. 40(9): p. 2493-505.

[67] Elahi, S., et al., *Galectin-9 binding to Tim-3 renders activated human CD4+T cells less susceptible to HIV-1 infection.* Blood, 2012. 119(18): p. 4192-204.

[68] Rahman, A.K.M.N., et al., *TIM-3 and its Immunoregulatory Role in HIV Infection.* J Clin Cell Immunol, 2012. S7: p. 007.

[69] Mahller, Y.Y., et al., *Molecular analysis of human cancer cells infected by an oncolytic HSV-1 reveals multiple upregulated cellular genes and a role for SOCS1 in virus replication.* Cancer Gene Ther, 2008. 15(11): p. 733-41.

[70] Yokota, S., et al., *Induction of suppressor of cytokine signaling-3 by herpes simplex virus type 1 confers efficient viral replication.* Virology, 2005. 338(1): p. 173-81.

[71] Channappanavar, R., B.S. Twardy, and S. Suvas, *Blocking of PDL-1 interaction enhances primary and secondary CD8 T cell response to herpes simplex virus-1 infection.* PLoS One, 2012. 7(7): p. e39757.

[72] Bryant-Hudson, K.M. and D.J. Carr, *PD-L1-expressing dendritic cells contribute to viral resistance during acute HSV-1 infection.* Clin Dev Immunol, 2012. 2012: p. 924619.

[73] Carr, D.J., P. Harle, and B.M. Gebhardt, *The immune response to ocular herpes simplex virus type 1 infection.* Exp Biol Med (Maywood), 2001. 226(5): p. 353-66.

[74] Wickham, S. and D.J. Carr, *Molecular mimicry versus bystander activation: herpetic stromal keratitis.* Autoimmunity, 2004. 37(5): p. 393-7.

[75] Reddy, P.B., et al., *Influence of galectin-9/Tim-3 interaction on herpes simplex virus-1 latency.* J Immunol, 2011. 187(11): p. 5745-55.

[76] Sehrawat, S., et al., *Role of Tim-3/galectin-9 inhibitory interaction in viral-induced immunopathology: shifting the balance toward regulators.* J Immunol, 2009. 182(5): p. 3191-201.

[77] Sehrawat, S., et al., *Galectin-9/TIM-3 interaction regulates virus-specific primary and memory CD8 T cell response.* PLoS Pathog, 2010. 6(5): p. e1000882.

[78] Kincaid, R.P. and C.S. Sullivan, *Virus-encoded microRNAs: an overview and a look to the future.* PLoS Pathog, 2012. 8(12): p. e1003018.

[79] Roberts, A.P. and C.L. Jopling, *Targeting viral infection by microRNA inhibition.* Genome Biol, 2010. 11(1): p. 201.

[80] Boldin, M.P., et al., *miR-146a is a significant brake on autoimmunity, myeloproliferation, and cancer in mice.* J Exp Med, 2011. 208(6): p. 1189-201.

[81] Bala, S., et al., *Increased microRNA-155 expression in the serum and peripheral monocytes in chronic HCV infection.* J Transl Med, 2012. 10: p. 151.

[82] El-Ekiaby, N., et al., *Repressed induction of interferon-related microRNAs miR-146a and miR-155 in peripheral blood mononuclear cells infected with HCV genotype 4.* FEBS Open Bio, 2012. 2: p. 179-86.

[83] Fognani, E., et al., *Role of microRNA profile modifications in hepatitis C virus-related mixed cryoglobulinemia.* PLoS One, 2013. 8(5): p. e62965.

[84] Bhanja Chowdhury, J., et al., *Hepatitis C virus infection modulates expression of interferon stimulatory gene IFITM1 by upregulating miR-130A.* J Virol, 2012. 86(18): p. 10221-5.

[85] Gupta, A., et al., *MicroRNAs, hepatitis C virus, and HCV/HIV-1 co-infection: new insights in pathogenesis and therapy.* Viruses, 2012. 4(11): p. 2485-513.

[86] Thibault, P.A., et al., *MicroRNA-122-dependent and-independent replication of Hepatitis C Virus in Hep3B human hepatoma cells.* Virology, 2013. 436(1): p. 179-90.

[87] Ouellet, D.L., et al., *Regulation of host gene expression by HIV-1 TAR microRNAs.* Retrovirology, 2013. 10(1): p. 86.

[88] Umbach, J.L., et al., *MicroRNAs expressed by herpes simplex virus 1 during latent infection regulate viral mRNAs.* Nature, 2008. 454(7205): p. 780-3.

[89] Bloom, D.C., *HSV LAT and neuronal survival.* Int Rev Immunol, 2004. 23(1-2): p. 187-98.

[90] Stevens, J.G., et al., *Prominence of the herpes simplex virus latency-associated transcript in trigeminal ganglia from seropositive hum*ans. J Infect Dis, 1988. 158(1): p. 117-23.

[91] Everett, R.D., ICP0, a regulator of herpes simplex virus during lytic and latent infection. Bioessays, 2000. 22(8): p. 761-70.

Chapter 5

Macrophages — Masters of Immune Activation, Suppression and Deviation

Andrew D. Foey

Additional information is available at the end of the chapter

http://dx.doi.org/10.5772/57541

1. Introduction

Immunostimulation is fundamental to efficient host responses to pathogens; a comprehensive understanding of which will inform the development of the next generation of vaccines. Integral to vaccine development is the mode of delivery to the appropriate host tissue. Mucosal tissue, with its ability to both tolerise and activate host immune responses, represents an ideal site for vaccine delivery. The continued study of such mucosal tissue with respect to its ability to exert immune activation, suppression and in deed deviation, will be of benefit to the design of next-generation vaccines.

Mucosal immunity is governed by the interaction of the barrier epithelial cells of the mucosal surface with the underlying immune cells. The most important immune cells, which are responsible for determining immune responsiveness at these surfaces, are those of the innate immune system; antigen presenting cells (APCs) such as dendritic cells (DCs) and macrophages (Mϕs). DCs play an important role in antigen processing and presentation, thus priming antigen-specific effector T cell responses by homing from the challenge site to the local lymph node. Mϕs, on the other hand, stay within the mucosal tissue at the forefront of the challenge site and play a major role in immune fate decision: activation, deviation or suppression. Under certain genetic, environmental and immunological conditions, these resident tissue macrophages are rendered dysfunctional and play a pivotal role in establishment and persistence of pathology. Taking into consideration their tissue residence and their potential to prime a wide range of immune responses, this review will focus on immunostimulation in the context of mucosal Mϕ function in both homeostasis and pathology in the oral mucosa and gastrointestinal tract (GIT). In addition, immunostimulation via Mϕ functionality can only fully be appreciated by considering the relative relationship of activation with both immune-deviation and suppression; such functionality will also be considered in this review.

2. Macrophages

Macrophages have long since been recognised to play a central role in the immune response. They are mononuclear phagocytic cells, which have been demonstrated to be involved in pathogen recognition, clearance, antigen processing and presentation, inflammation and tissue repair as well as pro-and anti-tumoral responses. Tissue Mφs perform a range of important homeostatic functions and exist in many different tissue-specific forms: microglia in the brain, alveolar Mφs in the lung, Kupfer cell in the liver, osteoclast in the bone, as well as splenic, intestinal, bone marrow and lymph node-associated subcapsular sinusoidal/ medullary Mφs. Thus, Mφs are central to innate immune inflammatory mechanisms and the priming of adaptive responses to both intracellular and extracellular pathogens as well as immune regulation and tumour surveillance; such diversity of effector functionality would suggest mucosal macrophages to be ideal targets for vaccine therapy.

2.1. Mφs exhibit distinct functional subsets

In general, Mφ functions are conferred by environmental stimuli, pre-programming or the route of differentiation. As such, Mφs exist in several subsets, which exhibit discrete functional and phenotypic traits. A certain level of confusion exists however, as to whether the Mφ subset has been generated by the use of distinct activation signals or as a consequence of longer-term culture/differentiation, or is even pre-programmed in the monocytes. There is some evidence to suggest that monocyte pre-programming is of some functional relevance, where there is a level of heterogeneity, and monocytes potentially exist as a classical ($CD14^{++}CD16^{-}HLA\text{-}DR^{+}$) subset and a pro-inflammatory subset ($CD14^{+}CD16^{+}HLA\text{-}DR^{++}$) [1,2] biased towards high level TNFα production and present in high numbers in inflammatory pathologies [3,4]. In its simplest guise, Mφ subsets have been described to exist as two functionally distinct forms, in particular associated with Th_1 or Th_2 adaptive responses: a pro-inflammatory subset (classically activated, type I or M1) and an anti-inflammatory/regulatory subset (alternative activation, type II or M2) [5,6], although further studies have suggested several subdivisions may exist within the M2 subset (reviewed in [7]).

M1 macrophages, also referred to as classically activated Mφs, are generally pro-inflammatory Mφs, which exhibit a functional phenotype that is anti-microbial (mediating resistance to intracellular pathogens), tissue destructive and anti-tumoral [8]. Upon activation, these Mφs express a plethora of pro-inflammatory cytokines (TNFα, IL-1β, IL-6, IL-12, IL-18, IL-23), chemokines (CXCL1, 2, 3, 5, 8, 9, 10, CCL2, 3, 4, 5, 11, 17 and 22)[9], proteases and ROS/RNS. As a consequence of this wide array of cytokines expressed, M1s play a pivotal role, not only in innate responses, but also adaptive, antigen-specific responses. As M1s secrete a high level of IL-12, they promote Th_1 differentiation, hence cell mediated immune mechanisms for the defence against intracellular pathogens [10,11]. In addition, Holscher et al., 2001, described the protective role of IL-12p40; this subunit is also common to IL-23, which is produced by M1s and is important in the differentiation and activation of Th_{17} cells [12,13]. Mφs can be polarised to the M1 phenotype in the presence of IFNγ and in combination with inflammatory stimuli such as LPS or TNFα. In addition, this M1 phenotype can also result from differentiation in the presence of GM-CSF [14,15] and further polarising signals such as anoxic environments [16], β-chemokines [17] and phorbol myristate acetate, PMA [18,19]. The presence and activation of pro-inflammatory M1s would have to be tightly controlled, as over-activation or dysregulation of M1s may result in uncontrolled pro-inflammatory pathology. The involvement of such a distinct Mϕ subset has been suggested to be central to the tissue-destructive pathology associated with the chronic inflammatory bowel disease, Crohn's disease [20].

In addition to the profile of factors listed in the paragraph above, the general profile of the M1 effector phenotype is IL-10^{lo} IL-12^{hi} IL-23^{hi} [21]. Associated with the M1-polarising stimuli, IFNγ and LPS, are distinct expression and activation profiles of intracellular signalling components. M1 polarisation is transduced via the transcription factors STAT-1 and NFkB, driving the expression of immune mediators characteristic of this subset, and via the activity of SOCS3 [22]. Finally, the M1-specific transcription factor, STAT-1, has been demonstrated to inhibit STAT-6 activation; this factor is required for M2 polarisation [23], thus an M1-associated transcription factor cross-regulates/suppresses M2 polarisation/activation. These observations alone were suggestive that there was a level of plasticity that existed between M1 pro-inflammatory Mϕs and the anti-inflammatory/regulatory M2 Mϕs.

M2 macrophages, which are also referred to as alternatively activated Mϕs, were found to exhibit a functionally distinct phenotype to that of M1s, originally via the ability of IL-4 to induce MR expression, followed by another Th_2 cytokine, IL-13 [24,25]. M2 functionality was generally described as an anti-inflammatory/immunoregulatory phenotype, which also mediates tissue remodelling and repair, resistance to parasites and tumour promotion, all of which was dependent on the activation/differentiation signals encountered [6,26]. Extensive research has found a wide range of M2 polarising signals to exist: these priming signals include IL4/IL13, IL-10, TGFβ, M-CSF, Vitamin D_3, immune complexes and the Th_2-derived cytokine, IL-21 [27] and reviewed in [28]. The versatility in polarising signals and effector functionality of M2 Mϕs resulted in the proposal that M2s exist in a variety of subsets: M2a (tissue repair), M2b (B cell IgG production) and M2c (anti-inflammatory/scavenging mechanisms) (reviewed in [7,26]) (refer to figure 1 below).

M2 polarisation is induced by a wealth of exogenous factors, presented above, which drive distinct signalling/transcription factor pathways as well as signature gene expression. There is an ever-increasing understanding of these endogenous molecular pathways initiated by polarising factors such as IL-4. Whereas p65 NFκB subunit expression is associated with M1 polarisation, M2 polarisation has been described to be orchestrated by p50 NFκB [30, 31], whereby p50 NFκB inhibits NFκB-dependent M1 polarisation. In addition, p50-deficient mice exhibit exacerbated M1-driven inflammatory responses with a concomitant suppression of M2-driven responses (allergy and anti-helminth immunity). In addition to p50 NFκB, M2-like differentiation/ polarisation has been demonstrated to be induced by agonists of PPARγ [32], CREB-controlled C/EBPβ [33] and epigenetic regulation of M2-defining gene products in mice (arginase-1, Ym1, FIZZ1 and mannose receptor) via the IL-4-STAT6-dependent histone demethylation of H3 by the histone demethylase, jmjd3 [34, 35]. Finally, signalling components not only positively regulate Mϕ differentiation and activation; the generation of alternatively activated (M2) Mϕs has been reported to be

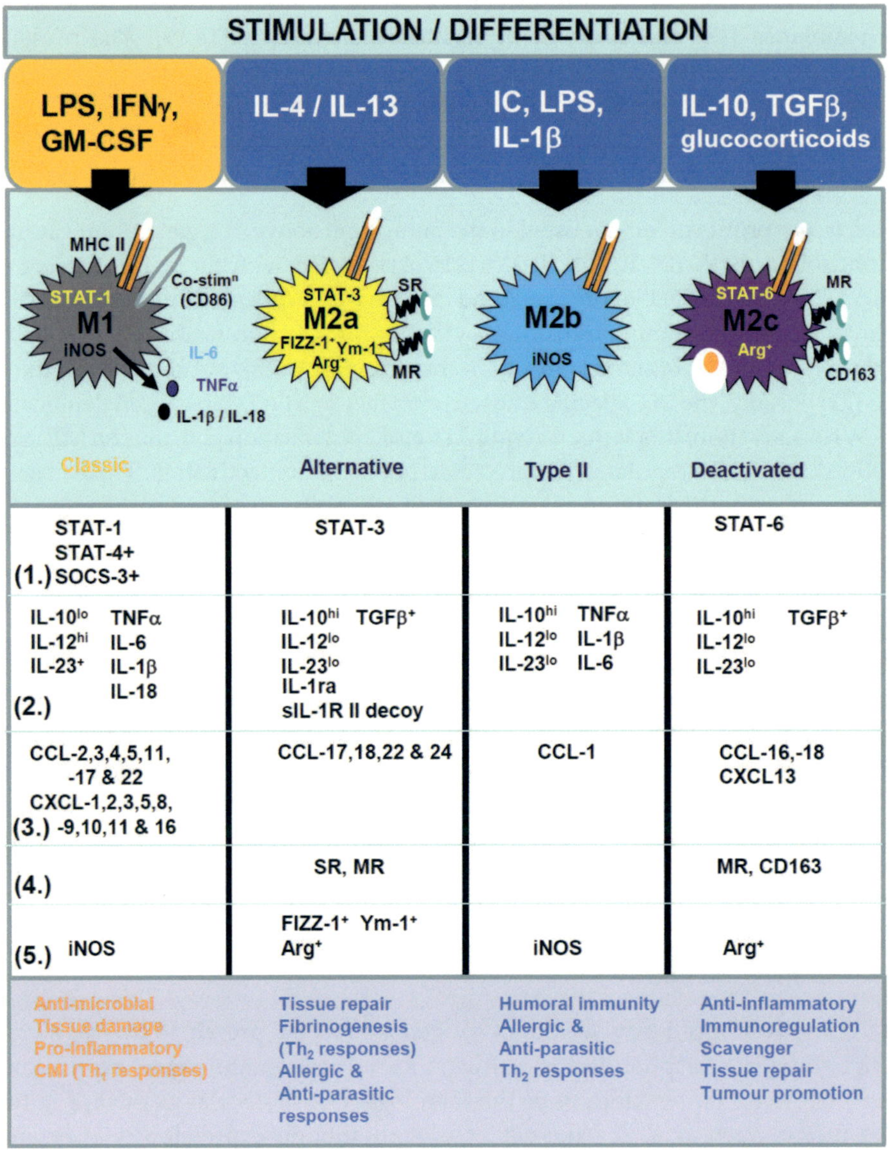

Figure 1. Activation and differentiation drive a range of functional macrophage phenotypes Mϕ effector subsets exist as pro-inflammatory M1 and regulatory or anti-inflammatory M2 phenotypes. M1s are elicited through activation by LPS and IFNγ and differentiated by GM-CSF, whereas M2s can be subdivided into M2a, M2b and M2c according to stimulation/differentiation and functional phenotype. Functional phenotype is characterised by a series of molecular markers listed in the incorporated table under the categories of (1.) signalling molecules, (2.) cytokine expression profile, (3.) chemokine profile, (4.) scavenger receptor expression and (5.) tryptophan metabolism (inducible nitric oxide synthase, iNOS, and arginase, Arg) and the poorly defined effector molecules, FIZZ-1 and Ym-1. The overall function of these Mϕ subsets is summarised in the lower segment of the table, ranging from pro-inflammatory, anti-tumour responses to anti-inflammatory, regulatory and tissue reparative responses. This figure is adapted from [28] and information presented in [7, 9, 23, 26, 29].

repressed by the negative regulator, src homology 2-containing inositol-5′-phosphatase, SHIP, a potent negative regulator of the PI3K pathway [36].

2.2. Functional and phenotypic plasticity of macrophages

Tissue-resident macrophages can thus express a wide variety of functional phenotypes, which is governed by the manner in which they are activated, differentiated or pre-programmed. This results in potentially two distinct opposing types; pro-inflammatory M1 Mϕ and anti-inflammatory/regulatory M2 Mϕ. If these subsets represent a terminally differentiated phenotype, then it is probable that Mϕs are incapable of functional plasticity. What is becoming clear however, is that M1 and M2 Mϕs do exhibit a level of plasticity and that tissue Mϕs are more likely represented on an intermediate sliding scale between pro-inflammatory/immune activatory and anti-inflammatory/regulatory functionality. Indeed, this functional plasticity and manipulation of Mϕ subset has been observed in many studies. A study focussing on bone marrow-derived Mϕs, observed that cytokine functional phenotypes could be altered/ reversed in the presence of Th_1 or Th_2 cytokines and that this plasticity in function was determined by changes to tissue microenvironment and whether these cytokines were encountered before or concomitantly with an activation stimulus [37]. This plasticity or reversal of Mϕ cytokine phenotype has recently been reinforced by the demonstration of a reversible, bi-directional differentiation of pro-inflammatory (M1) and anti-inflammatory (M2) monocyte-derived Mϕs in response to GM-CSF and M-CSF [38]. In addition, the control of these M-CSF and GM-CSF Mϕ and the invading monocyte populations has been demonstrated to be controllable via the use of neutralising antibodies to these differentiation factors in both homeostasis and inflammatory pathology of antigen-induced peritonitis and lung inflammation [39]. This study suggested that M-CSF-derived Mϕs played a non-reductant (M2-like regulatory) role whereas GM-CSF Mϕs maintained the inflammatory response (M1-like pro-inflammatory), contributing to prolonged monocyte and neutrophil infiltration. This is suggestive of the possibility of *in vivo* control of Mϕ effector phenotype through reduction in numbers and manipulation of plasticity.

Macrophage plasticity is not only determined by the differentiation factors but also by the local environmental stimulation factors, the intracellular signalling molecules activated and by the effector cytokines expressed/secreted by the macrophages. These environmental factors not only modulate Mϕ functional plasticity, the Mϕs themselves are able to cross-regulate each other thus moving or consolidating Mϕ effector response along this sliding scale of functionality between pro-inflammatory and anti-inflammatory/regulatory responses. These exogenous regulators include M1 and M2-associated cytokines (IFNγ, IL-12, IL-10, IL-4) which cross-regulate each other and immune complexes (ICs) which, through binding of their respective FcγR, can revert activation status or suppress/modulate cytokine expression, such as suppress IL-12 and induce IL-10 to an M2-like phenotype [40,41]. There is a wide range of intracellular signalling molecules, which play distinct roles in this cross-regulation and plasticity between M1 and M2 subsets. Pro-M1 responses can be mediated by SHIP-1 [42], p65 NFκB and IRF5 [43]; all of which, suppress M2s. On the flip-side, pro-M2 responses have been demonstrated to be mediated by tpl-2, p50 NFκB [31], STAT-6 [34], C/EBPβ and c-maf [33]; again, these molecules suppress the development of the other canonical Mϕ subset, M1s (reviewed in [44]). Indeed, the importance of the NFkB signalling pathway has been further consolidated by a study demonstrating that IKKβ played an anti-inflammatory role by suppressing classical Mϕ activation/M1 Mϕ phenotype via negative cross-talk with STAT-1, which is involved in the expression of IL-12, iNOS and MHCII [45] and via the maintenance of the IL-10^{hi}/IL12^{lo} functional phenotype [46].

Considering Mϕ subset phenotype, its environmental differentiation factors, activatory stimuli and effector cytokine profile; macrophage responses can be modulated by a wide range of factors which includes both positive and negative regulators. As such, the potential involvement of macrophages as an immunotherapeutic target for several pathologies can only be appreciated by a full understanding of both activatory and regulatory signals: immunostimulation, immunosuppression and immune deviation.

3. Stimulation and suppression of Mϕ effector responses

Macrophages exhibit a wide variety of receptors, which transduce a multitude of immunostimulatory signals. These activatory receptors are centred on responsiveness to conserved broad-spectrum molecular patterns associated with immune responsiveness to pathogens or endogenous, self-associated, danger signals. Pattern recognition receptors (PRRs) which stimulate or co-activate immune responses include the toll-like receptors (TLRs), NOD-like receptors (NLRs), C-type lectin receptors (CLRs) and scavenger receptors (SRs). In addition to these PRRs, Mϕs can also be activated by immune complex recognition via FcRs and cytokine stimulation through their cognate receptors.

Toll-like receptors respond to a wide repertoire of PAMPs, expressed on bacterial, viral, fungal and parasitic pathogens, and DAMPs; generally activating innate inflammatory-or anti-viral responses through the involvement of discriminatory utilisation of receptors, adaptor proteins and either NFκB-or IRF-dependent signalling pathways [47]. Indeed, the utilisation of such signalling pathways, in Mϕ polarisation, make it impossible to totally devolve consideration of polarisation, activation, cross-regulation and suppression. TLRs are expressed according to the localisation of pathogens; TLR2 (CD282), TLR1 (CD281), TLR6 (CD286), TLR4 (CD284) and TLR5 (CD285) being expressed on extracellular membranes, recognise extracellular pathogens, whereas TLR3 (CD283), TLR7 (CD287), TLR8 (CD288), and TLR9 (CD289) are expressed intracellularly, associated with endosomal membranes and recognition of intracellular resident pathogens. The extracellular facing TLRs were found to recognise a range of conserved PAMPs expressed by bacteria, including lipopeptides, LPS and flagellin, whereas TLRs 3, 7, 8 and 9 recognise dsRNA, dsDNA and hypomethylated CpG DNA motifs, respectively, expressed by viruses and bacteria.

TLRs activate a range of important signalling pathways and transcription factors, where their PAMPs activate MAPKs (ERK-1/2, p38 MAPK and JNK), which enhance gene expression and, in the case of p38, mRNA stability via AU-rich repeats present in the 3'UTRs. Activation of MAPK-dependent transcription factors along with other transcription factors are responsible for a wide repertoire of gene expression and immune functionality. Indeed, activation of TLR4 by LPS has been observed to activate ERK-1/2, JNK and p38 MAPKs as well as NFκB and IRF3; these signalling pathways give rise to a multitude of immune mediators which include TNFα, IL-1β, IL-6, IL-8, IL-12, iNOS, IL-10, MHC II. Macrophage activation can thus exhibit a wide range of functions, which include pro-inflammatory, anti-microbial responses, anti-inflammatory/regulatory responses and priming of adaptive immune responses through their capacity to process and present antigen.

Taking into consideration the previous sections, LPS and other PAMPs may be able to induce a wide variety of immune mediators; the expression of which will also be determined by other activatory stimuli, differentiation factors and both exogenous and endogenous suppressive molecules. TLR signals can be negatively regulated by a multitude of molecules (reviewed in [48]) which include; Myd88s, IRAK-M, IRF-4 [49,50], TREM-2, ST2 [51], Tollip, TRIAD3A, SOCS-1, SOCS-3, SHP1, SHP2, SIGIRR [52]. In addition to endogenous suppressors of TLR activation signals, it is becoming evident that TLRs can cross-regulate each other, resulting in suppression of distinct TLR signalling pathway or endotoxin tolerisation of Mϕs through homo-or hetero-tolerisation of distinct TLRs and their ensuing effector functionality (reviewed in [53]). Such mechanisms of tolerisation have been demonstrated to be differentially utilised, dependent on Mϕ subset as well as activation signal [54]. Such complex, inter-twined signalling pathways enable a level of innate "specificity" of anti-microbial activation response as well as a way in which these activatory signals are fine-tuned, suppressed or modulated.

NOD-like receptors (NLRs); due to their intracellular expression, originally thought to specifically respond to intracellular pathogens and their PAMPs, it has become apparent that NLRs are integral to the innate detection of both extracellular and intracellular-resident pathogens. The superfamily of NLRs consists of NOD1 and NOD2 which are intracellular receptors for peptidoglycan (D-γ-glutamyl-meso-DAP and muramyl dipeptide, respectively) [55]. NOD1 and NOD2 activate NFκB through the recruitment and activation of RIP2 and resulting activation of the IκB kinase complex [56]. As a result, NOD-signalling can induce pro-inflammatory, anti-microbial defences via the expression of a wide array of NF-κB-dependent gene products (reviewed in [57]).

In addition to the NFκB-activating NODs, the NLR family is also made up of a collection of receptors involved in the activation of caspases [58], specifically caspases 1 and 5 that are integral for the inflammasome construction, activation and processing of the pro-cytokines pro-IL-1β and pro-IL-18 into the mature and secretable IL-1β and IL-18. The inflammasome is activated by extracellular ATP and hypotonic stress, both representative of endogenous danger signals or DAMPs. ASC is an adaptor protein which recruits caspase-1 into an inflammasome activation complex; knock-out mice have demonstrated ASC to be essential for LPS-induced activation of caspase-1, where these mice failed to activate pro-caspase-1 or produce IL-1β and IL-18, even in the event of stimulation by both LPS and ATP (activation of the $P2X_7$ receptor) [59]. This requirement for inflammasome-mediated caspase-1 activation, hence IL-1β maturation and secretion, in response to LPS (a TLR4 ligand), emphasises a collaborative role for TLR and NLR pathways in the production of IL-1β and the ensuing inflammatory response. Other NLR family members, NALP1, NALP3 and Ipaf, have all been demonstrated to be associated with ASC in the inflammasome, playing an integral role in caspase-1-dependent activation of pro-inflammatory cytokines [60]. NLRs have also been reported to suppress both NFκB and caspase activation pathways. With respect to inhibition of NFκB, NALP10 and NALP12 display a suppressive activity, whereas NALP7 and NALP10 are suppressive for caspase activation (reviewed in [61]). Again, it is imperative to the direction of Mφ functional responses that the expression profile of NLRs be characterised, along with potential cross-communicating PRRs; this total profile gives scientists an insight of potential control of Mφ functionality as being activatory, suppressive or even being able to deviate/modify the cellular response.

RIG-like receptors (RLRs): are key intracellular innate immune sensors of viral infection. Whereas the predominant viral PRRs in DCs (particularly pDCs) are TLR3, TLR7, TLR8 and TLR9, RLR viral sensing and expression is predominant in Mφs [62]. Currently, the main RLRs are retinoic acid inducible gene-1 (RIG-1) and melanoma differentiation-associated gene (MDA)5; both of which detect dsRNA [63,64]. Similar to the viral-sensing TLRs, RLRs activate NFκB and IRF3 signalling pathways, resulting in gene expression of pro-inflammatory cytokine genes and anti-viral type I interferons (IFNα and IFNβ). Upon viral infection, these interferons exhibit a positive feedback loop which up-regulates RLR expression. MDA5 has been demonstrated to be important in the detection of picornovirus and polyinosine polycytidylic acid, poly(I:C)-induced IFNα production. On the other hand, the importance of RLRs to macrophage anti-viral responses is enforced by observations that RNA helicases eg. Lgp2, inhibits RIG1 signalling [65] and that an evasion mechanism utilised by hepatitis C virus is the production of RLR signalling inhibitory proteins [66,67]. This overlap in structure/functional relationships between TLRs and RLRs is suggestive that these receptor types function in tandem to provide ubiquitous anti-viral protection. Additionally, it is unclear as to whether RLRs also interact and mediate inflammasome activity, as a study by Johnston et al in 2005, has shown that a pox virus pyrin domain protein interacts with ASC-1 (NLR family member) and inhibits inflammatory and apoptotic inflammasome activity [68]. This viral escape mechanism, targeting NLR-mediated inflammasome activity, is also suggestive that RLRs cross-communicate with NLRs; thus efficient anti-viral protection is truly a trinity of innate reception between TLRs, NLRs and RLRs (reviewed in [61]).

Scavenger receptors (SRs) and C-type Lectin receptors (CLRs): this is a large group of receptors widely expressed on macrophage cells [69] which scavenge pathogenic material and cellular debris, initiating clearing responses through receptor-mediated endocytosis, phagocytosis or signals inflammatory responses. Responses elicited are dependent on patterns being recognised and combinations of PRRs being employed. The CLRs, being lectin receptors are generally sugar receptors, whereas SRs recognise and respond to a wider range of molecular patterns; however, there is a level of overlap, hence confusion between receptors of these families. Scavenger receptors are a broad family of PRRs, which involve both opsonin-mediated phagocytosis and opsonin-independent PRRs; the latter even including TLRs, lectins, complement receptors (CRs), CD14, CD36, scavengers of ACAMPs (see later section). Scavenger receptors include the SR-A class of receptors (SR-AI, SR-AII, MARCO), SR-B (CD36, SR-BI and Croquemort, CD163 – haemoglobin scavenger receptor), SR-C class (dSR-CI) and

SR-E (LOX-1) as well as other SR-A-like class members (SR-CLI – a potential CLR on the basis of C-type lectin domain expression), SR-D (macrosialin). In general, these scavenger receptors recognise a wide range of PAMPs including LTA, LPS, bacterial DNA, whole bacteria, sugar moieties and DAMPs, thus clearance of dead and dying host tissue, as well as pathogenic material (reviewed in [70]). The majority of the signalling scavenger receptors (Dectin-1, Dectin-2, Mϕ Mannose Receptor) are CLRs and will be covered in the next section.

CLRs play a major role in recognition and activation of anti-microbial immunity against a diverse range of pathogens, which include fungi, bacteria, viruses and parasites. They are receptors which contain one or more carbohydrate recognition domains (CRDs) which bind a wide variety of carbohydrate ligand moieties. Generally, CLRs can be categorised as either having a built-in endogenous signalling activity or requiring interaction with a partner adaptor protein which possesses signalling activity (reviewed in [71]). CLRs signal via integral ITAMs or partner ITAM-bearing adaptors such as FcγRs. Integral ITAM-bearing CLRs generally signal through a syk/CARD9 pathway which ultimately results in NFκB activation; such signalling CLRs include Dectin-1, Dectin-2 and Mincle. These CLRs are particularly prominent in mounting anti-fungal responses; Dectin-1 responds to β-glucans expressed in the fungal cell wall by initiating a variety of cellular responses which include phagocytosis, respiratory burst, activation of inflammasomes, cytokine production and the polarisation of adaptive responses to cell mediated immunity mediated by Th_1 and Th_{17} cells. In addition, Dectin-1 exhibits cross-talk with TLR2 and other myd88-dependent TLRs, thus again, co-operation of PRRs is critical for tailoring appropriate immune responses (reviewed in [72]). Dectin-2 and Mincle both recognise fungal α-mannans with Dectin-2 being associated with innate recognition and induction of Th_{17} responses. Of particular importance to the recognition and signal activation in response to fungal infection is the observation that Dectin-2 (signalling) can heterodimerise with Dectin-3, thus CLRs demonstrate a level of co-operativity with each other and fine-tuning of their responses to the fungal pathogen [71].

Bacterial sensing utilises Mincle, mannose receptor (MR) and DC-SIGN. MR has been shown to be involved in the recognition and responsiveness to *Klebsiella* and *Streptococcus* sp but so far, has not been recognised to contain a signalling motif. To initiate antibacterial responses, it is likely that the MR co-operates with other PRRs. Mincle however signals through the pathway detailed above, in order to activate NFκB-mediated responses required for innate and consequent cell mediated immune responses to Mycobacterial infection through recognition and binding of mycobacterial cord factor, trehalose-6,6′-dimycolate, TDM. Mycobacteria are also recognised and a response initiated through ManLam (mannosylated lipoarabinomannan) binding to DC-SIGN which is expressed by DCs; whether this CLR is expressed by Mϕs is yet to be definitively characterised [71]. DC-SIGN has also been described as being involved in viral recognition by binding to the gp120 envelope protein of HIV-1; this mechanism however may be more representative of a mode of viral transmission rather than anti-viral immunity. CLRs such as CLEC9A (DNGR-1) has been shown to be protective, by facilitating antigen cross-presentation, hence controlling infection of vaccinia virus and herpes simplex virus. Finally, both Dectin-2 and MR are involved in immunity to parasites, whereby Dectin-2 recognises Schistosoma mansonii egg antigen SEA resulting in the activation of the

NLRP3 inflammasome and alleviating Th_2 pathology. Of particular interest is the fact that Dectin-2 can also promote Th_2responsiveness, as opposed to suppressing it, when responding to the common allergen of house dust mite [71]. MR drives protective Th_2 responses during S.mansonii infection whereas enhances uptake of infectious circariae. These last few observations with respect to Dectin-2 and MR and their ability to drive Th_2 responses would appear to conform to the previously observed study of Mills et al, whereby M2 macrophages were associated with Th_2 immunity [5]; indeed, MR at least, has been assigned as an M2 marker. On the flip-side, Dectin-1 has been associated with initiation of Th_1 and Th_{17} anti-fungal responses; it would appear that any potential activation and modulation of specific immune responses would have to consider the role of pathogen associated carbohydrate expression and their respective CLRs expressed on host macrophages.

Siglecs: sialic acid-binding Ig-like lectins are members of the immunoglobulin superfamily involved in the recognition and reception of sialylated glycoconjugates, involved in endocytosis, positive and negative activation signals. Sialic acids are a family of nine-carbon sugars which are derivatives of neuraminic acid or keto deoxynonulosonic acid and appearing in different glycosidic linkages, typically at the exposed, non-reducing ends of oligosaccharide chains attached to proteins and lipids. It is thought that sialic acid residues either, mask subterminal sugars, prevent non-specific cell-cell interactions or act as ligands for modulating selective cell-cell interactions [73]. Currently, there are 13 Siglec family members expressed in humans and classified into two distinct subsets; siglecs 1 (CD169), 2 (CD22) and 4 are activatory receptors whereas siglecs 3 (CD33) and 5 (CD170) to 11, 14 and 16 (CD33-related siglecs) exhibit suppressive activity through two conserved ITIMs (immunereceptor tyrosine-based inhibition motif) in the cytoplasmic domain which are responsible for the recruitment of the signal suppressive phosphatase enzymes SHIP (lipid phosphatise), SHP-1 and SHP-2 (protein tyrosine phosphatises), which result in raised activation thresholds and antagonism of ITAM-dependent activation. More recently, tyrosine phosphorylation of CD33 and siglec-7 can recruit SOCS3 which leads to ubiquitination and proteosomal degredation of the Siglec; regulation of the negative regulator! [74,75]. Thus, expression and activation of distinct expression profiles of siglecs can either positively or negatively regulate immune and inflammatory responses. Monocytic cells have been shown to express Siglec-3 (CD33) and Siglecs-5,-7,-9 and-10, whereas generally, Mϕs express sialoadhesin (Siglec-1) and Siglecs-3 and-5 (reviewed in [76]), yet differentiation of monocytes to pro-and anti-inflammatory Mϕs using GM-CSF and M-CSF, respectively, showed retention of the monocyte Siglec phenotype [77]. This wide array of CD33-related siglec expression on monocytes and macrophages is suggestive of a degree of functional redundancy exists between these siglecs however, the specific expression profiles between cell types is indicative of specificity of function. More recently, research has uncovered more functional information regarding CD33-related siglecs; they may not just exert inhibitory responses through suppression of ITAM-dependent signals, as over-expression of siglec-9 in Mϕs both inhibits the TLR-induced expression of the pro-inflammatory cytokine, TNFα, but also induced the anti-inflammatory cytokine, IL-10 [78]. Again, as with other Mϕ receptors, the importance of a balance between positive and negative signals within the immune system is paramount.

FcγRs: are a family of receptors which bind the Fc region of IgG/IgG immune complexes and are responsible for mediating both activatory and suppressive responses by transducing their ligand-binding signal through either an endogenous cytoplasmic ITAM or ITIM motif, respectively. Three classes of FcγRs are expressed on immune cells such as Mϕs, these include the high affinity FcγRI (CD64) which binds monomeric IgG and the low affinity receptors FcγRII (CD32) and FcγRIII (CD16) that bind IgG immune complexes. Activatory receptors which possess cytoplasmic ITAM sequences include FcγRIIIa, FcγRI and FcγRIIa whereas the CD32 subtype, FcγRIIb is suppressive, containing a cytoplasmic ITIM sequence (reviewed in [79]). Thus recognition and clearance of IgG immune complexes may induce either an activatory or inhibitory signal which is dependent on expression profile of these FcRs and potential cross-talk with other PRRs. Ligation of FcγRIIIa induces the expression and secretion of Mϕ-derived TNFα, the mechanism of production and activation of which has been found to be associated with pathological inflammation [80]. Ligation of FcγRI however, was found to reverse Mϕ pro-inflammatory responses [81]. Indeed, taking into consideration the format of presentation of IgG, the immune response cell and their FcγR expression profile, Mϕs can be activated or inhibited with respect to inflammatory responses; differential FcγR-driven induction and suppression in collagen-induced arthritis model have resulted in this being considered as a realistic therapeutic regimen in the treatment of RA [82]. The final thing to consider with respect to FcγR-induced responses in Mϕs is the fact that these responses may differ between M1 and M2 subsets and that these responses may be deviated by manipulation of FcγR signalling or indeed exhibit suppression of inflammatory responses or manipulation of functional plasticity. Manipulation of these Mϕ receptors would represent a realistic option when considering their association with alternative activation, M2-like anti-inflammatory Mϕs.

Other macrophage suppressive receptors: Two further immunosuppressive molecules that control Mϕ functionality which are worthy of consideration are CD200R and SIRPα (CD172a); both members of the immunoglobulin superfamily (IgSF). CD172a interacts with a broadly expressed ligand, CD47, which results in the suppression of Mϕs through interaction with the tyrosine phosphatases, SHP1 and SHP2 [83] and reviewed in [84]). In addition, this interaction is made more complex by the observation of bi-directionality of signalling, where CD47 ligation has been found to selectively suppress monocyte IL-12 production, whereas TNFα, IL-1 and IL-6 was not suppressed. In contrast, the immunosuppressive cytokines, TGFβ and IL-10, were not altered by CD47 ligation; suppression of IL-12 was independent of TGFβ and IL-10 [85]. Thus, molecules such as CD172a and CD47 represent an attractive target couple for multi-mechanistic immune suppression. CD200R ligation, on the other hand, transduces a simpler immunological signal. CD200 (OX-2) is a cell surface glycoprotein containing Ig-like domains that interacts with CD200R expressed on Mϕs [86]. The human homologue of CD200R was characterised by Wright and colleagues who found that its cytoplasmic domain contained known signalling motifs [87]. The role of CD200R ligation was appreciated to be potentially suppressive where CD200-deficient mice were shown to display increased susceptibility to autoimmune disease models affecting joints. In accordance with this study, CD200Fc fusion protein was found to exhibit beneficial immunomodulation of arthritis and allograft rejection [88,89]. Indeed, the CD200Fc anti-arthritic response targeted pro-inflammatory cytokines in murine CIA, suppressing mRNA gene expression of TNFα, IL-1β, MMP13 but also IL-10 [90]. It is probable that CD200R represents a family of closely-related receptors; four homologues exist in the mouse, two of which, however, may exhibit activatory properties rather than suppressive, as they have been shown to pair with an ITAM-containing adaptor protein DAP12 [87]. Considering these early observations, it is likely that such IgSF members represent realistic therapeutic targets for immune suppression, activation and deviation of Mϕ-mediated pathological mechanisms associated with cancer, transplantation and inflammation.

Cytokine expression and responsiveness: Dysregulation and aberrant functionality of Mϕs is widely associated with pathology. Macrophages are central to phagocytosis and the modulation of inflammatory responses, through the induction and regulation of cytokine expression. Mϕs not only phagocytose pathogens and particulate material, they are important for the clearance of dead and dying host cells, utilising a wealth of scavenger receptors such as SRA, CD36, CD68, integrins, CD14, complement components and the phosphatidyl serine receptor (reviewed in [91]). Clearance of necrotic host cell material is generally associated with the induction of inflammatory responses, where necrotic cells are recognised by Mϕs and result in the production of TNFα and the driving of Th_1-mediated immune responses. In contrast, Mϕs recognise apoptotic cells [92], resulting in an anti-inflammatory environment, characterised by the production of TGFβ, PGE2 [93] and IL-10 [94]. In fact, the defective clearance of apoptotic cells has been linked with autoimmunity [95]. Recognition of apoptotic cells is thus important in immunoregulation modulated by Mϕs. Mϕs recognise and distinguish between apoptotic and necrotic cells via danger-associated molecular patterns (DAMPs) and apoptotic cell-associated molecular patterns (ACAMPs). This dichotomy in responsiveness is reflective of Mϕ subset functionality; indeed M2-like, alternatively activated Mϕs express a wide array of receptors for ACAMPs; it is likely that recognition of apoptotic cells will activate and programme M2 cells towards an anti-inflammatory and regulatory phenotype, whereas DAMPs and necrotic cells drive an immune activatory, pro-inflammatory response (reviewed in [96]).

Cytokines are not only induced by phagocytic recognition and clearance of dead and dying cells. They are produced by Mϕs and a wide variety of other immune cells as part of immune activatory or regulatory responses. As such, Mϕs are modulated by a variety of cytokines; the predominant Mϕ-modulatory cytokines include TGFβ, IL-10, IL-12, IL-4/IL-13, IFNγ and TNFα. IL-4/IL-13 and TGFβ/IL-10 have been described above to be associated with priming M2 Mϕ subset polarisation (M2a and M2c, respectively); whereas IL-12 and IFNγ play an important role in the polarisation and functionality of M1 cells and concomitantly, suppressing development and activation/functionality of M2s. The relative expression of these cytokines is thus imperative to subset functionality and cross-regulation.

TGFβ and IL-10 modulate Mϕ polarisation and functional plasticity to that of an M2c subset which exhibits a characteristic cytokine phenotype of IL-10^{hi}, IL-12^{lo}, IL-23^{lo} and TGFβ^{+}which is associated with anti-inflammatory responses, scavenging, immunoregulation, tissue repair and tumour promotion. Both TGFβ and IL-10 directly suppress immune activation via the down-regulation of the expression of MHC II, B7 costimulation (suppressing APC function) and pro-inflammatory cytokine production, with an indirect effect through cross-regulation of M1-derived cytokines and functionality. In contrast to this TGFβ-mediated suppression of Mϕ-driven functionality, pro-inflammatory cytokines such as TNFα modulate M1-driven responses, favouring anti-microbial killing, CMI and tissue-destructive pro-inflammatory responses. TNFα activates Mϕs following IFNγ priming, which results in a strong activation of NFκB and enhanced cell migration to inflammatory sites and consequent iNOS-mediated anti-microbial killing [97]. It also primes a sustained inflammatory response [98] and Mϕ survival, important to inflammation and to the pathology of sepsis [99]. TNFα and other pro-inflammatory cytokines such as IL-1β, not only play a pivotal role in the initiation and maintenance of the inflammatory response, but also modulate immunosuppressive mechanisms through the process of Mϕ endotoxin tolerance. Thus, the state of Mϕ activation, polarisation of subset functionality and the relative contribution of activatory, suppressive and immune-deviation signals associated with Mϕs, is of paramount importance in determining an appropriate immune response or pathological response as a consequence on Mϕ immune dysfunction (refer to figure 2 below). Finally, one last consideration regarding Mϕ functional responses to cytokines is that responsiveness has been demonstrated to be dysregulated, especially, with regards anti-inflammatory IL-10 signal transduction by IL-10 receptors in a chronic inflammatory environment [100]. Consideration of cytokine responsiveness of Mϕs can only be realistically appreciated when considering the local environment; homeostatic or pathogenic!

Macrophage functionality and inflammatory pathology: Mϕs are particularly abundant in mucosal tissues such as the oral cavity and the gastro-intestinal tract. Dysregulation of Mϕ functionality in such mucosal tissue has been shown to have grave impacts on mucosal function and to result in Mϕ-driven pathology. This section will focus on Mϕ dysregulation and impact on host tissue in the context of M1-and M2-driven responses associated with oral (chronic periodontitis and oral squamous cell carcinoma) and the GIT (Crohn's disease, ulcerative colitis and colorectal cancer) mucosal pathology. These pathologies display pathological mechanisms aligned to M1-or M2-like functional phenotypes; to fully appreciate these dysregulated responses, it is imperative to appreciate the functional phenotype of healthy, homeostatic mucosal macrophages. From studies focussing on the characterisation of gut mucosal Mϕs, in general mucosal Mϕs exhibit a functional phenotype similar to M2 Mϕs. Intestinal Mϕs express phagocytic scavenger receptors (CD33, CD36, CD68), HLA-DR, immunoregulatory receptors (CD200R and TGFβRI/RII) and immunoregulatory cytokines (IL-10, TGFβ) whereas fail to express the co-stimulatory molecules (CD40, CD80, CD86), pattern recognition receptors (CD14, TLRs), TREM-1, FcRs, CRs and the pro-inflammatory cytokines (TNFα, IL-1β, IL-6, IL-18). On the other hand, in general, inflammatory Mϕs express a wide variety of functional markers which include: PRRs (CD14, TLR2, TLR4, TLR5), FcRs (CD16, CD32, CD64, CD89), CRs, HLA-DR, co-stimulatory molecules, chemokine receptors (CCR5, CXCR4) and pro-inflammatory cytokines/markers (TREM-1, TNFα, IL-1β, IL-6, IL-18, CCL20) [28,101-103].

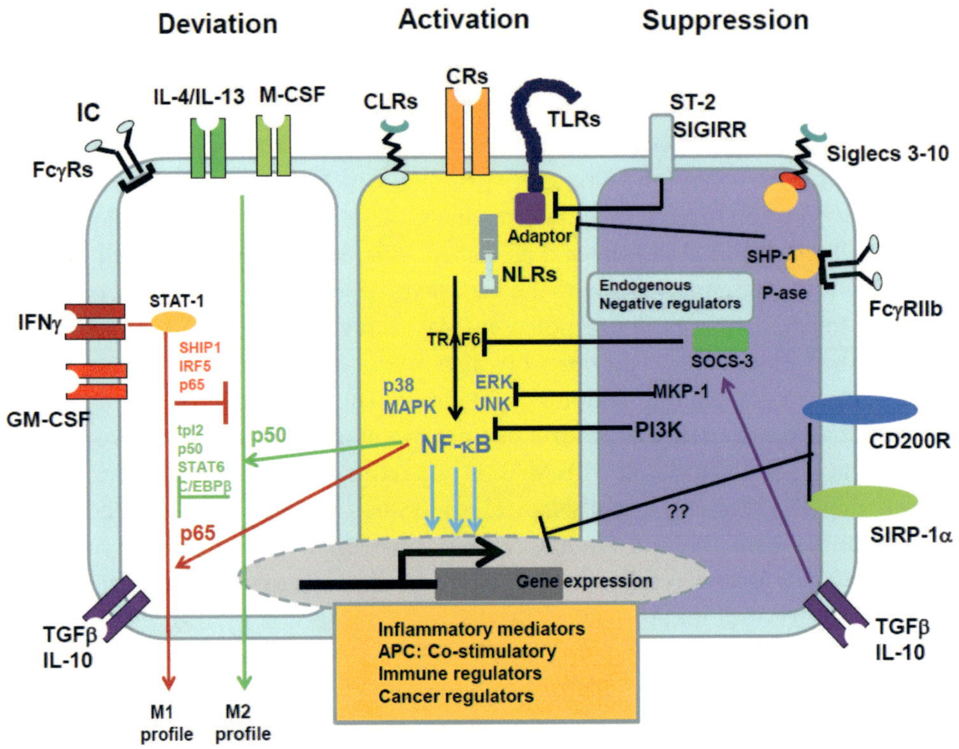

Figure 2. Macrophage effector functionality is determined by a variety of activation, suppression and deviation. Mϕ effector responses can be positively initiated by a range of receptors (yellow box) which include CLRs, TLRs, NLRs and complement receptors (CRs) which induce a range of activatory signalling pathways (p38, ERK and JNK mitogen activated protein kinases, MAPKs, and NFκB), resulting in specific gene expression. These positive signals can be suppressed (purple box) by a range of exogenous (SIGIRR, ST2, Siglecs, FcγRIIb, CD200R, SIRP-1α, TGFβR, IL-10R) and endogenous signals (SOCS3, MKP-1, PI3K, ITIM-associated SHP-1, SHP-2, SHIP-1). Finally, Mϕ functionality can deviate between M1 and M2 phenotype (white box), determined by exogenous factors (IL-4, IL-13, M-CSF, IFNγ, GM-CSF, TGFβ, IL-10) and internal signalling molecules (STAT1, STAT6, p65 NFκB, p50 NFκB).

3.1. M1-driven pathology

Crohn's disease (CD) is an inflammatory bowel disease (IBD) characterised by tissue-destructive transmural inflammatory skip lesions which present along the whole length of the GI tract. CD is characterised by dysfunctional innate immune responses, which result in a Th_1/Th_{17} axis of inflammatory destruction. This granulomatous inflammation is characterised by high expression of IL-12/IL-23, resulting in the predominance of Th_1/Th_{17} cells that produce IFNγ, TNFα and IL-17 [104]. This dysregulated pro-inflammatory response is believed to be associated with mutations to PRRs and pathogen sensing ability of the innate immune system. Genetic mutations in the CARD15 gene which encodes NOD2, an intracellular sensing receptor for bacterial peptidoglycan, are associated with CD Mϕs and have been demonstrated to modulate NFκB activation and up-regulate expression of the pro-inflammatory cytokines TNFα, IL-1β and IL-12 [105], whereas NOD2 activation would normally mediate anti-inflammatory signals induced through TLR2 [106]. In addition, NOD2 mutation also results in impaired recruitment of monocytes to mucosal tissue and their differentiation to a homeostatic intestinal Mϕ phenotype as well as impairment of Treg activity [107]. Thus, the combination of a dysregulated innate response in favour of pro-inflammatory cytokines, aberrant anti-inflammatory mechanisms, coupled with adaptive immune system bias towards a Th_1/Th_{17} cell mediated inflammatory response, result in the breaking of mucosal immune tolerance in favour of the tissue-destructive inflammatory mechanisms observed in the pathology of Crohn's disease and its perpetuation by both pathogenic and commensal luminal contents (reviewed in [108]). This loss in regulation results in a mucosal environment that is $IL\text{-}10^{low}$ $IL\text{-}12^{high}$, which induces M1-like Mϕ activation/differentiation and the up-regulation of expression of pro-inflammatory cytokines and co-stimulatory molecules [109].

The oral mucosa plays a significant role in tolerance induction; it is thought that dysregulation of mucosal Mϕ functionality contributes to the breaking of this tolerance and drives oral inflammatory pathologies such as oral lichen planus, recurrent aphthous stomatitis and chronic periodontitis [110]. Chronic periodontitis (CP) is a persistent inflammatory condition of the periodontal tissue, characterised by bouts of relapse and remission that, if left untreated, could result in destruction of periodontium and tooth loss. CP results from activation of host inflammatory response as a consequence of constant microbial challenge mounted to a dysbiotic microbial population present in the oral cavity, of which *Porphyromonas gingivalis* (PG) is a prominent member [111,112]. PG is an intracellular oral pathogen, which invades oral epithelial cells, dendritic cells and macrophages; clearance of such would require a Th_1-dependent cell mediated response [113,114]. PG-LPS subverts both host innate and adaptive responses away from clearing responses by low endotoxin activity along with preferential utilisation of TLR2 rather than TLR4 and by inducing Th_2-dependent humoral responses, respectively [115,116]. There is a dense population of Mϕs in the oral mucosa which react to PG by producing large amounts of pro-inflammatory cytokines (TNFα, IL-1α, IL-1β, IL-6, IL-8, IL-12, IL-18, IL-32, MCP-1) at the expense of anti-inflammatory cytokines (IL-10) [117]; displaying an M1 phenotype. What is a cause for concern, is that PG induces an M1-like response whereas deviates the adaptive response to one of a non-clearing Th_2-humoral response. This, coupled with the fact that PG differentially induces endotoxin tolerance in M1 and M2-like Mϕs [54], presents scientists with real problems with regards utilising Mϕs as therapeutic targets for the treatment of CP.

Less complicated is oral lichen planus (OLP); an inflammatory condition presenting as white striations or plaques in the buccal mucosa, tongue and gingiva [118]. This pathology is characterised by a dense T cell infiltrate with a corresponding destruction of basal membrane and recruited monocytes, which display an M1 cytokine expression phenotype, with high levels of GM-CSF, TNFα and IFNγ produced at the site of inflammation [118,119]. T cells associated with OLP have been described to produce IFNγ [120], as such, IFNγ can activate $CD8^+$cytotoxic T cells, NK cells and can feedback to activate M1 Mϕs and perpetuate their inflammatory effector response. These Mϕs are situated close to the basal membrane and can contribute to its inflammatory destruction, through the action of TNFα produced [121]. Therefore, M1 Mϕs drive the progression of OLP by activating a Th_1-mediated inflammatory response and perpetuation/exacerbation of this immunopathological response through a positive feedback mechanism.

3.2. M2-driven pathology

In contrast to CD, ulcerative colitis (UC or idiopathic proctocolitis) is an IBD where its site of involvement is confined to the large bowel (colon and rectum) and characterised by ulcerations in the mucosal lining layer. Patients with UC present with abdominal pain, bleeding anaemia and dietary restriction, resulting as a consequence of inflammatory destruction of the superficial mucosal layer, which is possibly driven by dysbiosis or inappropriate recognition and responsiveness to commensal gut organisms [122]. This pathology is driven by a M2/Th_2-mediated pathogenic mechanism resulting in a predominance of Th_2-derived IL-4, IL-5 and IL-13 cytokine production. These cytokines induce B cell class switching and the production of IgE with the consequent activation of mast cells and eosonophils, which degranulate toxic components upon cross-linkage of IgE and initiation of an ADCC response. As with CD, there is an increase in monocyte recruitment to the gut mucosa, where there is a high proportion of Mϕs expressing a less mature phenotype that are $CX3CR1^+TLR2^+CD33^+$[123]. These $CX3CR1^+$Mϕs have been described to suppress the severity of DSS-induced colitis and may represent a beneficial Mϕ subset with respect to inflammatory pathology [124]. Manipulation of this Mϕ phenotype may represent a realistic approach in controlling this M2/Th_2-driven inflammation. Thus there is a real need to characterise the inflammatory Mϕ subset which is involved in driving this disease. One observation that informs the scientific community with respect to Mϕ involvement in UC is the fact that CD1d-restricted type II NKTs induce colitis in mice [125]; it is probable that $CD1d^+$cells, where CD1d expression has been reported to be restricted to Mϕs, initiate or perpetuate this inflammatory pathology in humans. In addition to expression of IL-4, IL-13 and TNFα, serum levels of IL-23 have been associated with severity of disease in UC patients [126]; whereas CD pathology involved an immune axis of M1/Th_1/Th_{17}, the link with IL-23 production is suggestive of an M2/Th_2/Th_{17} axis driving UC immunopathological inflammation. In order for successful regimens to be adopted for the treatment of UC, it is imperative that this immunopathological axis is further characterised with respect to Mϕ functional phenotype and how these Mϕs can be modulated by expression analysis of both cell-associated immune activatory and suppressive molecules.

Macrophages have been realised to play a significant role in the immunopathology associated with tumorigenesis and the progression of solid tumours. Tumour initiation and development has been linked with NFκB activation and inflammation; indeed, it is now well established that tumour associated macrophages (TAMs) exhibit a pro-tumoral, anti-inflammatory and immunoregulatory M2 phenotype. As inflammation contributes to the progression of UC, links have been suggested between UC (an M2/Th_2 pathology) and the development of colorectal cancer (CRC). Comparisons exist between UC and CRC with respect to the up-regulation of both pro-inflammatory cytokines and the immunoregulatory cytokine, IL-10 [127], thus both pro-and anti-inflammatory mechanisms contribute to cancer progression. With respect to Mϕ functionality, NFκB activation through classical or alternative activation pathways (p65 versus p50 NFκB) exhibit functional plasticity where TAMs display pro-inflammatory, anti-tumoral M1-like responses or, conversely, anti-inflammatory, pro-tumoral M2-like behaviour [128].

In the case of oral mucosa, M1-driven chronic inflammatory pathology such as OLP and the resulting pro-inflammatory and anti-microbial environment (ROS/RNS) can induce mutagenesis and malignant transformation of oral epithelial cells resulting in oral cancer. One such oral cancer is oral squamous cell carcinoma (OSCC), characterised by a significant leukocyte infiltration of lymphocytes and particularly monocytes, recruited by MCP-1, which become TAMs [129]. These TAMs, facilitated by priming factors, such as M-CSF and IL-10, secreted by cancer cells, develop a pro-tumoral M2 phenotype (IL-10, EGF, FGF, PDGF, VEGF)[130] resulting in advanced stages of tumour progression [131,132]. This M2-like effector phenotype of TAMs results in an immunosuppressive, anti-inflammatory and tissue reparative environment, which benefits tumour growth. In addition to suppressing pro-inflammatory cytokines, activation of anti-tumour T cell responses through APC function is suppressed as the expression of MHC molecules is down-regulated and inhibitory co-stimulatory molecules, such as B7-H4, are up-regulated [133-135]. Finally, the M2 cytokines, IL-10 and TGFβ, can induce Tregs, which further strengthen the suppression of host anti-tumour responses [136]. Thus, TAMs modulate cancer cell survival/growth whereas the environment presented by the tumour cells influences the functional plasticity of the TAMs and that, through the bi-directionality of cellular interactions, it may be possible for the TAM plasticity to be harnessed in the control of tumour cell growth and even initiate tumour resolution.

4. Conclusions and future perspectives

Macrophages offer attractive drug targets for the treatment of a wealth of Mϕ-mediated diseases of the oral and gastrointestinal mucosa. The role of Mϕs in driving inflammatory diseases such as CD, OLP, CP, UC, and cancer (CRC and OSCC) is being extensively researched. With their role in the immunopathogenic mechanisms of these diseases, Mϕs are now a realistic candidate for "re-education" of their functional responses; either by immune activation, suppression or deviation. Mϕs exhibit pathogenic responses via M1-functionality, as is the case in CD, OLP and CP, whereas M2 effector phenotype drives UC, CRC and OSCC. These pathogenic immune cells express a wealth of immunoactivatory receptors (TLRs, NLRs, RLRs, CLRs, FcRs, SRs and cytokine receptors) and, as such, can be induced to exhibit pro-inflammatory responses, anti-inflammatory responses, anti-microbial killing responses as well as antigen processing and presentation, hence priming humoral and CMI adaptive responses against extracellular and intracellular pathogens. In addition, they also express immunosuppressive molecules (exogenous and endogenous PRR inhibitors, FcγRIIb, CD200R, SIRP-1α, Siglecs, NLR splice variants, IL-10, TGFβ) and may exhibit a sensitivity to endotoxin tolerance. Finally, Mϕs also possess receptors/molecules by which immune responses may be modulated or deviated; through FcRs, IL-4/IL-13/M-CSF/IL-10 and IFNγ/GM-CSF to the benefit of the host. Future aims of manipulating Mϕ effector functionality would focus on activation of M1 Mϕs to produce anti-tumour and pro-inflammatory cytokines, hence fostering a hostile anti-tumour innate environment as well as priming adaptive anti-tumour responses for the treatment of colorectal cancer and oral squamous cell carcinoma. In addition to immune activation of anti-tumour responses, harnessing immune receptors for immune deviation would appear to be a potentially effective approach; whereby the functional plasticity of M2-like TAMs was manipulated and re-programmed to a more anti-tumour setting by encouraging deviation of response to be M1-directed [137]. Although translatability of these approaches has proved, as yet, unsuccessful, this activation and re-programming approach has been appreciated for quite some time [138,139].

With the similarity and connectivity between cancer and inflammation, it would appear reasonable to use similar Mϕ-modulation approaches to the treatment of mucosal inflammatory pathology. With respect to CD, OLP and CP, the M1-driven pathologies, Mϕ-based immunotherapy is likely to focus on approaches that either suppresses, induce tolerance or deviate a response by encouraging a redressing of the balance between M1/M2 by immune-deviation towards an M2-driven response. Such a change towards M2 functionality can potentially be activated through M2-biassed signals through scavenger receptors or deviation via IC-FcγR, M-CSF or IL-4/IL-13 polarisation signals. More recently, this immune deviation can be encouraged by the introduction of products derived from M2-skewing extracellular pathogens such as helminth worms; the potential for medicine to travel full circle back to a more sophisticated look at old therapies! Finally, these destructive M1-driven inflammatory pathologies may warrant suppression. This can be achieved by manipulating mechanisms and molecules associated with endotoxin tolerance through chronic reception of pro-inflammatory cytokines or PAMPs through TLRs and through the induction of a range of intracellular negative regulators such as Tollip, SHP-1, SHIP1, p50 NFκB, PI3K, as well as extracellular/membrane-bound regulators (CD200R, SIRP-1α, ST-2, SIGIRR, IL-10R and TGFβR).

Through the presentation of the complex field of Mϕ biology with respect to Mϕ subsets; priming of monocytes through defined differentiation pathways, Mϕ effector phenotype and functional plasticity can be potentially manipulated in our favour for the treatment of M1-driven and M2-driven pathology. The future therapeutic regimens which focus on macrophage functionality in CD, OLP, CP, UC, CRC and OSCC can only hope to be successful from considering total Mϕ functionality with respect to immune activation, suppression and deviation.

Author details

Andrew D. Foey

School of Biomedical & Healthcare Sciences, University of Plymouth, Drake Circus, Plymouth, UK

References

[1] Zeigler-Heitbrock HWL, Fingerle G, Strobel M, Schraut W, Stetler F, Schutt C, Passlick B, Pforte A. The novel subset of CD14+/CD16+blood monocytes exhibits features of tissue macrophages. European Journal of Immunology 1993; 23(9):2053-2058.

[2] Zeigler-Heitbrock HWL. Heterogeneity of human blood monocytes: the CD14+CD16+subpopulation. Immunology Today 1996; 17(9):424-428.

[3] Belge K-U, Dayyani F, Horelt A, Siedlar M, Frankenberger M, Frankenberger B, Espevik T, Ziegler-Heitbrock L. The pro-inflammatory CD14+CD16+HLA-DR+ +monocytes are a major source of TNF. Journal of Immunology 2002; 168:3536-3542.

[4] Kawanaka N, Yamamura M, Aita T, Morita Y, Okamoto A, Kawashima M, Iwahashi M, Ueno A, Ohmoto Y, Makino H. CD14+CD16+blood monocytes and joint inflammation in rheumatoid arthritis. Arthritis and Rheumatism 2002; 46(10): 2578-2586.

[5] Mills CD, Kincaid K, Alt JM, Heilman MJ, Hill AM. M-1/M-2 macrophages and the Th1/ Th2 paradigm. Journal of Immunology 2000; 164:6166-6173.

[6] Anderson CF, Mosser DM. A novel phenotype for an activated macrophage: the type 2 activated macrophage. Journal of Leukocyte Biology 2002; 72(1):101-106.

[7] Mantovani A, Sica A, Sozzani S, Allavena P, Vecchi A, Locati M. The chemokine system in diverse forms of macrophage activation and polarisation. Trends in Immunology 2004; 25(12):677-686.

[8] Mosser DM. The many faces of macrophage activation. Journal of Leukocyte Biology 2003; 73(2):209-212.

[9] Van Ginderachter JA, Movahedi K, Hassanzadeh Ghassabeh G, Meerschaut S, Beschin A, Raes G, DeBaetselier P. Classical and alternative activation of mononuclear phagocytes: picking the best of both worlds for tumour promotion. Immunobiology 2006; 211:487-501.

[10] Louis J, Himmelrich H, Parra-Lopez C, Tacchini-Cottier F, Launois P. Regulation of protective immunity against Leishmania major in mice. Current Opinion in Immunology 1998; 10:459-464.

[11] Holscher C, Atkinson RA, Arendse B, Brown N, Myburgh E, Alber G, Brombacher F. A protective and agonistic function of IL-12p40 in mycobacterial infection. Journal of Immunology 2001; 167:6957-6966.

[12] Veldhoen M, Hocking RJ, Atkins CJ, Locksley RM, Stockinger B. TGF-β in the context of an inflammatory cytokine milieu supports de novo differentiation of IL-17-producing T cells. Immunity 2006; 24:179-189.

[13] Stockinger B, Veldhoen M. Differentiation and function of Th17 T cells. Current Opinion in Immunology 2007; 19 :281-286.

[14] Finnin M, Hamilton JA, Moss ST. Characterisation of a CSF-induced proliferating subpopulation of human peripheral blood monocytes by surface marker expression and cytokine production. Journal of Leukocyte Biology 1999; 66(6):953-960.

[15] Verreck FAW, de Boer T, Langenberg DML, van der Zanden L, Ottenhoff THM. Phenotypic and functional profiling of human pro-inflammatory type-1 and anti-inflammatory type-2 macrophages in response to microbial antigens and IFNγ-and CD40L-mediated co-stimulation. Journal of Leukocyte Biology 2006; 79:285-293.

[16] Albina J, Henry WL, Mastrofrancesca B, Martin BA, Reichner JS. Macrophage activation by culture in an anoxic environment. Journal of Immunology 1995; 155:4391-4396.

[17] Aliberti J, Machado FS, Souto JT, Campanelli AP, Teixeira MM, Gazzinelli RT, Silva JS. β-chemokines enhance parasite uptake and promote nitric oxide-dependent microbiostatic activity in murine inflammatory macrophages infected with *Trypanosoma cruzi*. Infection and Immunity 1999; 67:4819-4826.

[18] Kielian M, Cohn Z. Phorbol myristate acetate stimulates phagosome – lysosome fusion in mouse macrophages. Journal of Experimental Medicine 1981; 154:101-111.

[19] Green S, Phillips W. Activation of the macrophage respiratory burst by phorbol myristate acetate: evidence for both tyrosine-kinase-dependent and –independent pathways. International Journal of Biochemistry, Biophysics and Molecular Biology 1994; 1222:241-248.

[20] Grip O, Janciauskiene S, Lindgren S. Macrophages in inflammatory bowel disease. Current Drug Targets Inflammation Allergy 2003; 2:155-160.

[21] Mantovani A, Sica A, Locati M. New vistas on macrophage differentiation and activation. European Journal of Immunology 2007; 37:14-16.

[22] Liu Y, Stewart KN, Bishop E, Marek CJ, Kluth DC, Rees AJ, Wilson HM. Unique expression of suppressor of cytokine signalling 3 is essential for classical macrophage activation in rodents in vitro and in vivo. Journal of Immunology 2008; 180:6270-6278.

[23] Sica A, Bronte V. Altered macrophage differentiation and immune function in tumour development. Journal of Clinical Investigation 2007; 117:1155-1166.

[24] Stein M, Keshaw S, Harris N, Gordon S. Interleukin 4 potently enhances murine macrophage mannose receptor activity: a marker of alternative immunologic macrophage activation. Journal of Experimental Medicine 1992 ; 176:287-292.

[25] de Waal Malefyt R, Figdor CG, Huijbens R, Mohan-Peterson S, Bennett B, Culpepper J, Dang W, Zurawski G, de Vries JE. Effects of IL-13 on phenotype, cytokine production and cytotoxic function of human monocytes. Comparison with IL-4 and modulation by IFNgamma or IL-10. Journal of Immunology 1993; 151:6370-6381.

[26] Gordon S. Alternative activation of macrophages. Nature Reviews in Immunology 2003; 3:23-35.

[27] Pesce J, Kaviratne M, Ramalingam TR, Thompson RW, Urban JF, Cheever AW, Young DA, Collins M, Grusby MJ, Wynn TA. The IL-21 receptor augments Th2 effector function and alternative macrophage activation. Journal of Clinical Invesitgation 2006; 116(7):2044-2055.

[28] Foey AD. Mucosal macrophages: phenotype and functionality in homeostasis and pathology. 2012. In Handbook of macrophages: life cycle, functions and diseases. Takahashi, R., Kai, H., Eds. Nova Science Publishers Inc., New York, USA. Chapter 4, pp121-146.

[29] Martinez FO, Sica A, Mantovani A, Locati M. Macrophage activation and polarisation. Frontiers in Bioscience 2008; 13:453-461.

[30] Biswas SK, Gangi L, Paul S, Schioppa T, Saccani A, Sironi M, Bottazzi B, Doni A, Bronte V, Pasqualini F, Vago L, Nebuloni M, Mantovani A, Sica A. A distinct and unique transcriptional programme expressed by tumour-associated macrophages (defective NF-kappaB and enhanced IRF-3/STAT1 activation). Blood 2006; 107(5):2112-2122.

[31] Porta C, Rimoldi M, Raes G, Brys L, Ghezzi P, Di Liberto D, Dieli F, Ghisletti S, Natoli G, De Baetselier P, Mantovani A, Sica A. Tolerance and M2 (alternative) macrophage polarisation are related processes orchestrated by p50 nuclear factor kappaB. Proc. Natl. Acad. Sci. USA 2009; 106(35):14978-14983.

[32] Bouhlel MA, Derudas B, Rigamonti E, Dievart R, Brozek J, Harlon S, Zawadzki C, Jude B, Torpier G, Marx N, Staels B, Chinetti-Gbaguichi G. PPAR-gamma activation primes human monocytes into alternative M2 macrophages with anti-inflammatory properties. Cell Metabolism 2007; 6(2):137-143.

[33] Ruffell D, Mourkioti F, Gambardella A, Kirstetter P, Lopez RG, Rosenthal N, Nerlov C. A CREB-C/EBPbeta cascade induces M2 macrophage-specific gene expression and promotes muscle injury repair. Proceedings of the National Academy of Science USA 2009; 106:17475-17480.

[34] Welch JS, Escoubet-Lozach L, Sykes DB, Liddiard K, Greaves DR, Glass CK. Th2 cytokines and allergic challenge induce Ym-1 expression in macrophages by a STAT-6-dependent mechanism. Journal of Biological Chemistry 2002; 277:42821-42829.

[35] Ishii M, Wen H, Corsa CAS, Liu T, Coelho AL, Allen RM, Carson WF, Cavassani KA, Li X, Lukacs NW, Hogaboam CM, Dou Y, Kunkel SL. Epigenetic regulation of the alternatively activated macrophage phenotype. Blood 2009; 114(15):3244-3254.

[36] Rauh MJ, Ho V, Pereira C, Sham A, Sly LM, Lam V, Huxham L, Minchinton AL, Mui A, Krystal G. SHIP represses the generation of alternatively activated macrophages. Immunity 2005; 23:361-374.

[37] Stout RD, Jiang C, Matta B, Tietzel I, Watkins SK, Suttles J. Macrophages sequentially change their functional phenotype in response to changes in microenvironmental influences. Journal of Immunology 2005; 175:342-349.

[38] Xu W, Zhao X, Daha MR, van Kooten C. Reversible differentiation of pro-and anti-inflammatory macrophages. Molecular Immunology 2013; 53:179-186.

[39] Lenzo JC, Turner AL, Cook AD, Vlahos R, Anderson GP, Reynolds EC, Hamilton JA. Control of macrophage lineage populations by CSF-1 receptor and GM-CSF in homeostasis and inflammation. Immunology and Cell Biology 2011; 90(4):429-440.

[40] Grazio Cappiello M, Sutterwala FS, Trinchieri G, Mosser DM, Ma X. Suppression of IL-12 transcription in macrophages following Fc gamma receptor ligation. Journal of Immunology 2001; 166(7):4498-4506.

[41] Gerber JS, Mosser DM. Reversing lipopolysaccharide toxicity by ligating the macrophage Fc gamma receptors. Journal of Immunology 2001; 166(11):6861-6868.

[42] Weisser SB, McLarren KW, Voglmaier N, van Netten-Thomas CJ, Antov A, Flavell RA, Sly LM. Alternative activation of macrophages by IL-4 requires SHIP degradation. European Journal of Immunology 2011; 41:1742-1753.

[43] Krausgruber T, Blazek T, Smallie T, Alzabin S, Lockstone H, Sahgal N, Hussell T, Feldmann M, Udalova IA. IRF5 promotes inflammatory macrophage polarisation and Th1-Th17 responses. Nature Immunology 2011; 12:231-238.

[44] Martinez FO. Regulators of macrophage activation. European Journal of Immunology 2011; 41:1531-1534.

[45] Fong CHY, Bebien M, Didierlaurent A, Nebauer R, Hussell T, Broide D, Karin M, Lawrence T. An anti-inflammatory role for IKKβ through the inhibition of "classical" macrophage activation. Journal of Experimental Medicine 2008; 205(6):1269-1276.

[46] Hagemann T, Lawrence T, McNeish I, Charles KA, Kulbe H, Thompson RG, Robinson SC, Balkwill FR. "Re-educating" tumour-associated macrophages by targeting NF-kappaB. Journal of Experimental Medicine 2008; 205:1261-1268.

[47] O'Neill LAJ, Fitzgerald KA, Bowie AG. The Toll-IL-1 receptor adaptor family grows to five members. Trends in Immunology 2003; 24(6):286-289.

[48] O'Neill LAJ. When signalling pathways collide: positive and negative regulation of Toll-like receptor signal transduction. Immunity 2008; 29:12-20.

[49] Negishi H, Ohba Y, Yanai H, Takaoka A, Honma K, Yui K, Matsuyama T, Taniguchi T, Honda K. Negative regulation of Toll-like receptor signalling by IRF-4. Proceedings of the National Academy of Science USA 2005; 102(44):15989-15994.

[50] Honma K, Udono H, Kohno T, Yamamoto K, Ogawa A, Takemori T, Kumatori A, Suzuki S, Matsuyama T, Yui K. Interferon regulatory factor 4 negatively regulates the production of proinflammatory cytokines by macrophages in response to LPS. Proceedings of the National Academy of Science USA 2005; 102(44):16001-16006.

[51] Brint EK, Xu D, Liu H, Dunne A, McKenzie AN, O'Neill LA, Liew FY. ST2 is an inhibitor of interleukin 1 receptor and Toll-like receptor 4 signalling and maintains endotoxin tolerance. Nature Immunology 2004; 5(4):373-379.

[52] Wald D, Qin J, Zhan Z, Qian Y, Naramura M, Tian L, Towne J, Sims JE, Stark GR, Li X. SIGIRR, a negative regulator of Toll-like receptor-interleukin 1 receptor signalling. Nature Immunology 2003; 4(9):920-927.

[53] Biswas SK, Lopez-Collazo E. Endotoxin tolerance: new mechanisms, molecules and clinical significance. Trends in Immunology 2009; 30(10):475-487.

[54] Foey AD, Crean SJ. Macrophage subset sensitivity to endotoxin tolerisation by *Porphyromonas gingivalis*. PLoS ONE 2013; 8(7):e67955.

[55] Philpott DJ, Girardin S. The role of Toll-like receptors and Nod proteins in bacterial infection. Molecular Immunology 2004; 41(11):1099-1108.

[56] Abbott DW, Wilkins A, Asara JM, Cantley LC. The Crohn's disease protein, NOD2, requires RIP2 in order to induce ubiquitination of a novel site on NEMO. Current Biology 2004; 14:2217-2227.

[57] Strober W, Murray PJ, Kitani A, Watanabe T. Signalling pathways and molecular interactions of NOD1 and NOD2. Nature Reviews in Immunology 2006; 6:9-20.

[58] Chamaillard M, Girardin SE, Viala J, Philpott DJ. Nods, Nalps and Naip: intracellular regulators of bacterial-induced inflammation. Cellular Microbiology 2003; 5(9): 581-592.

[59] Mariathasan S, Newton K, Monack DM, Vucic D, French DM, Lee WP, Roose-Girma M, Erickson S, Dixit VM. Differential activation of the inflammasome by caspase-1 adaptors ASC and Ipaf. Nature 2004; 430:213-218.

[60] Martinon F, Tschopp J. Inflammatory caspases: linking an intracellular innate immune system to autoinflammatory diseases. Cell 2004; 117:561-574.

[61] Creagh EM, O'Neill LAJ. TLRs, NLRs and RLRs: a trinity of pathogen sensors that co-operate in innate immunity. Trends in Immunology 2006; 27(8):352-357.

[62] Kato H, Sato S, Yoneyama M, Yamamoto M, Uematsu S, Matsui K, Tsujimura T, Takeda K, Fujita T, Takeuchi O, Akira S. Cell-type specific involvement of RIG-1 in antiviral response. Immunity 2005; 23:19-28.

[63] Yoneyama M, Kikuchi M, Natsukawa T, Shinobu N, Imaizumi T, Miyagishi M, Taira K, Akira S, Fujita T. The RNA helicase RIG-1 has an essential function in double stranded RNA-induced innate anti-viral responses. Nature Immunology 2004; 5:730-737.

[64] Kang DC, Gopalkrishnam RV, Wu Q, Jankowsky E, Pyle AM, Fisher PB. Mda-5: an interferon-inducible putative RNA helicase with double stranded RNA-dependent ATPase activity and melanoma growth suppressive properties. Proceedings of the National Academy of Science USA 2002; 99:637-642.

[65] Rothenfusser S, Goutagny N, DiPerna G, Gong M, Monks BG, Schoenemeyer A, Yamamoto M, Akira S, Fitzgerald KA. The RNA helicase Lgp2 inhibits TLR-

dependent sensing of viral replication by RIG-1. Journal of Immunology 2005; 175:5260-5268.

[66] Meylan E, Curran J, Hofmann K, Moradpour D, Binder M, Bartenschlager R, Tschopp J. Cardif is an adaptor protein in the RIG-1 antiviral pathway and is targeted by hepatitis C virus. Nature 2005; 437:1167-1172.

[67] Li XD, Sun L, Seth RB, Pineda G, Chen ZJ. Hepatitis C virus protease NS3/4A cleaves mitochondrial antiviral signalling protein off the mitochondria to evade innate immunity. Proceedings of the National Academy of Sciences USA 2005; 102:17717-17722.

[68] Johnston JB, Barrett JW, Nazarian SH, Goodwin M, Riccioto D, Wang G, McFadden G. A poxvirus-encoded pyrin domain protein interacts with ASC-1 to inhibit host inflammatory and apoptotic responses to infection. Immunity 2005; 23:587-598.

[69] Peiser L, Gordon S. The function of scavenger receptors expressed by macrophages and their role in the regulation of inflammation. Microbes and Infection 2001; 3(2):149-159.

[70] Peiser L, Mukhopadhyay S, Gordon S. Scavenger receptors in innate immunity. Current Opinion in Immunology 2002; 14:123-128.

[71] Hardison SE, Brown GD. C-Type lectin receptors orchestrate anti-fungal immunity. Nature Immunology 2013; 13(9):817-822.

[72] Brown GD. Dectin-1: a signalling non-TLR pattern recognition receptor. Nature Reviews in Immunology 2006; 6:33-43.

[73] Kelm S, Schauer R. Sialic acids in molecular and cellular interactions. International Reviews in Cytology 1997; 175:137-240.

[74] Orr SJ, Morgan NM, Elliott J, Burrows JF, Scott CJ, McVicar DW, Johnston JA. CD33 responses are blocked by SOCS3 through accelerated proteosomal mediated turnover. Blood 2007a; 109:1061-1068.

[75] Orr SJ, Morgan NM, Buick RJ, Boyd CR, Elliott J, Burrows JF, Jefferies CA, Crocker PR, Johnston JA. SOCS3 targets siglec-7 for proteosomal degradation and blocks siglec-7-mediated responses. Journal of Biological Chemistry 2007b; 282(6):3418-3422.

[76] Crocker PR, Varki A. Siglecs, sialic acids and innate immunity. Trends in Immunology 2001; 22(6):337-342.

[77] Lock K, Zhang J, Lu J, Lee SH, Crocker PR. Expression of CD33-related siglecs on human mononuclear phagocytes, monocyte-derived dendritic cells and plasmacytoid dendritic cells. Immunobiology 2004; 209(1-2):199-207.

[78] Ando M, Tu W, Nishijima K, Lijima S. Siglec 9 enhances IL-10 production in macrophages via tyrosine-based motifs. Biochem. Biophys. Res. Commun. 2008; 369:878-883.

[79] Ravetch JV, Bolland S. IgG Fc receptors. Annual Reviews in Immunology 2001; 19:275-290.

[80] Abrahams VM, Cambridge G, Lydyard PM, Edwards JCW. Induction of tumour necrosis factor a production by adhered human monocytes. A key role for Fcg receptor type IIIa in rheumatoid arthritis. Arthritis and Rheumatism 2000; 43:608-616.

[81] Sutterwala FS, Noel GJ, Salgame P, Mosser DM. Reversal of proinflammatory responses by ligating the macrophage Fcgamma receptor type I. Journal of Experimental Medicine 1998; 188:217-222.

[82] Kleinau S, Martinsson P, Heyman B. Induction and suppression of collagen-induced arthritis is dependent on distinct Fcγ receptors. Journal of Experimental Medicine 2000; 191:1611-1616.

[83] Kharitonenkov A, Chen Z, Sures I, Wang H, Schilling J, Ullrich A. A family of proteins that inhibit signalling through tyrosine kinase receptors. Nature 1997; 386:181-186.

[84] Barclay AN, Wright GJ, Brooke G, Brown MH. CD200 and membrane protein interactions in the control of myeloid cells. Trends in Immunology 2002; 23(6):285-290.

[85] Armant M, Avice MN, Hermann P, Rubio M, Kiniwa M, Delespesse G, Sarfati M. CD47 ligation selectively downregulates human interleukin 12 production. Journal of Experimental Medicine 1999; 190(8):1175-1182.

[86] Wright GJ, Puklavec MJ, Willis AC, Hoek RM, Sedgwick JD, Brown MH, Barclay AN. Lymphoid/neuronal cell surface OX2 glycoprotein recognises a novel receptor on macrophages implicated in the control of their function. Immunity 2000; 13:233-242.

[87] Wright GJ, Cherwinski H, Foster-Cuevas M, Brooke G, Puklavec MJ, Bigler M, Song Y, Jenmalm M, Gorman D, McClanahan T, Liu M-R, Brown MH, Sedgwick JD, Phillips JH, Barclay AN. Characterisation of the CD200 receptor family in mice and humans and their interactions with CD200. Journal of Immunology 2003; 171:3034-3046.

[88] Gorczynski RM, Cattrall MS, Chen Z, Hu J, Lei J, Min WP, Yu G, Ni J. An immunoadhesin incorporating the molecule OX-2 is a potent immunosuppressant that prolongs allo-and xenograft survival. Journal of Immunology 1999; 163:1654.

[89] Gorczynski RM, Chen Z, Yu K, Hu J. CD200 immunoadhesin suppresses collagen-induced arthritis in mice. Clinical Immunology 2001; 101:328-334.

[90] Simelyte E, Criado G, Essex D, Uger RA, Feldmann M, Williams RO. CD200-Fc, a novel antiarthritic biologic agent that targets pro-inflammatory cytokine expression in the joints of mice with collagen-induced arthritis. Arthritis and Rheumatism 2008; 58(4): 1038-1043.

[91] Savill J, Dransfield I, Gregory C, Haslett C. A blast from the past: clearance of apoptotic cells regulates immune responses. Nature Reviews in Immunology 2002; 2:965-975.

[92] Savill J, Wyllie AH, Henson JE, Walport MJ, Henson PM, Haslett C. Macrophage phagocytosis of aging neutrophils in inflammation. Programmed cell death in the

neutrophil leads to its recognition by macrophages. Journal of Clinical Investigation 1989; 83(3):865-875.

[93] Fadok VA, Bratton DL, Konowal A, Freed PW, Westcott JY, Henson PM. Macrophages that have ingested apoptotic cells *in vitro* inhibit proinflammatory cytokine production through autocrine/paracrine mechanisms involving TGF-β, PGE2 and PAF. Journal of Clinical Investigation 1998; 101(4):890-898.

[94] Xu W, Roos A, Schlagwein N, Woltman AM, Daha MR, van Kooten C. IL-10-producing macrophages preferentially clear early apoptotic cells. Blood 2006; 107(12): 4930-4937.

[95] Taylor PR, Carugati A, Fadok VA, Cook HT, Andrews M, Carroll MC, Savill JS, Henson PM, Botto M, Walport MJ. A hierarchical role for classical pathway complement proteins in the clearance of apoptotic cells. Journal of Experimental Medicine 2000; 192:359-366.

[96] Albert ML. Death-defying immunity: do apoptotic cells influence antigen processing and presentation? Nature Reviews in Immunology 2004;4:223-231.

[97] Wesemann DR, Benveniste EN. STAT-1alpha and IFN-gamma as modulators of TNF-alpha signalling in macrophages: regulation and functional implications of the TNF receptor 1:STAT-1 alpha complex. Journal of Immunology 2003; 171(10):5313-5319.

[98] Yarilina A, Park-Min KH, Antoniv T, Hu X, Ivashkiv LB. TNF activates an IRF1-dependent autocrine loop leading to sustained expression of chemokines and STAT1-dependent type I interferon-response genes. Nature Immunology 2008; 9(4):378-387.

[99] Conte D, Holcik M, Lefebvre CA, Lacasse E, Picketts DJ, Wright KE, Korneluk RG. Inhibitor of apoptosis protein cIAP2 is essential for lipopolysaccharide-induced macrophage survival. Molecular and Cellular Biology 2006; 26(2):699-708.

[100] Avdiushko R, Hongo D, Lake-Bullock H, Kaplan A, Cohen D. IL-10 receptor dysfunction in macrophages during chronic inflammation. Journal of Leukocyte Biology 2001; 70:624-632.

[101] Rogler G, Hausmann M, Spottl T, Vogl D, Aschenbrenner E, Andus T, Falk W, Scholmerich J, Gross V. T cell co-stimulatory molecules are up-regulated on intestinal macrophages from inflammatory bowel disease mucosa. European Journal of Gastroenterology and Hepatology 1999; 11(10):1105-1111.

[102] Smith PD, Smythies LE, Mosteller-Barnum M, Sibley DA, Russell MW, Merger M, Sellers MT, Orenstein JM, Shimada T, Graham MF, Kubagawa H. Intestinal macrophages lack CD14 and CD89 and consequently down-regulated for LPS-and IgA-mediated activities. Journal of Immunology 2001; 167(5):2651-2656.

[103] Smythies LE, Sellers MT, Clements RH, Mosteller-Barnum M, Meng G, Benjamin WH, Orenstein JM, Smith PD. Human intestinal macrophages display profound inflammatory anergy despite avid phagocytic and bacteriocidal activity. Journal of Clinical Investigation 2005; 115(1):66-75.

[104] Strober W, Zhang F, Kitani A, Fuss I, Fichtner-Feigl S. Proinflammatory cytokines underlying the inflammation of Crohn's disease. Current Opinions in Gastroenterology 2010; 26:301-307.

[105] Maeda S, Hsu LC, Liu H, Bankston LA, Limura M, Kagnoff MF, Eckmann L, Karin M. Nod2 mutation in Crohn's disease potentiates NF-κB activity and IL-1β processing. Science 2006; 307:734-738.

[106] Netea MG, Kullberg BJ, de Jong DJ, Franke B, Sprong T, Naber THJ, Drenth JPH, van der Meer JW. NOD2 mediates anti-inflammatory signals induced by TLR2 ligands: Implications for Crohn's disease. European Journal of Immunology 2004; 34:2052-2059.

[107] Schenk M, Mueller C. Adaptations of intestinal macrophages to an antigen-rich environment. Seminars in Immunology 2007; 19:84-93.

[108] Hardy H, Harris J, Lyon E, Beal J, Foey AD. Probiotics, prebiotics and immunomodulation of gut mucosal defences: homeostasis and immunopathology. Nutrients 2013; 5:1869-1912.

[109] Bouma G, Strober W. The immunological and genetic basis of inflammatory bowel disease. Nature Reviews in Immunology 2003; 3:521-533.

[110] Merry R, Belfield L, McArdle P, McLennan A, Crean SJ, Foey AD. Oral health and pathology: a macrophage account. British Journal of Oral and Maxillofacial Surgery 2012; 50:2-7.

[111] Socransky SS, Hafferjee AD, Cugini MA, Smith C, Kent RL. Microbial complexes in subgingival plaque. Journal of Clinical Periodontology 1998; 25:134-144.

[112] Ezzo P, Cutler CW. Microorganisms as risk indicators for periodontal disease. Periodontology 2000 2003; 32:24-35.

[113] Yilmaz O, Watanabe K, Lamont RJ. Involvement of integrins in fimbrae-mediated binding and invasion by *Porphyromonas gingivalis*. Cellular Microbiology 2002; 4:305-314.

[114] Jotwani R, Cutler CW. Fimbriated *Porphyromonas gingivalis* is more efficient than fimbrae-deficient *P. gingivalis* in entering human dendritic cells *in vitro* and induces an inflammatory Th1 effector response. Infection and Immunity 2004; 72:1725-1732.

[115] Pulendran B, Kumar P, Cutler CW, Mohamadzadeh M, van Dyke T, Bancereau J. Lipopolysaccharide from distinct pathogens induce different classes of immune response in vivo. Journal of Immunology 2001; 167:5067-5076.

[116] Darveau RP, Pham TT, Lemley K, Reife RA, Bainbridge BW, Coats SR, Howald WN, Way SS, Hajjar AM. *Porphyromonas gingivalis* lipopolysaccharide contains multiple lipid A species that functionally interact with both Toll-like receptors 2 and 4. Infection and Immunity 2004; 72:5041-5051.

[117] Barksby HE, Nile CJ, Jaedicke KM, Taylor JJ, Preshaw PM. Differential expression of immunoregulatory genes in monocytes in response to *Porphyromonas gingivalis* and

Escherichia coli lipopolysaccharide. Clinical and Experimental Immunology 2009; 156:479-487.

[118] Sugerman PB, Savage NW, Walsh LJ, Zhao ZZ, Zhou XJ, Khan A, Seymour GJ, Bigby M. The pathogenesis of oral lichen planus. Critical Reviews in Oral Biology and Medicine 2002; 13:350-365.

[119] Yamamoto T, Osaki T, Yoneda K, Ueta E. Cytokine production by keratinocytes and mononuclear infiltrates in oral lichen planus. Journal of Oral Pathology and Medicine 1994; 23:309-315.

[120] Khan A, Farah CS, Savage NW, Walsh LJ, Harbrow DJ, Sugerman PB. Th1 cytokines in oral lichen planus. Journal of Oral Pathology and Medicine 2003; 32:77-83.

[121] Kono T, Tanii T, Furukawa M, Mizuno N, Taniguchi S, Ishii M, Hamada T. Effects of human recombinant tumour necrosis factor-alpha (TNF-alpha) on the proliferative potential of human keratinocytes cultured in serum-free medium. Journal of Dermatology 1990; 17:409-413.

[122] Gophna U, Sommerfeld K, Gophna S, Doolittle WF, Veldhuyzen van Zanten SJ. Differences between tissue-associated intestinal microfloras of patients with Crohn's disease and ulcerative colitis. Journal of Clinical Microbiology 2006; 44:4136-4141.

[123] Candia E, Diaz-Jiminez D, Langjahr P, Nunez LE, de la Fuente M, Farfan N, Lopez-Kostner F, Abedrapo M, Alvarez-Lobos M, Pinedo G, Beltran CJ, Gonzales C, Gonzales M-J, Quera R, Hermoso MA. Increased production of soluble TLR2 by lamina propria mononuclear cells from ulcerative colitis patients. Immunobiology 2012; 217(6): 634-642.

[124] Medina-Contreras O, Geem D, Laur O, Williams IR, Lira SA, Nusrat A, Parkos CA, Denning TL. CX3CR1 regulates intestinal macrophage homeostasis, bacterial translocation and colitogenic Th17 responses in mice. Journal of Clinical Investigation 2011; 121(12):4787-4795.

[125] Liao CM, Zimmer MI, Shanmuganad S, Yu HT, Cardell SL, Wang CR. Dysregulation of CD1d-restricted type II natural killer T cells leads to spontaneous development of colitis in mice. Gastroenterology 2012; 142(2):326-334.

[126] Mohammadi M, Hayatbakhsh MM, Zahedi MJ, Jalapour MR, Pakgohar A. Serum interleukin-23 levels in patients with ulcerative colitis. Iran Journal of Immunology 2011; 8(3):183-188.

[127] Szaradkiewicz A, Marciniak R, Chudzicka-Strgala I, Wasilewska A, Drews M, Majewski P, Karpinski T, Zwozdziak B. Proinflammatory cytokines and IL-10 in inflammatory bowel disease and colorectal cancer patients. Archives in Immunology and Therapeutic Experimentation 2009; 57:291-294.

[128] Karin M, Greten FR. NF-kappaB: linking inflammation and immunity to cancer development and progression. Nature Reviews in Immunology 2005; 5:749-759.

[129] Koide N, Nishio A, Sato T, Sugiyama A, Miyagawa S. Significance of macrophage chemoattractant protein-1 expression and macrophage infiltration in squamous cell carcinoma of the oesophagus. American Journal of Gastroenterology 2004; 99:1667-1674.

[130] Lalla RV, Boisoneau DS, Spiro JD, Kreutzer DL. Expression of vascular endothelial growth factor receptors on tumour cells in head and neck squamous cell carcinoma. Archives in Otolaryngology and Head and Neck Surgery 2003; 129:882-888.

[131] Sica A, Allavena P, Mantovani A. Cancer related inflammation: the macrophage connection. Cancer Letters 2008; 267:204-215.

[132] Kuropkat C, Dunne AA, Plehn S, Ossendorf M, Herz U, Renz H, Werner JA. Macrophage colony-stimulating factor as a tumour marker for squamous cell carcinoma of the head and neck. Tumour Biology 2003; 24:236-240.

[133] Kundu N, Fulton AM. Interleukin-10 inhibits tumour metastasis, downregulates MHC class I and enhances NK lysis. Cellular Immunology 1997; 180:55-61.

[134] de Waal Malefyt R, Haanem J, Spits H, Roncarolo MG, te Velde A, Figdor C, Johnson K, Kastelein R, Yssel H, de Vries JE. Interleukin 10 (IL-10) and viral IL-10 strongly reduce antigen-specific human T cell proliferation by diminishing the antigen-presenting capacity of monocytes via downregulation of class II major histocompatibility complex expression. Journal of Experimental Medicine 1991; 174:915-924.

[135] Kryczek I, Zou L, Rodriguez P, Zhu G, Wei S, Mottram P, Brumlik M, Cheng P, Curiel T, Myers L, Lackner A, Alvarez X, Ochoa A, Chen L, Zou W. B7-H4 expression identifies a novel suppressive macrophage population in human ovarian carcinoma. Journal of Experimental Medicine 2006; 203:871-881.

[136] Levings MK, Bacchetta R, Schulz U, Roncarolo MG. The role of IL-10 and TGF-beta in the differentiation and effector function of T regulatory cells. International Archives of Allergy and Immunology 2002; 129:263-276.

[137] Mantovani A, Sica A. Macrophages, innate immunity and cancer: balance, tolerance and diversity. Current Opinion in Immunology 2010; 22:231-237.

[138] Hennemann B, Beckmann G, Eichelmann A, Rehm A, Andreesen R. Phase I trial of adoptive immunotherapy of cancer patients using monocyte-derived macrophages activated with interferon gamma and lipopolysaccharide. Cancer Immunology and Immunotherapy 1998; 45(5):250-256.

[139] Guiducci C, Vicari AP, Sangaletti S, Trinchieri G, Columbo MP. Redirecting in vivo elicited tumour infiltrating macrophages and dendritic cells towards tumour rejection. Cancer Research 2005; 65(8):3437-3446.

Chapter 6

Immunostimulatory Effects of Triggering TLR3 Signaling Pathway — Implication for Cancer Immunotherapy

Mohamed Labib Salem, Said M. Hammad,
Mohamed R. El-shanshory, Mohamed A. Attia and
Abdel-Aziz A. Zidan

Additional information is available at the end of the chapter

http://dx.doi.org/10.5772/58575

1. Introduction

Immunostimulation based therapies hold promise of disease-specific interventions without the toxicity and other side effects, which are associated with traditional therapeutic modalities. Unfortunately, the exact manifestation of their therapeutic benefits and the mechanisms of their action are still pending for most immunotherapeutic strategies. Virtually, such kinds of treatments are ideal to establish standards of care and secure, as well as improve therapeutics outcomes. A growing interest for studying and understanding immunostimulation based therapeutics' strategies has increased since, it could stimulate different components of innate immunity and consequently stimulation of adaptive immunity [1-3].

These immunostimulation based therapies can be divided into two categories, nonspecific and specific immunotherapies. Nonspecific immunotherapy describes therapies that are designed to enhance the immune response without deliberately seeking to modulate the response to a particular antigen. These therapies include three main categories. The first depends on administration of certain agents that induces secretion of inflammatory cytokines that nonspecifically activate the immune system [4]. The second depends on administration of certain type of cytokine that can activate specific populations of immune cells. The third category include the administration of antibodies that block immune checkpoints or other suppressive pathways that are known to shut down the activity of immune system [5]. These nonspecific activation pathways are crucial for the initiation of fully functional immune responses encompassing both the innate and adaptive immune compartments [4].

Toll like receptors (TLRs) are a group of receptors that are expressed mainly in innate immune cells, including macrophages, monocytes, dendritic cells, natural killer cells and mast cells [6]. These TLRs specifically recognize microbes as well as different microbial components called TLR ligands. Interaction of TLR and TLR ligands trigger signaling pathways that lead to activation of innate immune cells through secretion of a plethora of inflammatory mediators including cytokines and chemokines [7, 8]. As such, different TLR ligands have been designed to be used as adjuvant system,

The inclusion of TLR ligands as a potential new class of adjuvants candidates has enabled the development of clinical effective vaccination strategies against many diseases [9, 10]. Polyinosinic-polycytidylic acid [Poly(I:C)] and its clinical grade poly-L-lysine (Poly-ICLC; Hiltonol®) represent important members of these immunostimulatory vaccine adjuvants as has been shown in several preclinical and clinical studies [11, 12]. In this review, we will introduce a brief description of the TLR family followed by a description of the signaling pathway of TLR and its role as a linker between innate and adaptive immunity. The structure, expression and function of Poly(I:C) will be reviewed along with its potential application in cancer vaccination, adoptive immunotherapy and chemo-immunotherapy in preclinical and clinical trials.

2. Toll-like receptors (TLRs) and their agonists

TLRs are a class of transmembrane signaling proteins that play a critical role in initiation and acceleration of innate and adaptive immune responses against different pathogen by recognizing these pathogens themselves or their products, including proteins, carbohydrates, lipids, and nucleic acids (single-and double-stranded RNA and DNA) [13]. TLRs were discovered in 1985 by Christiane Nüsslein-Volhard as factors involved in the embryonic development and resistance of the fly *Drosophila* to bacterial and fungal infection [14-16]. TLRs are pattern-recognition receptors (PRR) with an extracellular leucine-rich repeats (LRRs) domain and a conserved cytoplasmic domain homologous to that of the interleukin-1 receptor (IL-1R), termed the Toll/IL-1R homology (TIR) domain [17, 18]. Such structure of TLRs recognizes pathogen-associated microbial patterns (PAMPs) encoded in various pathogens. These products include lipopolysaccharide (LPS), peptidoglycan (PGN), flagellin, bacterial DNA, viral single and double stranded RNA and synthetic double-stranded RNA such as poly(I:C). TLRs also recognize danger-associated molecular patterns (DAMPs) that are endogenous molecules including intracellular proteins such as heat shock proteins (HSPs) and protein fragments from the extracellular matrix (HMGB1) released from necrotic or dead cells [10, 19]. Given this capability of TLRs to recognize a wide range of microbial products and their synthetic mimic, modulation of these receptors can significantly play a central role in shaping the outcomes of the anti-microbial immunity. Since cancer originates from self-cells resulting in a poor anti-tumor immunity if not tolerance, triggering TLR signaling pathways during cancer immunotherapy by their specific agonists can accentuate the resultant anti-tumor immunity.

TLRs expression profiles differ among tissues and cell types of the innate and adaptive immune system. TLRs are predominantly expressed on T cells, B cells, neutrophils, monocytes, NK cells, mast cells, and antigen-presenting cells (APCs), such as macrophages (MΦ) or dendritic cells (DCs). As such induction of TLR signaling activates APCs to provoke innate immunity and to induce adaptive immunity [6, 7, 20]. More recently, TLR have been found to be expressed on endothelial, epithelial cells and tumor cells, including melanoma [21]. TLRs are fundamentally located on the plasma membrane except TLR3, TLR7 and TLR9 that are located in the endoplasmic reticulum (ER) [22-24]. Mammalian TLRs include a large family consisting of ten to thirteen different types of TLRs that named simply TLR1 to TLR13 and each one of them recognize specific microbial components [25].

To date, ten human and thirteen murine TLRs have been identified; TLR1 to TLR9 are conserved between the human and mice. However, there are TLRs found in humans and not present in all mammals. For example, TLR10 in humans is present in mice. On the other hand, TLR11, TLR12 and TLR13 in mice are functional, but there is a stop codon in the human TLR11 TLR12 and TLR13 genes, which results in a lack of production of human TLR11 TLR12 and TLR13 [26, 27]. Signaling pathways of these TLRs can be triggered by their specific ligands. TLR ligands (TLRLs) are agents that bind to and activate TLRs. They are encoded in different types of organisms at the cell surface or at the internal cell compartments and they are expressed by different types of leucocytes and other cell types [28, 29].

TLRs/TLRLs bind results in a cascade of intra-cellular signaling pathways that induce the production of inflammatory cytokines and immune response [7, 8]. TLRLs are recognized by specific TLRs that are expressed on the surface of cells, for example, TLR2 is essential for the recognition of bacterial lipoproteins, lipomannans and lipoteichoic acids [30], while TLR5 detects bacterial flagellin [31]. TLR4 has been reported to recognize bacterial cell wall component lipopolysaccharide (LPS) [30], and TLR11 which recognize a profilin-like protein of *Toxoplasma gondii* [32] and uropathogenic *E.coli* [33]. In contrast, TLRs located within the endoplasmic reticulum (ER) can detect microbial nucleic acids, for example, TLR3 is required for response to virus-derived double-stranded RNA [34] and TLR9 recognize unmethylated CpG motifs [35]. Whereas, TLR7 and TLR8 could recognize small synthetic antiviral molecules [36], and single-stranded RNA [37].

3. TLRs Signaling pathways

Recent accumulating studies showed that TLRs signaling pathways can be divided into two signaling pathways, the MyD88-dependent pathway which is common to all the TLRs that resulted in the secretion of inflammatory cytokines, and TRIF-dependent pathway that is specific for TLR3 and TLR4 which associated with the stimulation of IFN-β and the maturation of dendritic cells [38-40].

3.1. MyD88-dependent pathway

The myeloid differentiation factor 88 (MyD88) dependent responses utilized by all TLRs except TLR3 and its occurring on hetero-or homo-dimerization of the TLRs receptor, upon activation by PAMPs or DAMPs. This dimerization induces the recruitment of adaptor proteins via the cytoplasmic TIR domain. These adaptor proteins include the TIR-domain containing proteins, TIRAP (TIR-associated protein), TRIF (TIR domain-containing adaptor protein-inducing IFN-β) and TRAM (TRIF-related adaptor molecule), MyD88, Mal (MyD88 adaptor-like protein), which triggers the TLR-mediated signaling pathways [41-45].

The transcription factor IRF7 is critical regulator for the production of IFN-α/β via MyD88 pathway. IRF7 presents in DCs is very low, and therefore TLR7, TLR8 and TLR9 operate mainly through the NF-κB–IRF5 pathway [10, 46, 47]. It is worth noting that the transducing ability of TLR7, TLR8 and TLR9 may change in favor of the IRF7 pathway. Whereas, TLR4 is located on the cell membrane, activation of TLR4 signal transduction through MyD88/TIRAP and TRAM/TRIF pathways leads to activation of innate immune responses, primarily through IRS serine phosphorylationI

3.2. TRIF-dependent pathway

The TLR3 ligand (dsRNA) and the TLR4 ligand (LPS) activate the TRIF-dependent pathway in which IRF-3 plays a key role. For TLR3 (dsRNA), activation of MyD88-independent pathways occurs via TRIF (TIR domain-containing adaptor protein-inducing IFN-β). Upon dsRNA binds within endosomes, TLR3 recruits the adaptor TRIF through a TIR–TIR interaction. TRIF, in turn, recruits RIP1 to activate NF-κB, via TRAFs and the IKK (IκB kinase) complex. TRIF also recruits protein kinases TBK1/IKKε and TRAF3 to activate IRF3/7. Since, IRF-3 can phosphorylate by TBK-1 and IKKε on C-terminal serines, leading to its dimerization and translocation into the nucleus. Active IRF-3 mediates transcription of genes from the IFN-β promoter. The secreted IFN-β binds to the IFN receptor (IFNR), and thus activates transcription of ISGs, such as IRF-7 [9, 48]. On the other hand, the intracellular dsRNA is recognized by the RNA helicase RIG-I (or MDA-5). Activation of the latter activates TBK-1 and IKKε via its CARD domain and activates IRF-3 as well. IRF-7 further stimulates transcription from the IFN-α and-β promoters in a positive feedback loop. Type I IFNs bind also to their receptors to trigger the JAK–STAT signaling pathway. Whereas, to induce inflammatory cytokines production. TLR4 activation is requires both the MyD88-dependent and independent pathways. This occurs via TIR domain containing adaptors TIRAP, MyD88, TRAM and TRIF, which in turn initiates activation of NFκB, MAPK, and IRF3 allowing its nuclear localization and production of IFN-β [40, 49].

The signaling pathway of TLRs is summarized in Figure 1. TLR7, TLR8 and TLR9 are present in endosomes, which are stimulated by viral ssRNA. Upon activation, TLR7, TLR8 and TLR9 signal through the adaptor MyD88, which in turn leads to phosphorylation and activation of IRF3. Following its activation, TLR3 signals through its adaptor TRIF, and thus activates non-canonical IKK kinases (TBK1/IKKε), which subsequently phosphorylate both IRF3 and IRF7. Active IRF-3 induces transcription from the IFN-β promoter. NF-κ β is also activated by TRIF mediated signaling through canonical IKK kinases (IKKα, β, and γ). RIG-I and MDA5 are located in cytoplasm and can recognize both ssRNA and dsRNA. Intracellular ssRNA and dsRNA are recognized by the RNA helicase RIG-I (or mda-5), which are expressed in most cells, activates TBK-1 and IKKε via its CARD domain through interaction with the mitochondrially located adaptor MAVS.

Different signal transducer and activator of transcription (STAT) family members can be activated by interferons (IFNs). As a response to both type I IFNs and type II IFN (IFNγ) stimulation, STAT1-STAT1 homodimers can be formed. These homodimers bind to IFNγ-activated site (GAS) enhancer elements in the promoters of IFN-stimulated genes, and these results in the induction of genes encoding pro-inflammatory cytokines and apoptotic factors. STAT1 and STAT2 heterodimers, which are activated by binding with IRF9, which in turn migrates to the nucleus to bind to IFN-stimulated response elements (ISREs) and activate antiviral and antibacterial genes.

4. Polyinosinic-polycytidylic acid [Poly(I:C)]

Although, several previous studies have been extensively studied poly(I:C) for over 35 years in humans [50, 51], it is receiving new interest as a crucial component in many new immunostimulatory combination therapeutic strategies. Poly(I:C) is a synthetic double-stranded RNA (dsRNA) that has recently been identified as a specific ligand for TLR3 [52-55]. dsRNA is a viral product produced by most viruses during their replication cycle, Both viral dsRNA and its artificial mimic, poly(I:C), are potent inducers of type I interferons (IFN-α/β) [56, 57], which is a crucial cytokines that exert anti-viral and immunostimulatory activities for both T and B lymphocytes [58, 59], DCs [11, 60] and activate monocytes to produce CSF, IL-1β, IL-12, and PGE_2 [61, 62].

Several studies have been shown that Poly(I:C) induces a strong innate immune response initiated by two types of PRRs; the TLRs and the RIG-I-like receptors (RLRs) which is a family of cytoplasmic RNA helicases that includes RIG-I and MDA-5 [63-67]. In addition, several studies have shown that Poly(I:C) transduces signals which activate the NF-κB and the IFN-β promoter [53, 54] and activates several nuclear and cytoplasmic enzyme systems such as oligoadenylate synthetase (OAS), the dsRNA dependent protein kinase R (PKR), RIG-I Helicase, and MDA5 (melanoma differentiation associated gene) which are implicated in antiviral and antitumor host defenses [7].

Poly(I:C) interact with TLR3, that is the specific intracellular recognition system that responds and signals to the intracellular presence of dsRNA and RNA virus infection [68]. TLR3 is mainly expressed on a broad range of antigen-processing cells (APCs), dendritic cell (DC) subsets, fibroblasts, intestinal epithelial [54, 69, 70] monocytes, macrophage (MΦ), mast cells, NK cells [71, 72], $CD4^+$and $CD8^+$T cells [6, 73]. Several prior studies have shown that poly(I:C) has potent pleiotropic immunostimulatory effects on several kinds of immune cells [74-76].

Poly(I:C), a synthetic dsRNA mimic copolymer, is a specific TLR3 agonist [13, 77]. Recently, we and others have reported that in vivo administration of the TLR3 agonist poly(I:C) into naïve mice induced rapid increases in the frequencies of NK cells mainly in the liver and that these effects associate with better antigen specific responses and antitumor efficacy [6, 78-81]. Consistent with earlier studies [81], we have demonstrated that the adjuvant effects of poly(I:C) to the antigen-specific CD8+T cell responses are partially dependent on NK cells through creation of a rapid beneficial cytokine milieu [82, 83]. Furthermore, in vitro treatment of highly purified NK cells with poly(I:C) significantly augmented NK cell-mediated cytotoxicity and up-regulated their expression of the activation marker CD69 [71]. Of particular interest, similar to viral infection, poly(I:C) treatment has been found to preferentially induce recruitment and activation of hepatic NK cells [79] and their trafficking to spleen coincided with enhanced cytokine expression [80]. These studies may explain the increased antitumor effects against metastasis observed in tumor models after poly(I:C) treatment [84].

5. Poly(I:C) and anti-tumor Immunity

A fundamental difference between tumor and microbes is that only the latter encode products (signatures) that are recognized as "danger signals" by pathogen recognition receptors (PPRs) expressed in the innate immune cells. [85] In most cases, immune system can mount vigorous immune responses against microbes, but not against cancer. Therefore, the challenge in cancer immunotherapy is how to manipulate the body's own immune system to fight cancer. [86] Mimicking the anti-microbial immunity, recent preclinical and clinical studies have established that provision of TLRL adjuvant system systemically or into tumor environment itself profoundly awaken the cross talk between innate and adaptive immunity, driving generation of efficacious anti-tumor immunity. [87] For instance, the addition of CpG DNA (typical TLR9L) to a melanoma vaccine resulted in effective cytolytic responses. [88] Imiquimod, a synthetic TLR7/8L, has been successfully used in the treatment of basal cell carcinoma [89, 90] and to enhance the immunogenicity of vaccine containing Flt3 ligand and a melanoma peptide. [91] MPL, a TLR4L, has been used as an adjuvant in clinical trials of vaccines against melanoma, glioma and pancreatic and colorectal carcinoma, inducing substantial tumor-specific immunity in response to vaccination [92, 93]. We have reported recently that co-administration of the TLR3L poly(I:C) in vivo with peptide vaccination established functional effector/memory responses [94] by induction of NK-driven beneficial cytokine milieu and DC activation. [81] Although the impact of both of TLRLs at the time of Ag priming has been the focus of several studies, their impacts at the time of Ag recall on the tumor-specific memory responses have not been actively investigated.

Since, cancer cells do not encode danger signals like virus, generation of anti-tumor memory T cells in the tumor setting would require a large pool of highly activated DCs. In response to TLRLs, resident immature DCs at the site of vaccination undergo a maturation program and migrate to the draining lymph nodes (LNs) [72, 95, 96]. Therefore, utilizing TLRLs is a potential approach to induce activation of immature DCs and maximize their contribution to memory cell responses. In line with this notion, recent studies have established the adjuvant effects of several TLRLs, in particular, TLR3L (poly(I:C), TLR7/8L (Imiquimod), and TLR9L (CpG) to the anti-tumor $CD8^{+}$T cell responses [81, 94, 97-101]. However, most of these studies tested the adjuvant effects of TLRLs in lymphodepleted hosts, and those few studies that utilized lymphodepleted hosts did not use adoptive cell therapy (ACT) system [98, 102-107].

Because the frequency of DCs in steady state condition is low, growth factors in particular Flt3L and G-CSF have been used to mobilize DCs in vivo [108-110]. With this regard, we have recently reported a rapid induction of type I IFNs and activation of DCs with decreases in the levels of T_{reg} cells after CTX treatment; resulting in augmented post vaccination responses which were further improved by addition of poly(I:C) to vaccination [111]. We have found also a marked expansion of immature DCs during the recovery phase after treatment with the anticancer drug cyclophosphamide (CTX), indicating to the mobilizing effect of CTX for DCs. Since DCs are equipped with TLRs that sense different microbial products such as poly(I:C), activation of these immature DCs in vivo may augment memory T cell responses. [85]. Recent studies, including ours have demonstrated the adjuvant effects of TLRLs to ACT in lymphodepleted hosts [112-114]. These studies suggest that combinatorial treatments with chemotherapy/immunotherapy and ACT can markedly improve memory T cell responses. Our observation of expansion of DCs post CTX therapy is a suitable model to dissect the optimal timing of the adjuvant effects of TLRLs to post vaccination responses of ACT in a lymphodepleted host.

Specifically, our recent studies showed that treatment of a recipient host with the non myeloablative dose of CTX augments post vaccination $CD8^{+}$T cell responses, which were associated with a quick activation of DCs in the lymphopenic phase [114]. We also found that CTX induces increases in the numbers of immature DCs during the recovery phase from days 9-16, peaking on day 12 [115]. These DCs demonstrated normal phagocytic ability in vitro and antigen uptake in vivo. Administration of poly(I:C) at the peak of DC expansion resulted in induction of rapid inflammatory milieu which associated with significant increases in the numbers of activated ($CCR7^{high}CD40^{high}$) DCs in lymph nodes.

Using the pmel-1 TCR transgenic mouse model, in which $CD8^{+}$T cells can recognize the natural tumor gp100 antigen on B16 melanoma, we demonstrated that vaccination of CTX-lymphodepleted mice with the MHC class-I melanoma gp100 peptide and poly(I:C) during the lymphopenic phase (day 2) and at the peak of DC expansion (day 12) resulted in significant augmentation in the number of activated DCs in lymph nodes with a temporal increase in the expansion of pmel-1 cells. Conditional depletion studies of DCs at day 12 before revaccination of CTX-treated recipient mice revealed that DCs are required for the optimal pmel-1 cell responses. Importantly, the therapeutic anti-tumor effects of the enhanced pmel-1 cell responses were demonstrated toward an advanced tumor of the poorly immunogenic B16 melanoma, indicating the clinical significance of our observation. Furthermore, we have found improvement in DCs expansion when CTX treatment was followed by a daily treatment with 5μg/mouse G-CSF for 5 days [6], without altering the efficacy of our prime-boost vaccination with hgp100/poly(I:C) [116].

T_{reg} cells express different TLRs [117] and can be activated by certain TLR agonists such as TLR4 [118-120], and TLR5 [121], and can be inactivated by TLR2 and TLR7/8 agonists [122, 123]. Indeed, total body irradiation and CTX-preconditioned hosts demonstrated that interference with T_{reg} cell activities can enhance tumor-specific T cell responses and anti-tumor immunity [124]' [125, 126]. Our preliminary studies and previous studies [105, 125-130], however, showed that although T_{reg} cells decrease in numbers during the lymphopenic phase after CTX treatment they recover to their normal levels at the recovery phase. These recovered T_{reg} cells may interfere with the efficacy of vaccination at recovery phase unless the vaccination is co-administered with a potent adjuvant that can block T_{reg} cell function. Indeed, induction of maturation of DCs by certain TLR agonists has been found to control T_{reg} cell function in vivo [122, 131, 132]. Therefore, it is possible that the enhanced pmel-1 cell expansion and anti-tumor effects of pmel-1 cells to peptide/poly(I:C) revaccination on day 12 post CTX treatment involve blocking of T_{reg} cell.

The potent anti-tumor efficacy of prime-boost vaccination with tumor antigen/poly(I:C) at precise time points post CTX therapy would lead to its potential application in the clinical setting. We would envision two treatment protocols for the clinical application of this prime-boost vaccination with tumor peptide and poly(I:C) on cancer (e.g. melanoma) patients. 1) Patients can be with a lymphodepletion dose of CTX followed by G-CSF to correct leucopenia, and vaccinate the patient with a candidate tumor Ag (gp100, MART, or TRP2) with co-administration of the clinical grade form of poly(I:C) such as Hiltonol®. Vaccination and Hiltonol® treatments can be repeated during the recovery from leucopenia (after 10-15 days of chemotherapy) when the numbers of DCs are increased. 2) The same as above but with adoptive transfer of peripheral blood mononuclear cells harvested from the cancer patient prior chemotherapy. These cells can be stimulated in vitro with 1ng/mL of the tumor antigens in the presence of 10ng/mL IL-12 for 3-5 days as we recently described in our preclinical model [133].

6. Poly(I:C) and antiviral immune response

The innate immune response is the first barrier against the invading pathogens and viruses and it responds through activating inflammatory and antiviral defense mechanisms by inducing IFNs-α/β against the viruses [134]. Several in vitro and in vivo studies have demonstrated that the main effects of poly(I:C) is the induction of IFNs-α/β, which play a crucial role in innate anti-viral response [135, 136].Several studies have been extensively demonstrated that poly(I:C) triggers the activation of PKR and other kinases which followed by the phosphorylation of the substrates of these enzymes that results in the subsequent translocation of transcription factors, NF-κB and IRF-3, to the nucleus where then they bind to the IFN-β promoter to form a transcription complex that induce IFN-β production [137-140]. It has been thought that the proximal inducer of IFNs-α/β is intracellular dsRNA generated as an intermediate during viral replication [53].

Recently, it has been shown that dsRNA and ssRNA molecules are recognized as intermediate by TLRs that is expressed on DCs, NK cells, MΦ and epithelium during virus replication [141]. Several studies have been extensively demonstrated that Poly(I:C) plays a critical role in inducing innate immune response against many viruses, such as influenza virus [142], human respiratory syncytial virus (RSV) [143], herpes simplex virus 2 (HSV-2) [144], and murine cytomegalovirus [25]. Several in vitro and in vivo studies have been shown that retinoic-acid-inducible gene I (RIG-I) and melanoma-differentiation-associated gene 5 (MDA-5), are the key in the detection of viral dsRNA and Poly(I:C) in the cytosol and subsequent eradication of the replicating viral genomes [66, 145, 146]. Treatment of animals with poly(I:C) results inactivation of the TLR3 receptor which in turn induces the activation of NF-κB and the production of type I interferons that induces strong antiviral and antineoplastic effects accompanied by activation of CD8+T and NK cells [53, 147]. In addition, poly(I:C) is shown to serve as an adjuvant to induce protective CD4+T cell responses against HIV [148].

7. Poly(I:C) and clinical trials

7.1. Hiltonol®

Hiltonol® or Poly-ICLC is a synthetic, nuclease-resistant, hydrophilic complex of polyinosinic and polycytidylic acid, stabilized with poly-L-lysine and carboxymethyl cellulose. Poly-ICLC is IFN-β inducer, which is known to steady the blood-brain-barrier (BBB) and minimize cellular infiltration into damaged brain regions following stroke [149, 150]. Several clinical trials were conducted to utilize poly-ICLC as an IFN inducer in cancer patients, the first clinical trial (phase 1) were conducted to determine the maximum tolerated dose (MTD) and it found that the MTD was (12 mg/m^2), which induced effective response in cancer patients [51]. Another study was conducted to determine the immunomodulatory effect of Poly-ICLC in cancer patients and it showed that there was no detectable serum IFN in patients that received 1 mg/m2 Poly-ICLC by IM injection [151]. In contrast, IFN was detectable in the serum of patients that received 4 mg/m^2 Poly-ICLC by IV injection. Then, phase I and II clinical trials were conducted in patients with many types of cancers including leukemia, lymphoma, brain tumors, myeloma, juvenile laryngeal papillomatosis, renal cell carcinoma, breast cancer, ovarian cancer, and melanoma [152-160].

In most of these early clinical trials, about 6 mg/m^2 Poly-ICLC was generally used intravenously. Fever, often with temperatures greater than 40°C, was a universal adverse event in the trials and was the primary dose-limiting factor. Other common adverse events reported in these trials included nausea, vomiting, hypotension, thrombocytopenia, leukopenia, arthralgia, myalgia, and fatigue. Additionally, very few objective responses were reported in these clinical trials. Due to its toxicity and relative ineffectiveness, utilizing Poly-ICLC was deserted after the availability of recombinant IFN. It was subsequently determined that lower doses (10 to 50 mg/kg) of Poly-ICLC resulted in a broader host defense stimulation, a potent adjuvant effect, and a specific antiretroviral effect mediated by the 2′5′OAS and PKR nuclear enzyme systems [161]. Consequently, Poly-ICLC is currently being developed for use only at doses up to 50 mg/kg. The poly-ICLC treatment prior to exposure to oxygen-glucose deprivation maintained the paracellular and transcellular transport across the endothelium and attenuated the drop in transendothelial electric resistance by enhancing IFN-β mRNA expression in astrocytes and microglia [162]. Recent study utilized poly-ICLC in activation of TLR3 signaling, which exerts a beneficial effect on NK cells, resulting in the increased cetuximab-dependent lysis of head and neck cancer (HNC) cells [163].

7.2. Ampligen®

Ampligen® is known as [poly(I)-poly(C12U)] that is composed of poly(IC) with a U mismatch at every 12th base of the C strand. The main effect of Ampligen® is the induction of Th1 response. This has been demonstrated in delayed-type hypersensitivity reactions and in current clinical studies with human immunodeficiency virus-infected patients. Other cells targeted are NK cells, cytotoxic $CD8^{+}T$ cells, and LAK-NK cells. Despite initial trials in the 1990s, little is known about Ampligen®, since; it is not routinely used in clinical practice. However, due to its notable and potent antiviral effects, Ampligen® has been generally well tolerated in randomized clinical trials [164, 165]. Since, Ampligen® did not consistently produce antiviral effects, but its antiviral activity was always seen after therapeutic treatment. Therefore, it was assumed that Ampligen have exquisite specificity for TLR3 [166, 167]. Early studies showed that treatment of chronically HBV-infected chimpanzees with polyICLC transiently reduced the levels of serum viral DNA, HBsAg and HBeAg [168]. In two independent studies, transient suppression of DHBV in ducks by Ampligen® was also observed [169, 170]. In vitro studies, Ampligen and zidovudine have combined: to act in synergy against HIV-1-infected cell lines [171, 172] and enabling restoration of the immune function in HIV-infected individuals. Wither through maintaining a stable or raising CD4 count, increasing delayed-type hypersensitivity reaction, and reducing rate of progression to AIDS [173].

More recently, Nicodemus et al (2010) evaluated polyIC12U and confirmed the potential of TLR3 stimulation with Ampligen® in enhancement bioactivity of cancer immunotherapies [166]. Their results revealed that Ampligen® is a potent inducer for the dendritic cell maturation and local cytokines producing in culture systems including IL-4, IL-6, IL-12p70, IFN g, MIP-1a and TNF α. Interestingly, treatment of wild-type mice with Ampligen® 24 hours following infection with a lethal viral inoculation was fully protective, whereas dosing 4 h prior to inoculation is ineffective in preventing mortality [167]. Intranasal Ampligen® administered to mice in conjunction with prototype avian flu vaccines, greatly enhances the cellular and humoral immunity achievable with the vaccine and also protects mice from lethal infection [174].

8. Conclusion

Since the discovery of the important role of TLRs in innate immunity and the initiation of an immune response that follows the activation of antigen-specific acquired immunity, rapid progress has been made on our understanding of the molecular mechanisms of TLRs. The inclusion of TLR ligands as a potential new class of adjuvants candidates has enabled the development of clinical effective vaccination strategies against many diseases. Poly(I:C) and Poly-ICLC represent two important member of these immunostimulatory vaccine adjuvants in mice, nonhuman primates and in human. TLR3 is specifically expressed in quite cell-type and species; it is expressed in specific myeloid cells, vascular endothelial cells and airway epithelial cells among others. Human TLR3 is highly expressed in immature DCs whereas

http://dx.doi.org/10.5772/58575

mouse TLR3 is highly expressed in macrophages, but in both species, its expression is induced by IFN.

Unlike other TLRs, TLR3 is unique, since, it is not required MyD88 for signaling, and instead, TRIF is the critical adaptor protein for its signaling. Whereas TLR3 displays a distinct intracellular localization compared with other TLRs, TLR7 and TLR9 trigger a quick, but short IFN response, whereas TLR3 might be more important for a prolonged response and the initiation of the adaptive immune response. Poly(I:C) interact with TLR3 that responds and signals to the intracellular presence of dsRNA and RNA virus infection. Poly(I:C), is strong inducers of IFN-α/β, which is a crucial cytokines that exert anti-viral and immunostimulatory activities for both T and B lymphocytes, DCs and activate monocytes to produce CSF, IL-1β, IL-12, and PGE2. It's also transduces signals which activate the NF-κB and the IFN-β promoter and activates several nuclear and cytoplasmic enzyme systems such as OAS, PKR, RIG-I Helicase, and MDA5 which are implicated in antiviral and antitumor host defenses.

The above mentioned pleotropic effects of the TLR3 agonist Poly(I:C) makes it as a candidate adjuvant system for anti-viral and anti-tumor immune responses, in particular its clinical forms Hiltonol® and Ampligen® induce similar immunomodulatory effects with accepted side effects.

Acknowledgements

The authors would like to thank Prof. Karolin K. Abdul-Aziz and Dr. Muobarak J. Tuorkey (Zoology Department, Faculty of Science, Damanhour University, Egypt) for their kind help during writing this chapter.

Author details

Mohamed Labib Salem[1,2*], Said M. Hammad[1,3], Mohamed R. El-shanshory[1,4], Mohamed A. Attia[1,3] and Abdel-Aziz A. Zidan[1,2]

*Address all correspondence to: mohamed.labib@science.tanta.edu.eg

1 Center of Excellence in Cancer Research (CECR), Tanta University Educational Hospital, Medical Campus, Tanta University, Egypt

2 Immunology and Biotechnology Unit, Zoology Department, Faculty of Science, Tanta University, Egypt

3 Clinical Pathology Department, Faculty of Medicine, Tanta University, Egypt

4 Pediatric Hematology and Oncology Unit, Faculty of Medicine, Tanta University, Egypt

References

[1] Pulendran, B. and R. Ahmed, *Translating innate immunity into immunological memory: implications for vaccine development.* Cell, 2006. 124(4): p. 849-63.

[2] Reed, S.G., et al., *New horizons in adjuvants for vaccine development.* Trends Immunol, 2009. 30(1): p. 23-32.

[3] Coffman, R.L., A. Sher, and R.A. Seder, *Vaccine adjuvants: putting innate immunity to work.* Immunity, 2010. 33(4): p. 492-503.

[4] Johnson, C.B., et al., *Tumours: Immunotherapy*, in *eLS*. 2001, John Wiley & Sons, Ltd.

[5] Belardelli, F. and M. Ferrantini, *Cytokines as a link between innate and adaptive antitumor immunity.* Trends Immunol, 2002. 23(4): p. 201-8.

[6] Salem, M.L., et al., *The TLR3 agonist poly(I:C) targets CD8+T cells and augments their antigen-specific responses upon their adoptive transfer into naive recipient mice.* Vaccine, 2009. 27(4): p. 549-57.

[7] Kawai, T. and S. Akira, *Innate immune recognition of viral infection.* Nat Immunol, 2006. 7(2): p. 131-7.

[8] Pichlmair, A. and C. Reis e Sousa, *Innate recognition of viruses.* Immunity, 2007. 27(3): p. 370-83.

[9] Beutler, B., *Inferences, questions and possibilities in Toll-like receptor signalling.* Nature, 2004. 430(6996): p. 257-63.

[10] Kawai, T. and S. Akira, *The role of pattern-recognition receptors in innate immunity: update on Toll-like receptors.* Nat Immunol, 2010. 11(5): p. 373-84.

[11] Longhi, M.P., et al., *Dendritic cells require a systemic type I interferon response to mature and induce CD4+Th1 immunity with poly IC as adjuvant.* J Exp Med, 2009. 206(7): p. 1589-602.

[12] Stahl-Hennig, C., et al., *Synthetic double-stranded RNAs are adjuvants for the induction of T helper 1 and humoral immune responses to human papillomavirus in rhesus macaques.* PLoS Pathog, 2009. 5(4): p. e1000373.

[13] Matsumoto, M. and T. Seya, *TLR3: interferon induction by double-stranded RNA including poly(I:C).* Adv Drug Deliv Rev, 2008. 60(7): p. 805-12.

[14] Anderson, K.V., G. Jurgens, and C. Nusslein-Volhard, *Establishment of dorsal-ventral polarity in the Drosophila embryo: genetic studies on the role of the Toll gene product.* Cell, 1985. 42(3): p. 779-89.

[15] Anderson, K.V., L. Bokla, and C. Nusslein-Volhard, *Establishment of dorsal-ventral polarity in the Drosophila embryo: the induction of polarity by the Toll gene product.* Cell, 1985. 42(3): p. 791-8.

[16] Lemaitre, B., J.M. Reichhart, and J.A. Hoffmann, *Drosophila host defense: differential induction of antimicrobial peptide genes after infection by various classes of microorganisms.* Proc Natl Acad Sci U S A, 1997. 94(26): p. 14614-9.

[17] Bowie, A. and L.A. O'Neill, *The interleukin-1 receptor/Toll-like receptor superfamily: signal generators for pro-inflammatory interleukins and microbial products.* J Leukoc Biol, 2000. 67(4): p. 508-14.

[18] Thompson, M.R., et al., *Pattern recognition receptors and the innate immune response to viral infection.* Viruses, 2011. 3(6): p. 920-40.

[19] Takahashi, K. and T. Kawai, *[Pathogen recognition by Toll-like receptor].* Nihon Rinsho, 2007. 65 Suppl 2 Pt. 1: p. 53-7.

[20] Uematsu, S. and S. Akira, *[Innate immune recognition of viral infection].* Uirusu, 2006. 56(1): p. 1-8.

[21] Salaun, B., et al., *Toll-like receptor 3 expressed by melanoma cells as a target for therapy?* Clin Cancer Res, 2007. 13(15 Pt 1): p. 4565-74.

[22] Nishiya, T. and A.L. DeFranco, *Ligand-regulated chimeric receptor approach reveals distinctive subcellular localization and signaling properties of the Toll-like receptors.* J Biol Chem, 2004. 279(18): p. 19008-17.

[23] He, X., et al., *Recognition of pathogen-associated nucleic acids by endosomal nucleic acid-sensing toll-like receptors.* Acta Biochim Biophys Sin (Shanghai), 2013. 45(4): p. 241-58.

[24] Akira, S., K. Takeda, and T. Kaisho, *Toll-like receptors: critical proteins linking innate and acquired immunity.* Nat Immunol, 2001. 2(8): p. 675-80.

[25] Tabeta, K., et al., *Toll-like receptors 9 and 3 as essential components of innate immune defense against mouse cytomegalovirus infection.* Proc Natl Acad Sci U S A, 2004. 101(10): p. 3516-21.

[26] Ariffin, J.K. and M.J. Sweet, *Differences in the repertoire, regulation and function of Toll-like Receptors and inflammasome-forming Nod-like Receptors between human and mouse.* Curr Opin Microbiol, 2013.

[27] Roach, J.C., et al., *The evolution of vertebrate Toll-like receptors.* Proc Natl Acad Sci U S A, 2005. 102(27): p. 9577-82.

[28] Pulendran, B., *Modulating vaccine responses with dendritic cells and Toll-like receptors.* Immunol Rev, 2004. 199: p. 227-50.

[29] Takeda, K. and S. Akira, *Toll-like receptors.* Curr Protoc Immunol, 2007. Chapter 14: p. Unit 14 12.

[30] Takeuchi, O., et al., *Differential roles of TLR2 and TLR4 in recognition of gram-negative and gram-positive bacterial cell wall components.* Immunity, 1999. 11(4): p. 443-51.

[31] Smith, K.D. and A. Ozinsky, *Toll-like receptor-5 and the innate immune response to bacterial flagellin.* Curr Top Microbiol Immunol, 2002. 270: p. 93-108.

[32] Lauw, F.N., D.R. Caffrey, and D.T. Golenbock, *Of mice and man: TLR11 (finally) finds profilin.* Trends Immunol, 2005. 26(10): p. 509-11.

[33] Zhang, D.M., et al., *[Down-regulation of Toll-like receptor 4 is related to the tolerance to lipopolysaccharide in rat alveolar macrophages].* Zhonghua Jie He He Hu Xi Za Zhi, 2003. 26(7): p. 411-4.

[34] Schulz, O., et al., *Toll-like receptor 3 promotes cross-priming to virus-infected cells.* Nature, 2005. 433(7028): p. 887-92.

[35] Sivori, S., et al., *CpG and double-stranded RNA trigger human NK cells by Toll-like receptors: induction of cytokine release and cytotoxicity against tumors and dendritic cells.* Proc Natl Acad Sci U S A, 2004. 101(27): p. 10116-21.

[36] Jurk, M., et al., *Human TLR7 or TLR8 independently confer responsiveness to the antiviral compound R-848.* Nat Immunol, 2002. 3(6): p. 499.

[37] Heil, F., et al., *Species-specific recognition of single-stranded RNA via toll-like receptor 7 and 8.* Science, 2004. 303(5663): p. 1526-9.

[38] Akira, S. and H. Hemmi, *Recognition of pathogen-associated molecular patterns by TLR family.* Immunol Lett, 2003. 85(2): p. 85-95.

[39] Adachi, O., et al., *Targeted disruption of the MyD88 gene results in loss of IL-1-and IL-18-mediated function.* Immunity, 1998. 9(1): p. 143-50.

[40] Kawai, T. and S. Akira, *TLR signaling.* Semin Immunol, 2007. 19(1): p. 24-32.

[41] Horng, T., et al., *The adaptor molecule TIRAP provides signalling specificity for Toll-like receptors.* Nature, 2002. 420(6913): p. 329-33.

[42] Fitzgerald, K.A., et al., *Mal (MyD88-adapter-like) is required for Toll-like receptor-4 signal transduction.* Nature, 2001. 413(6851): p. 78-83.

[43] Yamamoto, M., et al., *Cutting edge: a novel Toll/IL-1 receptor domain-containing adapter that preferentially activates the IFN-beta promoter in the Toll-like receptor signaling.* J Immunol, 2002. 169(12): p. 6668-72.

[44] Oshiumi, H., et al., *TICAM-1, an adaptor molecule that participates in Toll-like receptor 3-mediated interferon-beta induction.* Nat Immunol, 2003. 4(2): p. 161-7.

[45] Oshiumi, H., et al., *TIR-containing adapter molecule (TICAM)-2, a bridging adapter recruiting to toll-like receptor 4 TICAM-1 that induces interferon-beta.* J Biol Chem, 2003. 278(50): p. 49751-62.

[46] Keating, S.E., et al., *IRAK-2 participates in multiple toll-like receptor signaling pathways to NFkappaB via activation of TRAF6 ubiquitination.* J Biol Chem, 2007. 282(46): p. 33435-43.

[47] Kanayama, A., et al., *TAB2 and TAB3 activate the NF-kappaB pathway through binding to polyubiquitin chains.* Mol Cell, 2004. 15(4): p. 535-48.

[48] Takeda, K. and S. Akira, *TLR signaling pathways.* Semin Immunol, 2004. 16(1): p. 3-9.

[49] Kawai, T. and S. Akira, *Signaling to NF-kappaB by Toll-like receptors.* Trends Mol Med, 2007. 13(11): p. 460-9.

[50] Freeman, A.I., et al., *Pharmacologic effects of polyinosinic-polycytidylic acid in man.* J Med Virol, 1977. 1(2): p. 79-93.

[51] Levine, A.S., et al., *Initial clinical trials in cancer patients of polyriboinosinic-polyribocytidylic acid stabilized with poly-L-lysine, in carboxymethylcellulose [poly(ICLC)], a highly effective interferon inducer.* Cancer Res, 1979. 39(5): p. 1645-50.

[52] Cella, M., et al., *Plasmacytoid dendritic cells activated by influenza virus and CD40L drive a potent TH1 polarization.* Nat Immunol, 2000. 1(4): p. 305-10.

[53] Alexopoulou, L., et al., *Recognition of double-stranded RNA and activation of NF-kappaB by Toll-like receptor 3.* Nature, 2001. 413(6857): p. 732-8.

[54] Matsumoto, M., et al., *Establishment of a monoclonal antibody against human Toll-like receptor 3 that blocks double-stranded RNA-mediated signaling.* Biochem Biophys Res Commun, 2002. 293(5): p. 1364-9.

[55] Meusel, T.R., K.E. Kehoe, and F. Imani, *Protein kinase R regulates double-stranded RNA induction of TNF-alpha but not IL-1 beta mRNA in human epithelial cells.* J Immunol, 2002. 168(12): p. 6429-35.

[56] Levy, H.B., *Induction of interferon in vivo and in vitro by polynucleotides and derivatives, and preparation of derivatives.* Methods Enzymol, 1981. 78(Pt A): p. 242-51.

[57] Meurs, E., et al., *Molecular cloning and characterization of the human double-stranded RNA-activated protein kinase induced by interferon.* Cell, 1990. 62(2): p. 379-90.

[58] Kolumam, G.A., et al., *Type I interferons act directly on CD8 T cells to allow clonal expansion and memory formation in response to viral infection.* J Exp Med, 2005. 202(5): p. 637-50.

[59] Le Bon, A., et al., *Direct stimulation of T cells by type I IFN enhances the CD8+T cell response during cross-priming.* J Immunol, 2006. 176(8): p. 4682-9.

[60] Le Bon, A., et al., *Type i interferons potently enhance humoral immunity and can promote isotype switching by stimulating dendritic cells in vivo.* Immunity, 2001. 14(4): p. 461-70.

[61] Manetti, R., et al., *Polyinosinic acid: polycytidylic acid promotes T helper type 1-specific immune responses by stimulating macrophage production of interferon-alpha and interleukin-12.* Eur J Immunol, 1995. 25(9): p. 2656-60.

[62] Akiyama, Y., et al., *Differential ability of human blood monocyte subsets to release various cytokines.* J Leukoc Biol, 1985. 37(5): p. 519-30.

[63] Kok, K.H., et al., *The double-stranded RNA-binding protein PACT functions as a cellular activator of RIG-I to facilitate innate antiviral response.* Cell Host Microbe, 2011. 9(4): p. 299-309.

[64] Kawai, T. and S. Akira, *Antiviral signaling through pattern recognition receptors.* J Biochem, 2007. 141(2): p. 137-45.

[65] Koyama, S., et al., *Differential role of TLR-and RLR-signaling in the immune responses to influenza A virus infection and vaccination.* J Immunol, 2007. 179(7): p. 4711-20.

[66] Gitlin, L., et al., *Essential role of mda-5 in type I IFN responses to polyriboinosinic:polyribocytidylic acid and encephalomyocarditis picornavirus.* Proc Natl Acad Sci U S A, 2006. 103(22): p. 8459-64.

[67] Kato, H., et al., *Cell type-specific involvement of RIG-I in antiviral response.* Immunity, 2005. 23(1): p. 19-28.

[68] Matsumoto, M., et al., *Subcellular localization of Toll-like receptor 3 in human dendritic cells.* J Immunol, 2003. 171(6): p. 3154-62.

[69] Muzio, M., et al., *Differential expression and regulation of toll-like receptors (TLR) in human leukocytes: selective expression of TLR3 in dendritic cells.* J Immunol, 2000. 164(11): p. 5998-6004.

[70] Cario, E. and D.K. Podolsky, *Differential alteration in intestinal epithelial cell expression of toll-like receptor 3 (TLR3) and TLR4 in inflammatory bowel disease.* Infect Immun, 2000. 68(12): p. 7010-7.

[71] Schmidt, K.N., et al., *APC-independent activation of NK cells by the Toll-like receptor 3 agonist double-stranded RNA.* J Immunol, 2004. 172(1): p. 138-43.

[72] Banchereau, J., et al., *Dendritic cells: controllers of the immune system and a new promise for immunotherapy.* Novartis Found Symp, 2003. 252: p. 226-35; discussion 235-8, 257-67.

[73] Gelman, A.E., et al., *Toll-like receptor ligands directly promote activated CD4+T cell survival.* J Immunol, 2004. 172(10): p. 6065-73.

[74] Cella, M., et al., *Maturation, activation, and protection of dendritic cells induced by double-stranded RNA.* J Exp Med, 1999. 189(5): p. 821-9.

[75] Haines, D.S., K.I. Strauss, and D.H. Gillespie, *Cellular response to double-stranded RNA.* J Cell Biochem, 1991. 46(1): p. 9-20.

[76] Manetti, R., et al., *Polyinosinic acid: polycytidylic acid promotes T helper type 1-specific immune responses by stimulating macrophage production of interferon-alpha and interleukin-12.* Eur J Immunol, 1995. 25(9): p. 2656-60.

[77] Zhou, Y., et al., *Hepatitis C virus E2 envelope protein induces dendritic cell maturation.* J Viral Hepat, 2007. 14(12): p. 849-58.

[78] Wang, H., E. Rayburn, and R. Zhang, *Synthetic oligodeoxynucleotides containing deoxycytidyl-deoxyguanosine dinucleotides (CpG ODNs) and modified analogs as novel anticancer therapeutics.* Curr Pharm Des, 2005. 11(22): p. 2889-907.

[79] Dong, Z., et al., *Involvement of natural killer cells in PolyI:C-induced liver injury.* J Hepatol, 2004. 41(6): p. 966-73.

[80] Salazar-Mather, T.P., R. Ishikawa, and C.A. Biron, *NK cell trafficking and cytokine expression in splenic compartments after IFN induction and viral infection.* J Immunol, 1996. 157(7): p. 3054-64.

[81] Salem, M.L., et al., *The adjuvant effects of the toll-like receptor 3 ligand polyinosinic-cytidylic acid poly (I:C) on antigen-specific CD8+T cell responses are partially dependent on NK cells with the induction of a beneficial cytokine milieu.* Vaccine, 2006. 24(24): p. 5119-32.

[82] Salem, M.L., et al., *Vaccination using Toll-like receptor ligand (TLRL)-primed dendritic cells and TLR3L poly I:C administration leads to an augmentation of antigen-specific memory CD8+T cell responses..* 97th Annual Meeting for American Association of Cancer Research (AACR), Washington, DC., 2006.

[83] Alenzi, F.Q., et al., *Cellular and molecular aspects of Goodpasture syndrome.* Iran J Kidney Dis, 2012. 6(1): p. 1-8.

[84] Yang, Q., et al., *Antitumor activity of NK cells.* Immunol Res, 2006. 36(1-3): p. 13-25.

[85] Kowalczyk, D.W., *Tumors and the danger model.* Acta Biochim Pol, 2002. 49(2): p. 295-302.

[86] Seya, T., et al., *Role of toll-like receptors and their adaptors in adjuvant immunotherapy for cancer.* Anticancer Res, 2003. 23(6a): p. 4369-76.

[87] Okamoto, M. and M. Sato, *Toll-like receptor signaling in anti-cancer immunity.* J Med Invest, 2003. 50(1-2): p. 9-24.

[88] Speiser, D.E., et al., *Rapid and strong human CD8+T cell responses to vaccination with peptide, IFA, and CpG oligodeoxynucleotide 7909.* J Clin Invest, 2005. 115(3): p. 739-46.

[89] Smith, K.J., S. Hamza, and H. Skelton, *The imidazoquinolines and their place in the therapy of cutaneous disease.* Expert Opin Pharmacother, 2003. 4(7): p. 1105-19.

[90] Stockfleth, E., et al., *The use of Toll-like receptor-7 agonist in the treatment of basal cell carcinoma: an overview.* Br J Dermatol, 2003. 149 Suppl 66: p. 53-6.

[91] Shackleton, M., et al., *The impact of imiquimod, a Toll-like receptor-7 ligand (TLR7L), on the immunogenicity of melanoma peptide vaccination with adjuvant Flt3 ligand.* Cancer Immun, 2004. 4: p. 9.

[92] Baldridge, J.R., et al., *Taking a Toll on human disease: Toll-like receptor 4 agonists as vaccine adjuvants and monotherapeutic agents.* Expert Opin Biol Ther, 2004. 4(7): p. 1129-38.

[93] Stover, A.G., et al., *Structure-activity relationship of synthetic toll-like receptor 4 agonists.* J Biol Chem, 2004. 279(6): p. 4440-9.

[94] Salem, M.L., et al., *Defining the antigen-specific T-cell response to vaccination and poly(I:C)/TLR3 signaling: evidence of enhanced primary and memory CD8 T-cell responses and antitumor immunity.* J Immunother, 2005. 28(3): p. 220-8.

[95] Bachmann, M.F., M. Kopf, and B.J. Marsland, *Chemokines: more than just road signs.* Nat Rev Immunol, 2006. 6(2): p. 159-64.

[96] Shortman, K. and Y.J. Liu, *Mouse and human dendritic cell subtypes.* Nat Rev Immunol, 2002. 2(3): p. 151-61.

[97] Prins, R.M., et al., *The TLR-7 agonist, imiquimod, enhances dendritic cell survival and promotes tumor antigen-specific T cell priming: relation to central nervous system antitumor immunity.* J Immunol, 2006. 176(1): p. 157-64.

[98] Weigel, B.J., et al., *CpG oligodeoxynucleotides potentiate the antitumor effects of chemotherapy or tumor resection in an orthotopic murine model of rhabdomyosarcoma.* Clin Cancer Res, 2003. 9(8): p. 3105-14.

[99] Badovinac, V.P., et al., *Accelerated CD8+T-cell memory and prime-boost response after dendritic-cell vaccination.* Nat Med, 2005. 11(7): p. 748-56.

[100] Davila, E. and E. Celis, *Repeated administration of cytosine-phosphorothiolated guanine-containing oligonucleotides together with peptide/protein immunization results in enhanced CTL responses with anti-tumor activity.* J Immunol, 2000. 165(1): p. 539-47.

[101] Davila, E., R. Kennedy, and E. Celis, *Generation of antitumor immunity by cytotoxic T lymphocyte epitope peptide vaccination, CpG-oligodeoxynucleotide adjuvant, and CTLA-4 blockade.* Cancer Res, 2003. 63(12): p. 3281-8.

[102] Craft, N., et al., *The TLR7 agonist imiquimod enhances the anti-melanoma effects of a recombinant Listeria monocytogenes vaccine.* J Immunol, 2005. 175(3): p. 1983-90.

[103] Nowak, M., et al., *LPS-induced liver injury in D-galactosamine-sensitized mice requires secreted TNF-alpha and the TNF-p55 receptor.* Am J Physiol Regul Integr Comp Physiol, 2000. 278(5): p. R1202-9.

[104] Berraondo, P., et al., *Eradication of large tumors in mice by a tritherapy targeting the innate, adaptive, and regulatory components of the immune system.* Cancer Res, 2007. 67(18): p. 8847-55.

[105] Taieb, J., et al., *Chemoimmunotherapy of tumors: cyclophosphamide synergizes with exosome based vaccines.* J Immunol, 2006. 176(5): p. 2722-9.

[106] Garay, R.P., et al., *Cancer relapse under chemotherapy: why TLR2/4 receptor agonists can help.* Eur J Pharmacol, 2007. 563(1-3): p. 1-17.

[107] Adams, M., et al., *The rationale for combined chemo/immunotherapy using a Toll-like receptor 3 (TLR3) agonist and tumour-derived exosomes in advanced ovarian cancer.* Vaccine, 2005. 23(17-18): p. 2374-8.

[108] Berhanu, A., et al., *Combinational FLt3 ligand and granulocyte macrophage colony-stimulating factor treatment promotes enhanced tumor infiltration by dendritic cells and antitumor CD8(+) T-cell cross-priming but is ineffective as a therapy.* Cancer Res, 2006. 66(9): p. 4895-903.

[109] Koopman, G., et al., *Increase in plasmacytoid and myeloid dendritic cells by progenipoietin-1, a chimeric Flt-3 and G-CSF receptor agonist, in SIV-Infected rhesus macaques.* Hum Immunol, 2004. 65(4): p. 303-16.

[110] Maraskovsky, E., et al., *Dramatic numerical increase of functionally mature dendritic cells in FLT3 ligand-treated mice.* Adv Exp Med Biol, 1997. 417: p. 33-40.

[111] Salem, M.L., et al., *Defining the Ability of Cyclophosphamide Preconditioning to Enhance the Antigen-specific CD8+T-cell Response to Peptide Vaccination: Creation of a Beneficial Host Microenvironment Involving Type I IFNs and Myeloid Cells.* J Immunother, 2007. 30(1): p. 40-53.

[112] Paulos, C.M., et al., *Toll-like receptors in tumor immunotherapy.* Clin Cancer Res, 2007. 13(18 Pt 1): p. 5280-9.

[113] Paulos, C.M., et al., *Microbial translocation augments the function of adoptively transferred self/tumor-specific CD8 T cells via TLR4 signaling.* J Clin Invest, 2007. 117(8): p. 2197-204.

[114] Salem, M.L., et al., *Defining the ability of cyclophosphamide preconditioning to enhance the antigen-specific CD8+T-cell response to peptide vaccination: creation of a beneficial host microenvironment involving type I IFNs and myeloid cells.* J Immunother (1997), 2007. 30(1): p. 40-53.

[115] Salem, M.L., et al., *Recovery from cyclophosphamide-induced lymphopenia results in expansion of immature dendritic cells which can mediate enhanced prime-boost vaccination antitumor responses in vivo when stimulated with the TLR3 agonist poly(I:C).* J Immunol, 2009. 182(4): p. 2030-40.

[116] Rubinstein, M.P., et al., *Loss of T cell-mediated antitumor immunity after construct-specific downregulation of retrovirally encoded T-cell receptor expression in vivo.* Cancer Gene Ther, 2009. 16(2): p. 171-83.

[117] Kabelitz, D., *Expression and function of Toll-like receptors in T lymphocytes.* Curr Opin Immunol, 2007. 19(1): p. 39-45.

[118] Caramalho, I., et al., *Regulatory T cells selectively express toll-like receptors and are activated by lipopolysaccharide.* J Exp Med, 2003. 197(4): p. 403-11.

[119] Lewkowicz, P., et al., *Lipopolysaccharide-activated CD4+CD25+T regulatory cells inhibit neutrophil function and promote their apoptosis and death.* J Immunol, 2006. 177(10): p. 7155-63.

[120] den Haan, J.M., G. Kraal, and M.J. Bevan, *Cutting edge: Lipopolysaccharide induces IL-10-producing regulatory CD4+T cells that suppress the CD8+T cell response.* J Immunol, 2007. 178(9): p. 5429-33.

[121] Crellin, N.K., et al., *Human CD4+T cells express TLR5 and its ligand flagellin enhances the suppressive capacity and expression of FOXP3 in CD4+CD25+T regulatory cells.* J Immunol, 2005. 175(12): p. 8051-9.

[122] Sutmuller, R.P., et al., *Toll-like receptor 2 controls expansion and function of regulatory T cells.* J Clin Invest, 2006. 116(2): p. 485-94.

[123] Liu, P.T., et al., *Toll-like receptor triggering of a vitamin D-mediated human antimicrobial response.* Science, 2006. 311(5768): p. 1770-3.

[124] Antony, P.A., et al., *CD8+T cell immunity against a tumor/self-antigen is augmented by CD4+T helper cells and hindered by naturally occurring T regulatory cells.* J Immunol, 2005. 174(5): p. 2591-601.

[125] Wada, S., et al., *Cyclophosphamide augments antitumor immunity: studies in an autochthonous prostate cancer model.* Cancer Res, 2009. 69(10): p. 4309-18.

[126] Hirschhorn-Cymerman, D., et al., *OX40 engagement and chemotherapy combination provides potent antitumor immunity with concomitant regulatory T cell apoptosis.* J Exp Med, 2009. 206(5): p. 1103-16.

[127] Ghiringhelli, F., et al., *CD4+CD25+regulatory T cells suppress tumor immunity but are sensitive to cyclophosphamide which allows immunotherapy of established tumors to be curative.* Eur J Immunol, 2004. 34(2): p. 336-44.

[128] Hillebrands, J.L., et al., *A regulatory CD4+T cell subset in the BB rat model of autoimmune diabetes expresses neither CD25 nor Foxp3.* J Immunol, 2006. 177(11): p. 7820-32.

[129] Huleatt, J.W., et al., *Vaccination with recombinant fusion proteins incorporating Toll-like receptor ligands induces rapid cellular and humoral immunity.* Vaccine, 2007. 25(4): p. 763-75.

[130] Teitz-Tennenbaum, S., et al., *Radiotherapy combined with intratumoral dendritic cell vaccination enhances the therapeutic efficacy of adoptive T-cell transfer.* J Immunother, 2009. 32(6): p. 602-12.

[131] Fehervari, Z. and S. Sakaguchi, *A paragon of self-tolerance: CD25+CD4+regulatory T cells and the control of immune responses.* Arthritis Res Ther, 2004. 6(1): p. 19-25.

[132] Netea, M.G., et al., *Toll-like receptor 2 suppresses immunity against Candida albicans through induction of IL-10 and regulatory T cells.* J Immunol, 2004. 172(6): p. 3712-8.

[133] Diaz-Montero, C.M., et al., *Priming of naive CD8+T cells in the presence of IL-12 selectively enhances the survival of CD8+CD62Lhi cells and results in superior anti-tumor activity in a tolerogenic murine model.* Cancer Immunol Immunother, 2008. 57(4): p. 563-72.

[134] Le Bon, A. and D.F. Tough, *Links between innate and adaptive immunity via type I interferon.* Curr Opin Immunol, 2002. 14(4): p. 432-6.

[135] Koyama, S., et al., *Innate immune response to viral infection.* Cytokine, 2008. 43(3): p. 336-41.

[136] Kumar, A., J. Zhang, and F.S. Yu, *Toll-like receptor 3 agonist poly(I:C)-induced antiviral response in human corneal epithelial cells.* Immunology, 2006. 117(1): p. 11-21.

[137] Yoneyama, M., et al., *Direct triggering of the type I interferon system by virus infection: activation of a transcription factor complex containing IRF-3 and CBP/p300.* EMBO J, 1998. 17(4): p. 1087-95.

[138] Wathelet, M.G., et al., *Virus infection induces the assembly of coordinately activated transcription factors on the IFN-beta enhancer in vivo.* Mol Cell, 1998. 1(4): p. 507-18.

[139] Lin, R., et al., *Virus-dependent phosphorylation of the IRF-3 transcription factor regulates nuclear translocation, transactivation potential, and proteasome-mediated degradation.* Mol Cell Biol, 1998. 18(5): p. 2986-96.

[140] Juang, Y.T., et al., *Primary activation of interferon A and interferon B gene transcription by interferon regulatory factor 3.* Proc Natl Acad Sci U S A, 1998. 95(17): p. 9837-42.

[141] Sen, G.C. and S.N. Sarkar, *Transcriptional signaling by double-stranded RNA: role of TLR3.* Cytokine Growth Factor Rev, 2005. 16(1): p. 1-14.

[142] Guillot, L., et al., *Involvement of toll-like receptor 3 in the immune response of lung epithelial cells to double-stranded RNA and influenza A virus.* J Biol Chem, 2005. 280(7): p. 5571-80.

[143] Rudd, B.D., et al., *Differential role for TLR3 in respiratory syncytial virus-induced chemokine expression.* J Virol, 2005. 79(6): p. 3350-7.

[144] Ashkar, A.A., et al., *Toll-like receptor (TLR)-3, but not TLR4, agonist protects against genital herpes infection in the absence of inflammation seen with CpG DNA.* J Infect Dis, 2004. 190(10): p. 1841-9.

[145] Yoneyama, M., et al., *The RNA helicase RIG-I has an essential function in double-stranded RNA-induced innate antiviral responses.* Nat Immunol, 2004. 5(7): p. 730-7.

[146] Yoneyama, M., et al., *Shared and unique functions of the DExD/H-box helicases RIG-I, MDA5, and LGP2 in antiviral innate immunity.* J Immunol, 2005. 175(5): p. 2851-8.

[147] Akazawa, T., et al., *Antitumor NK activation induced by the Toll-like receptor 3-TICAM-1 (TRIF) pathway in myeloid dendritic cells.* Proc Natl Acad Sci U S A, 2007. 104(1): p. 252-7.

[148] Trumpfheller, C., et al., *The microbial mimic poly IC induces durable and protective CD4+T cell immunity together with a dendritic cell targeted vaccine.* Proc Natl Acad Sci U S A, 2008. 105(7): p. 2574-9.

[149] Veldhuis, W.B., et al., *Interferon-beta blocks infiltration of inflammatory cells and reduces infarct volume after ischemic stroke in the rat.* J Cereb Blood Flow Metab, 2003. 23(9): p. 1029-39.

[150] Kraus, J., et al., *Interferon-beta stabilizes barrier characteristics of brain endothelial cells in vitro.* Ann Neurol, 2004. 56(2): p. 192-205.

[151] Maluish, A.E., et al., *Immunomodulatory effects of poly(I,C)-LC in cancer patients.* J Biol Response Mod, 1985. 4(6): p. 656-63.

[152] Droller, M.J., *Immunotherapy of metastatic renal cell carcinoma with polyinosinic-polycytidylic acid.* J Urol, 1987. 137(2): p. 202-6.

[153] Hawkins, M.J., M. Levin, and E.C. Borden, *An Eastern Cooperative Oncology Group phase I-II pilot study of polyriboinosinic-polyribocytidylic acid poly-L-lysine complex in patients with metastatic malignant melanoma.* J Biol Response Mod, 1985. 4(6): p. 664-8.

[154] Krown, S.E., et al., *Phase I trials of poly(I,C) complexes in advanced cancer.* J Biol Response Mod, 1985. 4(6): p. 640-9.

[155] Lampkin, B.C., et al., *Phase II trial of a complex polyriboinosinic-polyribocytidylic acid with poly-L-lysine and carboxymethyl cellulose in the treatment of children with acute leukemia and neuroblastoma: a report from the Children's Cancer Study Group.* Cancer Res, 1985. 45(11 Pt 2): p. 5904-9.

[156] Levine, A.S. and H.B. Levy, *Phase I-II trials of poly IC stabilized with poly-L-lysine.* Cancer Treat Rep, 1978. 62(11): p. 1907-12.

[157] Nakamura, O., et al., *Phase I-II trials of poly(ICLC) in malignant brain tumor patients.* J Interferon Res, 1982. 2(1): p. 1-4.

[158] Rettenmaier, M.A., M.L. Berman, and P.J. DiSaia, *Treatment of advanced ovarian cancer with polyinosinic-polycytidylic lysine carboxymethylcellulose (poly(ICLC)).* Gynecol Oncol, 1986. 24(3): p. 359-61.

[159] Stevenson, H.C., et al., *A phase I evaluation of poly(I,C)-LC in cancer patients.* J Biol Response Mod, 1985. 4(6): p. 650-5.

[160] Theriault, R.L., et al., *Evaluation of polyinosinic-polycytidylic and poly-L-lysine in metastatic breast cancer.* Cancer Treat Rep, 1986. 70(11): p. 1341-2.

[161] Ewel, C.H., et al., *Polyinosinic-polycytidylic acid complexed with poly-L-lysine and carboxymethylcellulose in combination with interleukin 2 in patients with cancer: clinical and immunological effects.* Cancer Res, 1992. 52(11): p. 3005-10.

[162] Gesuete, R., et al., *Poly-ICLC preconditioning protects the blood-brain barrier against ischemic injury in vitro through type I interferon signaling.* J Neurochem, 2012. 123 Suppl 2: p. 75-85.

[163] Ming Lim, C., et al., *TLR3 agonists improve the immunostimulatory potential of cetuximab against EGFR head and neck cancer cells.* Oncoimmunology, 2013. 2(6): p. e24677.

[164] Strayer, D.R., et al., *A controlled clinical trial with a specifically configured RNA drug, poly(I).poly(C12U), in chronic fatigue syndrome.* Clin Infect Dis, 1994. 18 Suppl 1: p. S88-95.

[165] Thompson, K.A., et al., *Results of a double-blind placebo-controlled study of the double-stranded RNA drug polyI:polyC12U in the treatment of HIV infection.* Eur J Clin Microbiol Infect Dis, 1996. 15(7): p. 580-7.

[166] Nicodemus, C.F. and J.S. Berek, *TLR3 agonists as immunotherapeutic agents.* Immunotherapy, 2010. 2(2): p. 137-40.

[167] Gowen, B.B., et al., *TLR3 is essential for the induction of protective immunity against Punta Toro Virus infection by the double-stranded RNA (dsRNA), poly(I:C12U), but not Poly(I:C): differential recognition of synthetic dsRNA molecules.* J Immunol, 2007. 178(8): p. 5200-8.

[168] Purcell, R.H., et al., *Modification of chronic hepatitis-B virus infection in chimpanzees by administration of an interferon inducer.* Lancet, 1976. 2(7989): p. 757-61.

[169] Ijichi, K., et al., *In vivo antiviral effects of mismatched double-stranded RNA on duck hepatitis B virus.* J Med Virol, 1994. 43(2): p. 161-5.

[170] Niu, J., et al., *The use of ampligen alone and in combination with ganciclovir and coumermycin A1 for the treatment of ducks congenitally-infected with duck hepatitis B virus.* Antiviral Res, 1993. 21(2): p. 155-71.

[171] O'Marro, S.D., et al., *The effect of combinations of ampligen and zidovudine or dideoxyinosine against human immunodeficiency viruses in vitro.* Antiviral Res, 1992. 17(2): p. 169-77.

[172] Gillespie, D., et al., *Synergistic inhibition of AZT-resistant HIV by AZT combined with poly(I):poly(C12U), without synergistic toxicity to bone marrow progenitor cell elements.* In Vivo, 1994. 8(3): p. 375-81.

[173] Carter, W.A., et al., *Mismatched double-stranded RNA, Ampligen (poly(I): poly(C12U), demonstrat*es antiviral and immunostimulatory activities in HIV disease. Int J Immunopharmacol, 1991. 13 Suppl 1: p. 69-76.

[174] Ichinohe, T., et al., Intranasal immunization with H5N1 vaccine plus Poly I:Poly C12U, a Toll-like receptor agonist, protects mice against homologous and heterologous virus challenge. Microbes Infect, 2007. 9(11): p. 1333-40.

Section 3

Local Immunity

Chapter 7

Immune Regulation of *Chlamydia trachomatis* Infections of the Female Genital Tract

Louise M. Hafner, Trudi A. Collet and
Danica K. Hickey

Additional information is available at the end of the chapter

http://dx.doi.org/10.5772/57542

1. Introduction

Tubal infertility and reproductive damage, preeclampsia and preterm births may potentially occur in many of the 50 million women who are annually infected with *Chlamydia trachomatis* [reviewed in 1; 2- 4]. *C.trachomatis* infections of the genital tract are also reported to increase the risk of human immunodeficiency virus type 1(HIV-1) susceptibility and viral shedding in the genital tract either directly by pro-inflammatory signalling pathways or indirectly by their effects on genital epithelial cells [5]. A dramatic increase in the number of HIV-1 chemokine co-receptor CXCR4- and CCR5-positive T cell targets has also been reported in the endocervix of *C. trachomatis*-positive women [6].

Gynecological cancer development is also suggested to be linked with Chlamydial genital tract infections. Epidemiological reports have proposed that *C.trachomatis* may act as a co-factor in the development of human papilloma virus (HPV)-induced squamous cell carcinomas (SCC), with an association between distinct serovariants of *C. trachomatis* (B, D, E, G, I, and J) and SCC being reported [7,8]. It is also likely that *C. trachomatis* co-infections of the lower genital tract (LGT) play a role in carcinogenesis of the female upper genital tract (UGT), particularly epithelial ovarian and type II carcinomas [9,10]. To explain the epidemiological associations of Chlamydial infections cervical and ovarian cancer development it has been hypothesised that the pathogen perhaps triggers epigenetic changes in host chromatin and impairs host DNA repair pathways [11] or that it changes host cell survival pathways by disrupting DNA damage signalling pathways associated with tumorigenesis [12].

The majority (70-80%) of genital tract infections in women are asymptomatic and are not diagnosed or treated and persistent or "silent" infections are reported as occurring years after initial acquisition of *Chlamydia* with 50% of women continuing to shed the organism one year after infection is diagnosed [13]. Left untreated the organisms can ascend to the uterus and Fallopian tubes to cause pelvic inflammatory disease (PID). Inflammation of the Fallopian tubes can lead to scarring and fibrosis which can then lead to ectopic pregnancy (EP), subfertility and infertility with repeated or multiple infections increasing the chances of disease sequelae [14-17]. Additionally, infections during pregnancy may result in peripartum transmission of *Chlamydia* to newborns potentially resulting in neonatal conjunctivitis and late-onset pneumonia [18, 19].

Globally it is estimated that over 100 million adults were infected with *C. trachomatis* in 2008 [20]. The annual direct medical cost of sexually transmitted diseases (including *Chlamydia* and those caused by HIV) has been estimated at $US16.9 billion [21]. Despite continued improvements in diagnostic and screening procedures for *Chlamydia* the incidence of infection continues to increase with a significant increase, particularly in the rates of EP [22]. Even though azithromycin is available to treat uncomplicated lower genital tract infections [23], antibiotic therapy will not always be efficacious and one hypothesis is that *Chlamydia* treatments may in fact attenuate protective immunity in some patients [24]. Recent evidence has shown that although spontaneous resolution of infection before treatment occurred in 22% of naturally infected women, following azithromycion treatment, 16.5% of women were re-infected and this rate was higher (19.9%) in those women with persistent infection when compared with the rate (5%) in women who spontaneously cleared the infection [25]. Repeat infections are thought to be one of the primary causes of ongoing transmission of *Chlamydia*. Development of a vaccine that can either prevent infection or disease is therefore of vital importance for *Chlamydia* [26, 27].

1.1. The organism: *C. trachomatis*

*Chlamydia*e are small (0.5μm and genomes of 1.05Mb) gram negative intracellular bacteria and the human pathobiotype, *C. trachomatis* comprises non-invasive biovars that infect squamo-columnar epithelial cells of the female genital tract [28-30]. *C.trachomatis* replicates within non-acidic vacuoles of these genital tract cells, acquiring essential lipids from the host cell during infection to survive and replicate [31]. Based on serologic differences elicited by variable domain (VD) regions of the Chlamydial major outer membrane protein A (OmpA), *C.trachomatis* biovars currently are classified into 19 serovars with serovars D-K causing urogenital infections [32-37].

Urogenital isolates of *C.trachomatis* may also contain a highly conserved 7.5 kB non-integrative plasmid that has a role in the pathobiology of these organisms [38, 39]. The plasmid functions as a significant virulence factor in the murine model of genital tract disease [40] with plasmid loss resulting in failure to induce upper genital tract pathology in this model [41]. Within clinical isolates of *C.trachomatis*, carriage of the 7.5 kB plasmid is almost universal, although a few naturally-occurring, plasmid deficient strains have been reported that are not associated with increased disease severity [42-45]. Recently it was reported that naturally-occurring plasmid-free urogenital isolates of *C.trachomatis* serovar F also had reduced infectivity and virulence in a murine model [46].

1.2. Developmental cycle

Chlamydia undergoes a unique biphasic developmental cycle that encompasses two forms of reproduction; an intracellular phase of non-infectious metabolically active and replicative forms of reticulate bodies (RBs) and the extracellular phase of infectious elementary bodies (EBs) that attach to and invade epithelial cells [47; reviewed in 48, and 49 and 50].

Chlamydial infection of superficial columnar cervical cells in the FGT is initiated by the attachment and endocytosis of the EB into these mucosal epithelial cells. EB containing endosomes then are internalised within host-derived membranes where the pathogen then hijacks both vesicular and non-vesicular mediated pathways of the host to obtain host-derived membrane lipids, including sphingomyelin (SM) and cholesterol, for intracellular growth and development [reviewed in 51]. Once resources such as sphingomyelin are obtained from the host cell and the vesicle expands, the EBs differentiate into the metabolically active, non-infectious and larger (0.8μm) reticulate bodies (RB) in the normal developmental cycle. Transformation of the metabolically-inactive EBs into the metabolically-active RBs occurs at approximately 3 h post-infection (pi), and replication by binary fission over a 24-48h time period then is initiated [52]. The RB containing endosome expands and produces a microscopically-visible Chlamydial microcolony referred to as an "inclusion" [53]. RBs then use host cell ATP and other metabolites to grow and replicate by binary fission within the Chlamydial inclusion.

Many inducers of persistence (including Interferon gamma (IFN-g), amino acid starvation and antibiotics) will result in deviation from the 'normal developmental cycle', resulting in a viable but non-cultivable growth stage and the formation of large, abnormal developmental forms termed aberrant bodies (ABs) also known as aberrant RB, or persistent bodies [54]. In normal development, RBs will continue to divide undergoing between 8-12 rounds of replication. Later in the infectious process, the RBs asynchronously begin to differentiate back into EBs, there is evidence of intermediate bodies (IBs) at this stage and the EBs accumulate within the inclusion. Depending upon the Chlamydial species, at 30-80h post-infection the infectious EB's that have matured from the RBs are released either by host cell lysis or by a packaged-release mechanism called extrusion, allowing the EBs to infect neighbouring cells for successive rounds of infection.

1.3. Intracellular survival strategies

C. trachomatis is proficient at maintaining enduring relationships with its host by modulating and evading the immune system using a multitude of mechanisms [55]. These include inhibiting IFN-g–inducible major histocompatibility complex (MHC) class II expression [56] that in human endocervical cells is known to be mediated by direct and indirect (soluble) factors [57]. The multiple potential mechanisms used by *Chlamydia* to dampen immune responses recently have been summarized [58].

To modulate host signal transduction cascades and allow their developmental cycles to take place Chlamydiae are known to secrete up to sixteen anti-host (effector) proteins (reviewed in 59; 60). They also recruit proteins from the host and the first identified host proteins to be recruited into the Chlamydial inclusion include the eukaryotic nuclear protein ZNF23, a pro-apoptotic factor that potentially allows *Chlamydia* to inhibit host cell apoptosis thus enabling bacterial survival in the host [61].

1.4. Chlamydial infections and disease sequelae

1.4.1. Infections in women

Significant reproductive morbidity can occur in women following infection of the LGT with *C. trachomatis*. In the estimated 20% of women with symptoms, *C.trachomatis* infection of the columnar epithelial cells of the endocervix can result in cervicitis [62-64; reviewed in 65] and urethritis [66]. Severe complications of untreated LGT Chlamydial infections in women, whether symptomatic or asymptomatic can result in ascension of the organism from the lower to the UGT. Endometritis represents an early stage in the continuum from LGT infection through to salpingitis, a Fallopian tube disease also confirmed to be associated with *C.trachomatis* infection. Since a critical source of Fallopian tube inflammation is infection with *C.trachomatis,* it has been hypothesized that *C.trachomatis* infection may be involved in chronic tubal inflammation and subsequent fimbrial carcinogenesis and hence could perhaps be the origin of some ovarian cancers [67]. Interestingly, a recent retrospective analysis of 34 cases of serous pelvic carcinomas (which are the most frequent histologic type of ovarian cancers) reported that 70% of cases did in fact involve the Fallopian tubes [68].

Chlamydial infection of the pelvis can lead to symptomatic pelvic inflammatory disease (PID) that can result in Fallopian tube inflammation [69] and salpingitis is reported to occur in 20-40% of women with untreated or repeated Chlamydial infections [70,71]. A recent model predicts that annual screening would prevent 61% of *C.trachomatis*-related PID in women who became infected in their LGTs with *Chlamydia* [72]. In addition to salpingitis the long-term consequences of PID can also include chronic pelvic pain and ectopic pregnancy (EP). It has been proposed that since *C.trachomatis* infection increases tubal expression of prokineticin receptor (PROKR2) mRNA this expression then predisposes to ectopic implantation in the Fallopian tube [73]. Recent papers have reported that one third of EPs could be attributable to Chlamydial infection [74] and have also reviewed the pathogenesis of *Chlamydia*-induced tubal EP [75].

PID is caused by infection of the female genital tract with many microorganisms including *C. trachomatis* [reviewed in 16] and following symptomatic PID of polymicrobial etiology up to 18% of women may develop tubal factor infertility (TFI), which is amongst the leading causes of infertility accounting for 7-9.8% of all female factor infertilities [76-80]. Testing for serum antibody to the Chlamydial 60kDa Heat shock protein (i.e.cHSP60 antibody) is an accurate means for predicting *Chlamydia*-associated TFI [81] and elevated levels of anti-Chlamydial caseinolytic protease P (ClpP) antibodies were recently identified in 21 TFI patients [82]. Prolonged exposure to *Chlamydia* due to a chronic persistent infection or frequent re-infection has also been associated with chronic inflammation and TFI [83-85]. It has been reported that 9.5% women developed PID over 12 months in women who tested positive for *Chlamydia* at baseline [86].

1.4.2. *Ophthalmia neonatorum and infant pneumonia*

The high prevalence of Chlamydial infections of the cervix in women of child-bearing age results in annual exposure of an estimated 100,000 neonates to *Chlamydia* infections [87] and neonatal Chlamydial infections are generally acquired during passage through an infected birth canal. A Chlamydial cause should be considered for all infants aged ≤30 days who have conjunctivitis and, if positively diagnosed, appropriate treatment initiated for the infant, mother and her sex partner(s).

Chlamydia infections of neonates have been reported to be at 18 percent for ophthalmia neonatorum and 16 percent for pneumonia for infants exposed to *C. trachomatis* in vaginal secretions in the birth canal, with up to 60% of these infants showing serological evidence of Chlamydial infection [88]. Using data pooled from studies since 1977 it has been estimated that the incidence of ophthalmia neonatorum caused by exposure of the neonate to *C.trachomatis* at birth is actually around 15 percent and that of pneumonia is around 7 percent [89].

Neonatal infection with *C. trachomatis* involves the mucous membranes of the neonatal eye, oropharynx, urogenital tract, and rectum and when symptomatic can result in a number of diseases in the first few months of life such as inclusion conjunctivitis, pneumonia or both [90,91; reviewed in 92; 93). Ophthalmia neonatorum has been reported as developing from 5-14 days post-delivery in up to 50% of infants of *C.trachomatis* infected mothers [94] and perhaps even as late as 42 days after birth [94] with between 5-30% of perinatally-infected infants also having nasopharyngeal infection [reviewed in 95]. A recent prospective study from Brazil estimated the prevalence of rate of *Chlamydia* among pregnant women (<30 years) in their third trimester as 72.7% and reported that 50% of 16 newborn babies had respiratory symptoms within the first 60 days of life [96].

Afebrile pneumonia may be seen in infants colonised in the respiratory tract with *C.trachomatis* and this may/may not be associated with inclusion conjunctivitis. After three or more weeks following Chlamydial infection of the infants a subacute, afebrile pneumonia with onset at ages 1–3 months develops in approximately seven percent of these cases [97, 92, 19]. Clinical characteristics have been described for infant pneumonia caused by *C.trachomatis* in infants with nasopharyngeal shedding and in around half of the infected infants conjunctivitis was recorded, with middle ear abnormalities recorded in more than half of the *Chlamydia*-positive infants and wheezing an unusual finding in these infants [98]. A more recent study has also highlighted that *C. trachomatis* is an important cause of lower respiratory tract infection in infants in India below six months of age [99].

1.5. Immunopathogenesis and immunoprotection

The host inflammatory response to *C.trachomatis* is involved in immunity but also the pathology that leads to serious morbidities of chronic pelvic pain, EP and tubal infertility following female genital tract infection. Protective responses to *C.trachomatis* infections of the female genital tract are elicited to clear primary infection and to resist re-infection and include both innate and adaptive (particularly CD4+ T cell) cells and immune responses. Cells of both the innate and adaptive immune systems are found in the FGT in Fallopian tubes, uterus, cervix and vagina [100] and we have recently reviewed the localisation of T lymphocyte populations in the female upper (UGT) and lower (LGT) genital tracts over the menstrual cycle [101].

Effector cells of the innate (non-specific) immune response found in the FGT include epithelial cells, monocytes, macrophages, granulocytes (neutrophils, eosinophils and basophils), dendritic cells (DCs) and Natural Killer (NK) cells conferring protection through chemokines, cytokines and phagocytosis. Innate (non-specific) host defense particularly in the lower genital tract (LGT) is also provided by the vaginal microbiota maintained in a healthy equilibrium (reviewed in [102] as well as by the myriad of antimicrobial peptides (AMPs) and protease inhibitors of cervicovaginal fluid [103] including elafin, lysozyme and cathelicidins, amongst others and reviewed in (Wira and Fahey, 2004). The AMPs and pathogen recognition receptors (PRRs) such as toll-like receptors (TLRs) are key intermediaries of innate immunity in the FGT [104-107]. The innate immune cells (especially neutrophils) elicit inflammation to protect against infections however these inflammatory responses are usually inefficient and repeated Chlamydial infections are common [108].

The rapid innate immune response is the first line of defence against a *C. trachomatis* infection of columnar epithelial cells. PRRs recognise the pathogen and TLRs play a vital role in the host immune system by recognizing pathogenic components (pathogen associated molecular patterns (PAMPs) and danger associated molecular patterns (DAMPs)) and inducing a protective immune response to the pathogen [109]. Data indicate that host genetic factors may contribute up to 40% to the variation in clinical course of *Chlamydia* infection [110]. Host genetic variants in TLRs have been found to influence *Chlamydia* LGT infections in women [111]. For example protection against tubal disease following a *C.trachomatis* infection has been reportedly associated with single nucleotide polymorphisms (SNPs) in the innate immune (TLR) gene, TLR2 [112]. SNPs in TLR4 have also been reported to play a role in making women more prone to subfertility (i.e. no pregnancy after 1 year) as a late complication of *Chlamydia* infection [113] and worldwide estimates are that 10-15% of all couples are subfertile [114]. SNPs in other pathogen recognition receptors including nucleotide-binding oligomerization domain receptors (NODs) have been reported to influence susceptibility and severity of *Chlamydia* infections [115]. Taken together these observations have lead to the recent suggested potential translational and clinical value of adding diagnostic host genetic marker profiles on the basis of infection and inflammation to the current clinical management of subfertility [116].

The more gradual adaptive immune response to Chlamydial infection is mediated through antibodies and/or T cells and is a very specific recognition and response to foreign antigens. Cervical cell production of IFN-g and interleukin-12 (IL-12) in response to stimulation with *C.trachomatis* EBs has a positive correlation with fertility in *C.trachomatis* seropositive patients [117]. Recruitment and activation of B cell (humoral) and T cell (cell-mediated/adaptive) immunity is also coordinated by the release of these factors. The initiation of this adaptive response may lead to spontaneous resolution of natural infection in some populations [25] although chronic infections in women indicate that rarely does this response to *C.trachomatis* result in clearance of the infection; nor does it adequately protect against re-infection. The cellular components of this specific immunity include T lymphocytes expressing $\alpha\beta$- and $\gamma\delta$-T cell receptors (TCR) and immunoglobulin (Ig) producing B lymphocytes [reviewed in 101].

During active primary genital infections in women, serum and genital mucosal IgA and IgG antibodies to Chlamydial EBs and specific Chlamydial proteins including heat-shock (HSP) and plasmid proteins are usually detected [118]. AntiChlamydial antibodies are not sufficient to protect infected females from re-infections [119].

Once *Chlamydia* has established intracellular infection, cells of the adaptive immune system, and particularly T helper 1 (Th1) type CD4+ T cells secreting IFN-g are required for clearance of primary infection and to protect from re-infection [120]. It has been observed from human data that MHC Class II-restricted CD4+T cells of the Th1 phenotype are critical for the recovery from primary Chlamydial infection and also have a role in protecting from disease sequelae [121,122]. Other major lineages of activated CD4+ T cells that play critical roles in Chlamydial infections include the Th2 cells, Th17 cells (producing IL-17 and IL-23) and Tregulatory (Treg) cells [123,124]. Additional T cells involved in adaptive immunity include intraepithelial lymphocytes (γδ T cells) and cytotoxic T lymphocytes (CD8+ T cells) that are known to induce apoptosis of infected Chlamydial cells [125].

Disease outcomes are dependent upon the complex interactions between virulence factors of, and evasion strategies used by, *C.trachomatis* and host immune responses including variants in genetic markers associated with infection and inflammation. Host factors and cellular immune responses associated with susceptibility to, or protection from Chlamydial infection and/or diseases have recently been reviewed [126].

2. Chlamydial genital tract infection and immune regulation by sex hormones

The FGT comprises several immune compartments found in the UGT (endocervix, ovaries, Fallopian tubes and uterus) and LGT (ectocervix, and vagina). The UGT is lined with a single layer of columnar epithelium and the LGT with is lined with stratified squamous epithelium [100]. The transitional zone where squamous epithelium changes to columnar epithelium is the most immunologically active site of the FGT [127].

The human FGT contains components of the innate and adaptive mucosal immune responses that are found in various distributions at different sites throughout the tract. In the FGT the major lymphocyte components are Natural Killer (NK) cells and T lymphocytes including CD3+ T lymphocytes that are present in all tissues of the tract. In the LGT the CD8+ and CD4+ are dispersed throughout the stroma whilst lymphoid aggregates of these cells are formed in the uterus [128]; granulocytes are present and these are principally located in the Fallopian tubes. Finally, relative to T lymphocytes, smaller numbers of monocytes and B lymphocytes are found throughout all tissues of the FGT [129].

Host protection of the FGT is afforded by two arms of defense comprising innate (non-specific) and acquired (specific) immunity. The cellular components of the specific immune responses at this site are T lymphocytes expressing αβ- and γδ-T cell receptors (TCR) and immunoglobulins (Ig) producing B lymphocytes [130]. Effectors of non-specific responses include epithelial cells, monocytes, macrophages, granulocytes (neutrophils, eosinophils and basophils), dendritic cells (DCs) and Natural Killer (NK) cells that confer protection due to chemokines, cytokines and phagocytosis. Cells of both the innate and adaptive immune systems are found in Fallopian tubes, uterus, cervix and vagina [131].

Both innate and adaptive mucosal immunity in the FGT are regulated by the female sex hormones estrogen (E2) and progesterone (pregn-4-ene3,20-dione) or (P4) and have been reviewed [130, 132, reviewed in 101]. Hormones regulate the transport of Igs, levels of cytokines, expression of Toll-like receptor (TLR) genes [133,134] and the distribution of immune cells and antigen presentation in the genital tissues during the reproductive cycle. Estradiol regulates the structure and function of the FGT via the classic model of steroid action ('i.e. genomic regulation) which is mediated by activated nuclear receptors including estrogen receptors (ER)-α and ER-β [131,135]. Estradiol can also exert rapid "non-classic" steroid effects on diverse signalling pathways and second messenger systems that occur independently of transcriptional or classic genomic regulation [136]. These rapid responses are often referred to as 'non-genomic' steroid effects and they can affect genital tract cells and innate and humoral immunity at this site which may alter the pathogens ability to infect the genital tract [137].

The recruitment and function of immune components of the FGT are precisely regulated by hormonal changes during the menstrual cycle by the sex steroids that co-ordinate cell trafficking and immune activation at this mucosal site. Female sex hormones E2, progestins and androgens are produced by ovarian cells with levels of estradiol (17β-estradiol) and P4 varying in accordance with fluctuations in the menstrual cycle [130]. In the menstrual/ovarian cycle of humans the endometrium develops and follicles grow until ovulation in the Proliferative/ Follicular phase. The Secretory/Luteal phase is characterised by high levels of progesterone from the corpus luteum to maintain the endometrium. Finally, corpus luteum regression and menstruation occurs during the menstrual phase At menstruation, serum estradiol levels measure typically <50pg/ml. Gradually increasing amounts of estradiol are found in the follicular (proliferative) phase of the adult female menstrual cycle with serum levels at a pre-ovulatory stage (day 14) ranging from 110-410 pg/ml and dropping briefly at ovulation. Levels of estradiol (20-160pg/mol) and P4(>5ng/ml) are present during the luteal (secretory) phase from days 14-28 of the menstrual cycle typically peaking at day 21 of the cycle. At the end of the secretory phase estradiol levels return to their menstrual levels.

The innate response is triggered by PRRs (including TLRs and non-TLRs such as NOD-like receptors) expressed predominantly by innate immune effector cells such as macrophages, neutrophils and DCs that are found in the genital mucosa. Human oviduct epithelial cells (ECs) express Toll-like receptor 3 and E2 has been reported to suppress the TLR-3-induced cytokine and chemokine production in human endometrial epithelial cells [138].The effects of E2 on the differentiation and function of antigen-presenting cells (APCs) *in vitro* has been reviewed (see [139; 132]. Much of the current evidence shows that E2 can activate dendritic cells and differentially regulate adaptive immune responses through direct effects on DC functions [140] via E2 receptor (ER) ligands [141]. These include TLR4 and its co-receptor Cluster of Differentiation (CD) 14 (Chlamydial LPS and Chlamydial HSP60) [142; 143; 144] TLR2 (Chlamydial HSP60) [145,146] and NOD protein, Nod2 (rudimentary proteoglycan motif produced by *C. trachomatis* and *C.muridarum*) [147]. Expression of TLR genes 2,3,4,5,6,9 and 10 is reportedly significantly higher in human endometrial tissue during the secretory phase (when P4 is the predominant hormone) compared to all other phases of the menstrual cycle [148].

Changes in the populations of DC and macrophage cells in the murine FGT occur due to varying levels of ovarian steroid hormones at this site in the model [149], and in women, changes in these cell populations occur due to the varying stages of the menstrual cycle, noting that the frequencies of macrophages and immature DCs are higher in the menstrual phase when compared to all other phases of the cycle [150, 151]. CD16-expressing macrophages and monocytes are also key components of the innate immune system of the FGT and are cells that are capable of producing cytokines and chemokines upon activation. These cells are also known to be profoundly affected by E2 [reviewed in 152]. Studies have shown that E2 uses both estrogen receptor (ER) alpha (ERα) and ER beta (ERβ) to decrease CD16 expression on monocytes and hence to alter monocytic cytokine release following CD16 receptor activation [153].

T lymphocytes present in the FGT, specifically CD4+ and CD8+ T cells, and immune mediators of cell-mediated immunity are found distributed within distinct regions of the female LGT. The normal vaginal mucosa contains T cells and APCs with the few immune cells present consisting primarily of CD1a+ DCs and CD8+ intraepithelial lymphocytes (IELs) [154]. The tissues in the UGT have been found to express a greater number Th1-associated chemokines than the tissues in the LGT comprising the cervical-vaginal region [153]. The menstrual cycle and menopause have been reported to have no apparent effect on cellular localization or abundance of T lymphocyte subsets and APCs in any of the lower genital tract tissues [127]. In humans, expansion of human CD4+CD25+ regulatory T cells (Tregs) has been reported to occur in the late follicular (proliferative) phases of the menstrual cycles of fertile women [124].

Levels of IgG and IgA antibodies in FGT fluids are also known to be modulated by the stage of the menstrual cycle in women. E2 up-regulates the *in vitro* expression in the FGT of secretory component (SC) increasing transport of IgA into the lumen [154] and transport of polymeric IgA (pIgA) into FGT tissues is significantly decreased by ovariectomy, although this decline can be reversed by addition of E2 but not P4 [155]. The effects of ovarian hormones on immunoglobulin secreting cells (ISC) function in healthy women were also investigated and it was reported that ISC frequency in peripheral blood mononuclear cells (PMBC) was highest during the peri-ovulatory stage of the menstrual cycle [156].

2.1. Sex hormones and chlamydial infection

It is becoming increasingly well documented that sex hormones E2 and P4 regulate host susceptibility, as well as innate and adaptive immune responses to the sexually transmitted pathogen *Chlamydia* infecting the mucosal surfaces of the FGT [reviewed in 101].

Data from several animal models of genital tract Chlamydial infection have shown that Chlamydial infection may be influenced by timing of exposure and the steroid status of the mucosal epithelium. In the murine model of *C.muridarum* infection pre-exposure of the animals to P4 is required to achieve maximal infection outcomes in the animals [157]. However, treatment of female guinea pigs with E2 resulted in *Chlamydia caviae* infections of greater intensity and longer duration [157-160] an effect that it also observed following oral contraceptive administration to these animals [161]. In the female reproductive tract rat model it was reported that no Chlamydial inclusions were detected in either the uterus or vagina in rats that had been infected with *C. trachomatis* (mouse pneumonitis strain MoPn) at estrus and diestrus without prior P4 priming [162]. In rat studies it has also been reported that when ovariectomized animals were administered estradiol, progesterone, or a combination of both and infected with *Chlamydia trachomatis* via the intrauterine route no Chlamydiae were found vaginal secretions of E2-treated animals nor were there any signs of uterine or vaginal inflammation in these animals [163].

Additionally, the use of *in vitro* cell lines to investigate *C. trachomatis* infection have produced data showing that the hormonal status of the epithelium can influence the outcome of Chlamydial infections in these models. It was shown that E2 treatment of HeLa cells pre-infection with *C.trachomatis* (serovar K or L1) enhanced both of adherence of EBs to the cells as well as Chlamydial inclusion formation; post-infection, the presence of E2 was required for the enhancement of inclusion formation [164]. Using a hormone responsive human endometrial cell line an association between repeated Chlamydial infections in women and high levels of E2 has been reported [165]. More recently it has been reported that the sex hormones E2 and P4 can directly modulate Chlamydial genes associated with persistence (the viable but non-culturable state in the Chlamydial developmental cycle) in the host. It is likely, however, that the major effects of these hormones on Chlamydial infection are indirect via the host cells [166]. The outer membrane complex B (*omcB)* and tryptophan B (*trpB*) genes are two of several reliable markers for Chlamydial persistence [167,168]. It was reported that in E2-supplemented cultures of *C.trachomatis* serovar D infections of a hormone-responsive human endometrial cell line, an up-regulation of the *omcB* and *trpB* genes was observed suggesting a stress response indicative of Chlamydial persistence; morphological changes (aberrant, enlarged RBs) were also observed in these cultures consistent with a persistence response [166]. P4-supplemented cultures resulted in a general up-regulation of genes encoding amino acid and carbohydrate metabolism pathways [166].

Chlamydia trachomatis infection of the female LGT stimulates innate immune cells by activation of TLR2/TLR4 [reviewed in 169]. TLRs 2 and 4 have been found at the highest expression levels in endometrium and Fallopian tube tissue [170] with the predominant expression of TLR4 and its co-receptor CD14 in the Fallopian tubes proposed to play an important role in the innate host defence mechanism against ascending *C. trachomatis* infections [169,171]. In a recent study *C.trachomatis*-infected women have been reported to express higher TLR2, TLR4 and inducible nitric oxide synthase (iNOS) in their cervical monocytes compared to controls. It is thought that TLR4 initiates the innate immune response to Chlamydial infection, activation of TLR2 leads to expression of inflammatory cytokines whilst iNOS contributes to Chlamydial clearance from this mucosal site [172]. Recently it has been reported that E2 reduces TLR4 expression of human monocyte derived Dendritic cells and suggested that this may increase host susceptibility to *C. trachomatis* infections [173].

Studies of *C.trachomatis* infections of the FGT have reported many effects of hormones on infection and immunity to the pathogen at this mucosal site. For example significant increases in the sensitivities of cervical epithelial cells to infection with *C.trachomatis* occur in the later stages of the female menstrual cycle [174]. It has been reported that Chlamydial infection occurring in the early E2-dominant phases of the cycle was a significant predictor for development of salpingitis [175]. Clinical findings have also reported on the enhancing effects of E2 on Chlamydial infection and disease sequelae in the infected female genital tract. It has been reported that women are more susceptible to Chlamydial infection under the influence of E2 [165]. In women with fertility disorders (n= 115) and in women with *C.trachomatis* mucopurulent cervicitis (n=86) a significantly positive correlation was recorded between Chlamydial load and E2 levels [117].

Chemokine receptors direct T lymphocytes to the site of mucosal infection, including infection of genital tract epithelial cells with *C.trachomatis* and these receptors can be modulated by E2. In a study examining samples from human patients it was reported that CCR5 (chemokine (C-C motif) receptor 5) expression increased followed *C. trachomatis* genital infections [125].

Reproductive hormones may potentially act with cytokines to regulate immune responses in the FGT to Chlamydial genital tract infections *in vivo*. Significant negative correlation has been reported between E2 levels in women with primary Chlamydial genital infections and cervical wash concentrations of IL-10, IL-1beta and IL-6 cytokines. Significant negative correlations were also recorded between IL1-beta cytokines and P4 levels in women with recurrent Chlamydial infections [176]. Thus it would appear that Chlamydial infection of the human FGT is modulated in part by the combined actions of cytokines with E2 and P4. More recent investigations reveal that levels of E2 were significantly higher in *Chlamydia*-positive women with fertility disorders when compared to fertile women suggesting that this sex hormone contributes to development of disease sequelae to *C.trachomatis* infection of the FGT[165].

E2 has been reported to exacerbate Chlamydial infections in women following administration of oral contraceptives [177] an observation also noted for female guinea pigs [161]. A prospective study on oral contraceptive pills or depo medroxyprogesterone acetate and sexually transmitted disease acquisition reported that women using oral contraceptive pills were at increased risk for acquisition of *Chlamydia* [178]. Hormonal contraceptive use in women, particularly depo medroxyprogesterone (DMPA), has also been reported in observational studies to be associated with a four-fold increase in Chlamydial genital tract infections [179].

3. Immunopathogenesis — chlamydial infections, tubal factor infertility, ectopic pregnancy and pid

A primary Chlamydial infection of the FGT can elicit host immune responses that are involved both in immunity to infection and in pathology of disease. Innate immune responses constitute the first line of defence against pathogens and include TLRs that are expressed in the FGT. Further, although the host immune response affords protection against infection *via* means of rapid and efficient bacterial destruction, resultant inflammatory responses may lead to tissue damage and/or persistent infection.

In reaction to Chlamydial entry in host cells, innate immune responses occur at the infected mucosal site 1-2 days post infection [180]. Intense inflammation and predominant mucosal infiltration of phagocytes, neutrophils and macrophages ingest and enzymatically destroy the bacteria. In conjunction with the production and subsequent activation of phagocytic cells, others, crucial to infection resolution are also activated [181]. Natural killer (NK) cells are activated in direct response to *C. trachomatis* infection or indirectly by macrophagic stimulation of IL-12, a potent NK cell-triggering cytokine. Once activated, NK cells produce IFN-g which stimulate macrophages, further promoting phagocytosis. Innate immunity may impede infection, however, the inaccessibility of *Chlamydia* to circulating antibodies whose sole purpose is elimination necessitates adaptive immune effector mechanisms of both humoral and cell-mediated immunity.

Activation of cell-mediated immunity post infection is demonstrated by the proliferative response ratio of peripheral blood lymphocytes to Chlamydial EBs. T cells, which functionally differentiate into Th1 or Th2 subtypes based upon cytokine secretion profiles, also amass at the infection site [182]. Further, interaction of *C. trachomatis* with the cytokine network is a key component for resolution of infection and one in which a cytokine response is elicited either through direct infection of epithelial cells or by host cell interaction. In concert with the inflammatory process, tissue repair, comprising the removal of dead cells and the ingrowth of fibroblasts, leads to scar formation and potential impairment of Fallopian tube function [183]. Moreover, all three tubal layers i.e. interstitial, muscular and serosal may be implicated in scar development. Infection of the serosal layer elicits an inflammatory exudate, present on the peritoneal surface, thereby adhering all adjacent surfaces and structures. Although the innate and adaptive immune responses systematically co-ordinate their efforts to ultimately resolve infection, the immune response to Chlamydial infection can cause deciliation of tubal epithelium, intralumineal adhesions, tubal occlusion and peritubal adhesions. As a result, such gross anatomical and pathological changes may lead to infertility, EP and possible spontaneous abortion [184].

Primary Chlamydial infections of the FGT thus induce both innate and adaptive host immune responses that contribute to clearance of the infections. However, results from a 5-year study of natural genital Chlamydial infections in women strongly suggested that *C. trachomatis* infection was cleared from the cervix epithelium in only 54% of the women at 12 months [185]. This low clearance rate is due, in part, to the organism's ability to utilise various mechanisms with which to evade the host immune system. In fact rarely do host immune responses to *Chlamydia* induce a total clearance of genital infections. Indeed, the women remaining infected in the genital tract with *C. trachomatis* are unable to mount strong adaptive immune responses to clear the pathogen hence they become asymptomatic and remain undiagnosed with a persistent Chlamydial infection. Chronic inflammation resultant from a persistent *C. trachomatis* infection can lead to a wide spectrum of disease manifestations. In persistently-infected *Chlamydia*l host cells, inflammatory cytokines are released in response to the latent infection to aid in the eradication of the pathogen. Unfortunately, these cytokines, which act as immunomodulators may in fact, induce and sustain tissue damage and host inflammatory responses. Compounded with repeated infections, the continued production of cytokines may cause serious disease sequelae such as PID, TFI, chronic pelvic pain or EP. Chlamydial Hsp60 (cHsp60), a known potent inducer of host inflammatory responses, may protect against Chlamydial infections [186]; paradoxically, however, cHsp60 is also able to induce pro-inflammatory responses, which can lead to tissue damage in women infected with *C. trachomatis* [187-189].

Recent data from a prospective study of 30 women diagnosed with a ruptured EP demonstrated that anti-cHsp60 immunity confers a higher risk of EP [190]. Furthermore, in those women who were positive for anti-cHsp60 antibodies and suffered an EP, all had significantly lower IL-1β levels than Chlamydial sero-negative EP cases [190]. Importantly, high serum concentrations of IL-1β in the Fallopian tubes correlated with successful uterine implantation of embryos [191-192]. Data obtained from a prospective cohort of women at high risk for *C. trachomatis* infection demonstrated that a Th1 response i.e. the release of IFN-g to cHSP60 was associated with protection against the bacterial infection [186]. In contrast, it was also shown that an IL-10 response to the same Chlamydial antigen increased infection risk. In a study that investigated cytokine responses of cervical mononuclear cells obtained from 153 women all serologically positive for *C. trachomatis*, it was found that exposure to cHsp60 and cHsp10 may drastically affect the host's mucosal immune function by increasing the production and subsequent release of IFN-g, IL-10 and tumour necrosis factor-α (TNF-α) [193] thereby potentiating further tissue damage and disease sequelae.

TLRs are responsible for initiation of the adaptive immune system, thereby leading to the ultimate destruction of foreign microbes. Moreover, since they recognise structurally conserved molecules from various bacteria, they play a vital role in host defence. Chlamydial-induced PID was investigated and it was reported that among women clinically diagnosed with PID, those who carried variants in TLR 1 and TLR 4 genes had significantly increased odds of *C. trachomatis* infection [191]. In a more recent study, it was concluded that racial variation in TLR variants amongst women with PID may alter signalling pathways subsequent to microbial recognition, thus causing an increase in associated inflammation [194]. An investigation of pregnant women positive for *C. trachomatis* showed that those with serological evidence of prenatal *C. trachomatis* infections were more likely to develop pre-eclampsia [192].

Polymorphic membrane proteins (Pmps) represent 13.6% of *C. trachomatis'* entire coding genome [195], therefore inferring a potential role in Chlamydial biology and virulence. In a group of 40 *C. trachomatis*-infected women with clinically diagnosed mild to moderate PID, antibody levels of PmpA, PmpD and PmpI were evaluated. Interestingly, those women with PmpA antibodies were less likely to fall pregnant (p=0.042) and achieve a live birth (p=0.005) compared with those sero-negative for PmpA [196] suggesting that the immunopathological damage may indeed be a result of PmpA virulence. Further, it was also reported that women who were sero-positive for PmpI antibodies had a higher incidence of upper genital tract infection (p=0.026). However, antibodies to PmpD and PmpI did not alter the risk of FGT inflammation or sequelae.

One of the most important and common long-term complications of Chlamydial PID is TFI. Numerous studies have demonstrated serological evidence of prior *C. trachomatis* infection is associated with TFI [197-201]. An investigation conducted by the World Health Organisation (1995) of TFI rates as a consequence of *C. trachomatis* or *N. gonorrhoeae*-induced PID showed that *C. trachomatis*-induced PID was associated with a higher incidence of TFI when compared to PID caused by *N. gonorrhoeae*. A retrospective study of 1844 women all laparascopically diagnosed with PID due to *C. trachomatis* showed that 209 (16%) failed to conceive [202]. Of these, confirmed TFI was established in 141 patients with PID. Importantly, the rate of infertility was directly associated with the number and severity of PID infections. Specifically, every subsequent episode of PID approximately doubled the rate of TFI i.e. 8% upon one *C. trachomatis* infection, to 19.5% from two exposures resulting in infection and an increase to 40% resultant from three or more exposures.

In a more recent study that evaluated cHsp60-specific antibody and cell-mediated responses as predictors for TFI [201] it was reported that *C. trachomatis*-specific IgG antibodies were more common in TFI patients (43.2%) when compared to the control group (13.5%), thus suggesting *C. trachomatis* may play a significant pathogenic role in the development of TFI. To elucidate the clinical variability of TFI caused by *C. trachomatis*, functional polymorphisms in various cytokines were assessed [203]. The study showed that allelic variation in IL-10 and TNF-α increased the risk of severe tubal damage in women diagnosed with infertility caused by *C. trachomatis*. Similarly, a more recent study demonstrated that variation in the IL-12B gene was associated with increased susceptibility and TFI severity [204]. Interestingly, polymorphic changes in IL-10 and IFN-g appear to be linked with a more intensive lymphocytic proliferation in response to *C. trachomatis* antigens [205]. Antibody production following cHSP60 exposure was found to be significantly higher in those women (n=21) clinically diagnosed with TFI [206]. Furthermore, elevated antibody levels to caseinolytic protease P, a proteolytic subunit of the ATP-dependent Clp protease complex involved in the degradation of aberrant proteins, was also demonstrated in TFI patients. Serum levels of IgG1 and IgG3 antibodies against chlamydial major outer membrane protein (MOMP) and cHSP60 were shown to be elevated in women (n=70) with TFI compared with the control group (n=92; normal Fallopian tubes and sero-negative for *Chlamydia*) (p=<0.001) [207]. A study that evaluated the potential association of anti-Chlamydial IgM antibodies and TFI showed that of the 50 women assessed, 60% were sero-positive [208]. Of these, 52% presented with bilateral tubal blockage, which was more commonly detected in the ampullary portion (36%) of the Fallopian tube.

4. Immune responses, protection and pathology of chlamydial genital tract infections

Chlamydia (serovars D-K) infects epithelial cells lining the FGT with primary infection establishing in the endocervix [209]. If not controlled, primary infection can ascend the reproductive tract leading to the establishment of infection within the endometrium and Fallopian tubes. The kinetics of ascension of *Chlamydia* to the URT is unclear. Although *Chlamydia* can be transported via attachment onto sperm, the demonstration that small particles (the size of sperm) when deposited into the vaginal vault, rapidly ascend up into the uterus within 2 mins suggests as the general flow of fluids within the FGT may facilitate ascending infection [210, 211. For most women natural immunity appears to take a long time to acquire - if at all. As previously noted in a study by Molano and colleagues, it was demonstrated that 50% of women continue to shed the organism one year after infection is first documented, and 5 to 10% continue shedding even 3 years later [13]. There is limited evidence to suggest that the generation of natural immunity occurs in some individuals. A number of studies have reported that in around 20% of cases, spontaneous resolution of infection occurs [212,213]. As mentioned previously, Giesler and colleagues showed that women with spontaneously resolved genital infections were less likely to be re-infected within twelve months [25]. The host's immune factors associated with the spontaneous resolution of infection are yet to be elucidated. Unfortunately, any natural immunity induced following primary infection appears to be short-lived and serovar-specific resulting in many re-infections [214-217]. Animal models of Chlamydial genital tract infection have shown that the generation of Th1 cell mediated immunity is characterized by a strong IFNγ and TNFα cytokine production and that this strong response is essential for clearance of primary Chlamydial genital infections [218-220]. The observation that B cell deficient mice can resolve a primary infection suggests that antibodies play a non-critical role in protection [100]. However, B cell responses are important in resolving secondary infections. The generation of *Chlamydia* specific antibodies that are able to neutralize bacteria preventing infection have been reported in various cell lines *in vitro* [221-223] and *in vivo* [224]. $CD4^+$ T helper cells induced during primary infection mediate affinity maturation of antibodies, Ig class switching, and B cell memory responses during subsequent infection. Therefore, B cell memory and antibody production in the presence or absence of $CD4^+$ cells is critical for the prevention of *Chlamydia* reinfection [225-227] In addition, results from murine studies show the infiltration of immune cells, including CD8+ T cells, B cells, neutrophils and dendritic cells is associated with clearance both of intracellular and of extracellular Chlamydial bodies [228, 117, 229,230]. Using cytobrush sampling of women, an increase in neutrophils, dendritic cells and lymphocytes (CD4+ and CD8+) was reported during *Chlamydia* infections in these woemn [125,231].

Chlamydia infection of endocervical cells results in an increase in pro-inflammatory cytokine and chemokine production such as IL-1, IL-8, IL-12, IL-6[232, 233, 209]. Live *C. trachomatis* is innately recognized by pattern recognition receptors (PRRs) including Toll-like receptors and nucleotide-binding oligomerization domain (NOD)-like receptors. Both TLR2 and TLR4 are highly expressed in female genital tissues and have shown to be activated by live *Chlamydia* [234]. The myeloid differentiation primary response gene (MyD)88 is essential for nuclear factor–κ-β (NF$\kappa\beta$) signalling and transcription of pro-inflammatory cytokines and along with TLR2, MyD88 has been shown to co-localize within the intracellular Chlamydial inclusion during infection [235]. Mouse TLR2 knockout animals produce lower TNFα and macrophage inflammatory protein-2 (MIP-2) and report a significant decrease on oviduct pathology and hydrosaphinx, suggesting a major role for TLR2 in pathogenesis [236]. The direct activation of another PPR NOD-1 by *Chlamydia* results in the production of IL-8, which is produced at high concentrations during infection and recruit neutrophils to the genital tract [237, 238]. Overall, cytokine production during infection mediates the recruitment of innate immune cells that secrete IFNγ and TNFα. These include natural killer (NK), Dendritic cells and neutrophils [239, 229]. The recruitment of innate immune cells and cytokine production is linked to upper reproductive tract pathology and scaring leading to the development of tubal infertility and ectopic pregnancy. In particular, Hvid and colleagues reported that during a *C.trachomatis* infection the production of IL-1 from Fallopian tubes biopsies led to the destruction ciliated epithelium. Furthermore IL-1 production additionally induced IL-8 production from Fallopian tube epithelial cells thereby potentially meditating the recruitment of neutrophils to this site [232]. The development of a chronic or persistent *Chlamydia* infection would induce continued production of innate immune mediators perpetuating cellular recruitment leading to epithelial damage, scaring and disease. The innate immune cell generation of immunopathogenesis and disease is termed the cellular paradigm [182].

Following clearance of a primary *Chlamydia* infection, re-infections are common in women; moreover, re-infections are strongly associated with development of pathology in these women. Results from animal models of Chlamydial infection have shown that during re-infection T cells are present within the URT at a higher magnitude than in primary infection [240]. *Chlamydia* has shown to act as both an immunizing and sensitizing infection. Non-human primate vaccine trials have shown that immunization with whole cell organisms led to hypersensitivity and an increase immunopathogical response leading to greater scaring in an ocular model. This suggests a specific role for adaptive responses in pathology and this is termed the immunological paradigm. Although the specific mechanism or causative antigen in unknown, it is hypothesized that during re-exposure pathogenesis is associated with either delayed-type hypersentitivity (DTH) or molecular mimicry causing autoimmunity [241]. DTH is hypothesized to be associated with persistent Chlamydial infection. During latent infections, low level antigen specific immune stimulation is believed to contribute to chronic inflammatory cell infiltration [242]. A role for antigenic sensitivity associated with DTH has been observed in animal models. Guinea pigs sensitized with Triton-X-100 soluble EBs and monkeys sensitized through immunization with a whole Chlamydial vaccines both reported the generation greater inflammation and DTH during re-exposure compared to un-sensitized controls [243,244]. In additon to DTH, autoimmunity may play a role in pathogenesis through the mechanism of molecular mimicry. Chlamydial HSP-60 (cHSP60) shares similar homology to self HSP-60 with recent evidence showing that C. trachomatis HSP-60 contains four T-cell epitopes that display identity with human HSP-60 [245, 246].T cell stimulation by self HSP-60 when pre-immunized with cHSP60 is characterized by the production of pro-inflammatory IFN-g. In contrast, pre-immunization and and re-exposure with self HSP60 results in the production of the anti-inflammatory cytokine IL-10 [247] although previous studies have shown that T cells isolated from patients with PID and TFI respond to cHSP-60 stimulation, and the presence of cHSP-60 specific antibodies correlate with the severity of PID and TFI pathology [248,188]. A recent study by Ness *et al.,* showed that increased cHSP60 antibody titres are not associated with the development of PID [249]. Further the presence of strong cHSP60 T cell IFN-g has more recently been shown to predict protection rather than pathology during reinfection [250]. The conflicting association of cHSP60 with protection or pathology is indicative of a balance between specific cell mediated responses leading to protection or pathogy.

Recent evidence has shown that the Chlamydial plasmid may play a role in generating pathology during infection. As mentioned earlier, almost all *C. trachomatis* isolates contain a 7.5 kB cryptic plasmid although plasmid-free isolates have been shown in genital serotypes L2, D and E [43-45]. During infection of mice with plasmid-cured *C. muridarum* strains a strong Th-1 cell response is induced however immune pathology and tissue damge is not observed [41] Further, plasmid cured *C. muridarum or C. trachomatis* strains do not stimulate the production of cytokines though TLR2-dependent activation *in vivo* and *in vitro* respectively [251]. In contrast, Frazer *et al* showed that in the guinea pig model, a plasmid cured *C. caviae* strain both signals through TLR-2 and induced post infection pathology suggesting that the association of the *Chlamydial* plasmid with virulence is not universally conserved among Chlamydial species [252]. Importantly, murine studies have shown that previous infection with plasmid-free is protective against the development of immunopathology with subsequent infection with a virulent strain [41]. This has lead to the use of plasmid-cured strains as attenuated Chlamydial vaccines in mouse and primate models of infection [41, 253].

Overall, the natural history of Chlamydial infections in women varies in which some untreated individuals with untreated infections persist for long periods asymptomatically and progress to cause pathology and disease, while others spontaneously resolve infection. Although the mechanisms are yet to be fully elucidated, there are currently two proposed mechanisms for the development of pathology in the female reproductive tract; the cellular and the immunological paridigms that are associated with innate and adaptive responses respectively. Further, these mechanisms are not mutually exclusive and may both play a role in the development of upper reproductive tract pathology and disease during primary and subsequent infections. The recent identification of plasmid-free strains associated with induced protection against immunopathology may provide a mechanism for immune stimulation leading to pathology and disease.

5. Past and present treatments, how to improve local immunity and future vaccine developments

5.1. Antibiotic treatment

Chlamydia infection of the FGT is largely asymptomatic with approximately 80% of women observing no reported symptoms [254]. Whilst there are no specific genital symptoms associated with Chlamydial cervical infection, 37% of women who develop cervicitis observe mucopurulent discharge and in 19%, hypertrophic ectopy (Distinctive oedema of the columnar epithelium in the female endocervix) [29, 62, 255]. Due to the asymptomatic nature of infection in the reproductive tract many infections remain undetected and therefore, untreated. Chlamydial infections, if symptomatic, can be treated through the administration of antibiotics. The current recommended antibiotic for treatment are either a single dose (1g) azithromycin or 7 day treatment with doxycycline (2x100mg per day)[256]. Other drug treatment programs used to treat *Chlamydia* infections in humans include erythromycin base, (4x500mg per day for 7 days), or erythromycin ethylsuccinate (4x800mg per day for seven days).

Erythromycin is effective against *Chlamydia* infection in the FRT however its use is associated side effects that may limit compliance [256]. Likewise, Levofloxacin (1x500mg per day for 7 days) and ofloxacin (2x300mg per day for 7 days) are effective for treating *Chlamydia* infections but are expensive compared to other alternatives [256]. Following antibiotic treatment it is recommended that treated persons abstain from sexual intercourse for 7 days to prevent spreading the infection to partners which may lead to subsequent re-infections [41]. Partner notification and partner treatment are also important targets to halt re-infections.

Although antibiotics are an effective treatment option, they have been shown to be less effective in cases of well-established chronic Chlamydial infections. Early reports determined that the current treatment of azithromycin and doxycycline are more that 95% effective at clearing *Chlamydia* genital tract infection [257, 259]. However, recent strong evidence suggests that antibiotic treatment failure could be greater than the 5% previously reported when accounting for re-infection [260]. A major hurdle in measuring the rates of antibiotic treatment failure is the inability to distinguish between recurrent infections and re-infection from infected untreated or new sexual partners [261]. Discrepancies in the proportion of treatment failures have been directly associated with testing methods used. Most of the published work investigating treatment failure involved tissue culture as a means to detect infection, which has now been predominately replaced with nucleic acid amplification testing (NAAT). Tissue culture is less sensitive and has shown to be less effective at identifying small numbers of persistent bacteria leading to an over estimation of successful *Chlamydia* eradication following treatment [257,262]. In a recent study by Batteiger *et al* (2010) investigating post treatment infection in adolescent girls, it was observed that 7.9% of those sampled developed recurrent infections following azithromycin treatment which was not attributed to reinfection [263]. Similarly, Goldern et al (2005) study in women without the risk for re-infection showed a recurring infection rate of 8% following azithromycin at 3-19 week follow-up representing treatment failure.[264]. Current studies argue that previous rates of antibiotic treatment failure of less than 5% were underestimated due to the available information at the time and that a true rate of treatment failure of may be greater than 8%. One major concern associated with increasing antibiotic failure is the development of antibiotic resistance. However, unlike other organisms such as *Staphylococcus,* to date there is no evidence of natural and stable antibiotic homotypic resistance (genetically inherited) *in vivo* in Chlamydial strains collected from human genital tract infections [265].

Contributing to antibiotic treatment failure in *Chlamydia* infections is the phenomenon called heterotrophic antimicrobial resistance. Heterotrophic resistance refers to the replication of heterogeneous population containing both resistant and susceptible bacteria from a subculture of a single resistant organism propagated on antimicrobial-containing medium, that is not genetically inherited [266]. It is hypothesized that at high bacterial loads a small population of *Chlamydia* organisms survive, potentially due to an innate ability to establish a latent/persistent infection [266]. Importantly these isolates at low loads do not show altered antibiotic susceptibility or increased resistance due to genetic changes [267]. Latent, non-replicating, non-infectious aberrant RBs associated with persistence can survive within host cells for extended periods of time at which infectious organism can not be isolated or able to be cultured.

However, latent bodies can revert to infectious organisms leading to a recurrent infection. *In vivo* persistent infections in women are supported by the observation that some positive samples obtained using *Chlamydia*-specific DNA or antigen specific testing do not report the presence live infectious EBs via cell culture [268-270]. Furthermore, alternating infectious and persistent phases of Chlamydial growth correlate with acute and chronic infections *in vivo* [271]. During Chlamydial infection in women, a large variation in bacterial load has been observed in the genital tract and antibiotic failure due to heterotrophic resistance is associated with high bacterial loads [272, 273]. West *et al* (2005) showed that 91% of individuals with a low load at baseline observed no infection at follow up (2 months), whereas 74% percent of individuals with high bacterial load reported no follow up infection [274]. The development of persistent bodies *in vivo* during high bacterial load may be an important mechanism driving antibiotic failure, as these slow growing aberrant forms of *Chlamydia* may be less susceptible to antibiotic therapy. *In vitro* studies have shown that antibiotic treatment directly induces the presence of non-cultivable *Chlamydia* that can be reactivated with the withdrawal of treatment. *In vivo* the re-emergence of the active infectious form from persistence may take a number of weeks or months in which previous short term (<3 weeks) follow up testing via culture methods would provide a false negative result. Likewise false positive results may arise post-treatment due to persistent DNA detected through NAAT testing [275]. As such, one recommendation is that follow up screening > 5weeks post treatment is implemented for screening programs to determine treatment failure [259]. Estimating a true rate of treatment failures is complicated as many re-current infections remain unreported due to the asymptomatic nature of infections coupled with a lack of follow up testing in many screening and treatment programs.

5.2. Are screening and treatment programs leading to arrested *Chlamydia* immunity?

In many western countries, screening and antibiotic treatment programs for early detection of *Chlamydia* have been implemented over the past ten years. The goal of these programs is to reduce *Chlamydia* transmission leading to the long-term prevention of disease sequelae, including PID and infertility. *Chlamydia* infections are most common among young people accounting for approximately 80% of all infections. The United States Center for Disease Control (US CDC) estimates that in the United States alone, one in 15 sexually active females aged 14-19 years has *Chlamydia*. Due to this high burden, the US CDC recommends annual screening for all sexually-active women under 26 years of age [276]. As such, most programs have been specifically targeted towards young women with a focus to identify and treat asymptomatic infections. In addition, these programs seek to promote partner notification and treatment to prevent subsequent re-infection. Although screening and treatment programs coupled with aggressive education and health programs have been implemented in many countries for over a decade, *Chlamydia* rates have continued to increase. For example, the US CDC reported an increase of 9.7% of *Chlamydial* infections between 2007 and 2008 [277]. This increasing trend has also be reported in many countries where long term screening and treatment programs have been in place including Sweden, Canada, the United Kingdom and Australia [278-281. Interpreting this increased prevalence or incidence of *Chlamydia* in the population requires caution and some argue that increases are directly associated with increased testing rates and detection associate with easy home sampling and the development of the more sensitive nuclear acid amplification test in the 1990's.

However, it has been hypothesized that an increase in *Chlamydia* prevalence worldwide at a time of aggressive screening and testing programs is associated with 'arrested immune hypothesis' [24]. The 'arrested immune hypothesis' states that early detection and treatment of *Chlamydia* actually impairs the development of natural immunity in these antibiotic treated individuals. A recent study by Giesler *et al* (2013) supports the concept of antibiotic treatment may attenuate protective immunity against reinfection. This work showed that women with spontaneous resolution of *Chlamydia* infection were four times less likely to be re-infected compared to women with infections cleared by azithromycin treatment [25]. The potential hampering of protective immunity development through antibiotic treatment is believed to be the associated an increased *Chlamydia* re-infections. In the province of British Columbia, Canada, *Chlamydia* screening and treatment programs have been in place since 1991. Here they have reported a 5% increase in the re-infection rate over the course of the program [282]. Moreover, re-infection rates were reported to be greatest in young women and potential increased risk of development Chlamydial disease sequelae. The emergence of antibiotic resistant organisms, development of persistence, poor patient compliance and high re-infection rates has highlighted the need for an efficacious vaccine to halt the spread of infection throughout the population.

5.3. Chlamydia vaccine development

The development of an efficacious vaccine is the greatest potential to prevent infection and the subsequent development of disease. According to the World Health Organization a vaccine for the common STI "would have a significant impact on the spread of the disease". An ideal prophylactic Chlamydial vaccine would target immune responses to each of the two stages of the Chlamydial life cycle; (1) Antibodies directed against infectious extracellular elementary bodies preventing cell-adhesion; and (2) T cell mediated immune responses targeting infection cells during early to mid Chlamydial replication. Both responses require the activation of CD4-T cells, which have been shown through mouse models to be essential for clearing *Chlamydia* in the genital tract [283]. A number of considerations are required when designing vaccines; choice of antigen and adjuvant, administration route, the potential target of the vaccine (who to vaccinate?) and the purpose of the vaccine, prophylactic or therapeutic.

Early attempts in the 1950's and 1960's to develop a Chlamydial vaccine were based on the Pasteurian principle of isolate, inactivate and inject [284].However, although this has been a useful principle in the development of vaccine for veterinary field leading to a commercial vaccine for feline Chlamydial infections [285] a human whole-cell vaccine has been unsuccessful. Although crude whole cell vaccine trials in against ocular Trachoma in humans had observed short-term protection in 70% of vaccinated individuals, the development of strong pro-inflammatory immune responses to bacterial components led to adverse side effects in vaccinated individuals. Furthermore, vaccine trials using primates reported the generation of hypersensitivity leading to increased inflammation and extensive ocular scarring in vaccine recipients therefore whole *Chlamdyia* vaccine trials in humans subsequently were abandoned

[286]. This work suggested that specific antigens within the *Chlamydia* proteome are associated with protection while others mediate immunopathology that may be shared between Chlamydial strains. The recent development of genomic and proteomic technology has provided an unbiased approach to antigen discovery for the generation of a sub-unit *Chlamydia* vaccine [287]. Antigen discovery approaches have included; (1) 2D gel elctrophoresis combined with immunoblotting or radio-immunprecipitation for the discovery of antibody specific antigens [288-290]; (2) Genome-wide protein expression to discover both antibody and T cell antigens [291]; (3) Antigen discovery using of T cell clone lines [292] and; (4) Immunoproteomic approach to identify peptides presented to CD4+ T cells on class II MHC molecules [293].

Sub-unit vaccines provide safer alternatives to whole cell preparations and a number of *Chlamydia* antigen candidates have been investigated [294]. A number of antigens have been used unsuccessfully in animal trials that include cHsp60 and Chlamydial lipopolysaccharide (cLPS). Chlamydial Hsp60 is an important pathogenicity factor for the development of human Chlamydial infection-associated disease sequelae [295]. Although *Chlamydia* specific immunity is generated, cHsp60 as an antigen was associated with the induction of inflammation limiting the potential as a vaccine antigen. Chlamydial LPS was a prime antigen candidate due to its localization to the outer cell membrane. Unfortunately, immunization with LPS does not induce the production either of post-immunization or of post-infection antibodies and does not confer protection following live bacterial challenge in primate ocular infection models [296]. Immunization with surface exposed membrane proteins have proved more successful in animal models. These include the Chlamydial major outer membrane protein (MOMP) and the polymorphic membrane protein family (Pmps). The 40kDa MOMP constitutes 50-60% of the outer membrane of the bacterium [297-299]. To date, Chlamydial MOMP has been the leading vaccine antigen candidate investigated in animal models, including non-human primate models. Within the many serovars of the *C. trachomatis* species a large amount of primary structural homology is observed, however, antigenic properties of MOMP are related to the serovar specific surface exposed variable domain (VD) regions. For example, serological studies have shown cross reactivity between the Chlamydial L2 and D serovars, but the G, H and I serovars differ significantly [300]. Therefore the use of Chlamydial MOMP from one serovar results in only serovar-specific immunity and this alone is not sufficient for an effective, protective, multi-serovar vaccine. Combining multiple MOMP proteins from specific serovars in a multi sub-unit vaccine may potentially protect against the most common human genital tract infections. Recently with the aid of immunproteomics Brunham and colleagues identified the expression of several Pmps which when used in mouse *C. muridarum* infection model led to the production of neutralizing antibodies *in vitro* and partial protective immunity *in vivo* [301, 302]. Pmp antigens have also been reported to be immunogenic in human infections [303]. In contrast to EB membrane-bound antigens, Chlamydial secreted proteins have been used as antigen targets. During intracellular *Chlamydia* replication, proteins are secreted from the inclusion body into the host cytosol and may therefore be available for processing and packaging on MHC molecules, thus specifically inducing T cell immunity. The secreted proteins known as Inclusion proteins (Inc) and Chlamydial proteasome/protease-like activity factor (CPAF) have been shown to be potential vaccine targets in mouse models [304, 305]. During Chlamydial infection of humans, both CPAF and Inc antigen specific responses are observed supporting their potential as antigens in a human vaccine [305, 306] [305]. A number of Chlamydial antigens trialled as vaccine candidates have recently been reviewed by Hafner et *al.* [27].

Although sub-unit vaccines provide safer alternatives to the use of live or attenuated organisms, they are poorly immunogenic. Adjuvants are required to direct the immune response to a co-administrated antigen. For *Chlamydia*, a balance of Th2 driven neutralizing antibodies and Th1 cytokine production characterized by strong IFN-g within the FGT mucosae is required. A number of adjuvants have been developed for use experimentally in trials for Chlamydial vaccines. These include live viral vectors [307], immunostimulating complexes such as DDA and ISCOMs [308, 309, liposomes [310], detergent/surfactant-based adjuvants [311, Lipid formulations [312,313, *Vibrio cholerae* ghosts [314, unmethylated 1.7.4.1CPG-ODN bacterial motifs [308,222] and cytokines [315]. In addition to antigen and adjuvant combinations, the route of immunization is an important component of vaccination strategies. Historically most vaccines are delivered through injection that is either sub-cutaneous (S.C) or intra-muscular (I.M). Although effective in generating strong systemic immunity, the generation of mucosal immunity has shown to be varied and limited when using systemic immunization routes. However, these methods have shown in animal models to generate partial protection against *Chlamydia* infections. A recent study by Eko et al. (2011) using I.M. vaccination of *Chlamydia* antigens expressed by Vibrio Cholerae Ghosts (VVG) has shown to be effective in reducing the duration of infection in mice; however, sterilizing immunity was not observed in this trial [316]. Another approach is targeting the mucosal immune system directly with needle free mucosal routes. Not only are mucosal immunization regimes able to generate immunity and multiple mucosal surfaces, the needle free nature of delivery has the advantage of being safe and inexpensive to deliver. Immunization with candidate Chlamydial vaccines via mucosal routes such as oral [312], intranasal [223,317], intravaginal [318 and transcutaneous [222,223,313] have shown to target protective immunity in the female reproductive tract; again, however sterilizing immunity has not yet been achieved using these vaccine approaches.

Over the past 60 years since the first crude whole cell Chlamydial vaccines were investigated, a number of technologies such as gemomic sequencing have enhanced the forward movement of the development of a protective Chlamydial vaccine. In light of the continued increased infection and re-infection rates, even with aggressive screening and treatment programs, the need for an efficacious Chlamydial vaccine is essential. Mathematical modeling that simulates transmission of *Chlamydia* in a heterosexual population has been developed to determine the impact of an efficacious vaccine regime [319]. The model tracks the infection time course, disease progression, and dynamic infectiousness of infected individuals and the transmission to others. This model determined that a fully protective vaccine administered prior to sexual debut could eradicate Chlamydial epidemics within 20 years. Furthermore, the specific targeting of women (100% vaccine coverage) would have an increased impact in reducing epidemiology than vaccination 50% of the male and female population together. However, currently no vaccine has been shown to generate sterilizing immunity. Modelling reports that in the absence of a sterilizing vaccine, a *Chlamydia* vaccine effective for at least 10 years would provide order to lead to population-level eradication. Furthermore, a non-sterilizing vaccine could protect individuals by raising the infectiousness threshold and secondary reduce the peak load and the duration of the infection in vaccinated individuals. Animal models have shown that some experimental vaccines, although not producing sterilizing immunity in these models, may reduce the development of pathology e.g. hydrosalphinx in the murine model. This suggests that a therapeutic vaccine could potentially be given to women a past or even current infection to prevent the development of pathology. Although little work has been undertaken in this area, Carey et al. reported that in the mouse *C. muridarum* model vaccination during or after infection reduction in the strength of the immune response was observed. This work demonstrates that a therapeutic vaccine could be used to limit an uncontrolled host response leading to immunopathology during re-infection [320]. In light of the fact that there currently is no vaccine to prevent Chlamydial genital tract infections in women we believe that a vaccine designed to reduce bacterial burden and prevent disease may be a more rational target for future research.

6. Summary/conclusions

In this Chapter we have presented current knowledge of immune regulation during infections of the female genital tract caused by the intracellular bacterial pathogen, *Chlamydia trachomatis*. Our review has highlighted the following information regarding Chlamydial infections of the FGT:

- Tubal infertility and reproductive damage, preeclampsia and preterm births may potentially occur in many of the 50 million women who are annually infected with *Chlamydia trachomatis*
- Gynecological cancer development is also suggested to be linked with Chlamydial genital tract infections.
- The majority (70-80%) of genital tract infections in women are asymptomatic
- The annual direct medical cost of sexually transmitted diseases (including *Chlamydia* and those caused by HIV) has been estimated at $US16.9 billion
- Urogenital isolates of *C.trachomatis* may also contain a highly conserved 7.5kB non-integrative plasmid that has a role in the pathobiology of these organisms
- *Chlamydia* infections of neonates have been reported to be at 18 percent for ophthalmia neonatorum and 16 percent for pneumonia for infants exposed to *C. trachomatis* in vaginal secretions in the birth canal
- The host inflammatory response to *C.trachomatis* is involved in immunity but also the pathology that leads to serious morbidities of chronic pelvic pain, EP and tubal infertility following female genital tract infection
- Disease outcomes are dependent upon the complex interactions between virulence factors of, and evasion strategies used by, *C.trachomatis* and host immune responses including variants in genetic markers associated with infection and inflammation

- It is becoming increasingly well documented that sex hormones E2 and P4 regulate host susceptibility, as well as innate and adaptive immune responses to the sexually transmitted pathogen *Chlamydia* infecting the mucosal surfaces of the FGT
- In light of the continued increase in infection and re-infection rates even with aggressive screening and treatment programs, a need for an efficacious vaccine is essential.
- Finally, since there currently is no vaccine to prevent Chlamydial genital tract infections we consider that a vaccine designed to reduce bacterial burden and prevent disease pathology may be a rational target for future Chlamydial research.

Author details

Louise M. Hafner, Trudi A. Collet and Danica K. Hickey

Institute of Health and Biomedical Innovation, (IHBI), Queensland University of Technology (QUT), Australia

References

[1] Stamm WE. *Chlamydia trachomatis* infections: progress and problems.J Infect Dis. 1999;179 Suppl 2:S380-3.

[2] Starnbach MN, Roan NR. Conquering sexually transmitted diseases. Nature Reviews Immunology 2008; 8(4):313-317.

[3] Haggerty, C.L., Panum, I., Uldum, S.A., Bass, D.C., Olsen, J., Darville, T., Eastman, J.M., Simhan, H.N., Roberts, J.M., Ness, R.B. *Chlamydia trachomatis* infection may increase the risk of preeclampsia. Pregnancy Hypertension: An International Journal of Women's Cardiovascular Health, 2013; 3:28-33.

[4] Rours GI, Duijts L, Moll HA, Arends LR, de Groot R, Jaddoe VW, Hofman A, Steegers EA, Mackenbach JP, Ott A, Willemse HF, van der Zwaan EA, Verkooijen RP, Verbrugh HA. *Chlamydia trachomatis* infection during pregnancy associated with preterm delivery: a population-based prospective cohort study. Eur J Epidemiol. 2011a;26(6): 493-502.

[5] Ferreira, V.H., Nazli, A., Khan, G., et al. Endometrial epithelial cell responses to coinfecting viral and bacterial pathogens in the genital tract can activate the HIV-1 LTR in an NF{kappa}B-and AP1-dependent manner. J Infect Dis. 2011; 204(2):299-308.

[6] Schust, D.J., Ibana, JA., Buckner, LR., Ficarra, M., Sugimoto, J., Amedee, AM and Quayle AJ Potential mechanisms for increased HIV-1 transmission across the endocervical epithelium during *C.trachomatis* infection. Curr HIV Res, 2012; 10(3): 218-27.

[7] Madeleine, M., Anttila, T., Schwartz, S. et al. Risk of cervical cancer associated with *Chlamydia trachomatis* antibodies by histology, HPV type and HPV cofactors Int J Cancer 2007; 120(3): 650-655.

[8] Deluca GD, Basiletti J, Schelover E, Vásquez ND, Alonso JM, Marín HM, Lucero RH, Picconi MA. *Chlamydia trachomatis* as a probable cofactor in human papillomavirus infection in aboriginal women from northeastern Argentina. Braz J Infect Dis. 2011; 15(6):567-72.

[9] Shanmughapriya S, Senthilkumar G, Vinodhini K, Das BC, Vasanthi N, Natarajaseenivasan K. Viral and bacterial aetiologies of epithelial ovarian cancer. Eur J Clin Microbiol Infect Dis. 2012;31(9):2311-7.

[10] Idahl A, Lundin E, Jurstrand M, Kumlin U, Elgh F, Ohlson N, Ottander U. *Chlamydia trachomatis* and *Mycoplasma genitalium* plasma antibodies in relation to epithelial ovarian tumors. Infect Dis Obstet Gynecol. 2011; Volume 2011, Article ID 824627, 10 pages. doi:10.1155/2011/824627.

[11] Chumduri C, Gurumurthy RK, Zadora PK, Mi Y, Meyer TF. *Chlamydia* infection promotes host DNA damage and proliferation but impairs the DNA damage response. Cell Host Microbe. 2013;13(6):746-758.

[12] Padberg I, Janßen S, Meyer TF. *Chlamydia trachomatis* inhibits telomeric DNA damage signaling via transient hTERT upregulation. I Int J Med Microbiol. 2013 pii: S1438-4221(13)00080-5. doi: 10.1016/j.ijmm.2013.06.001.

[13] Molano M, Meijer CJ, Weiderpass E, Arslan A, Posso H, Franceschi S, et al. The natural course of *Chlamydia trachomatis* infection in asymptomatic Colombian women: a 5-year follow-up study. J Infect Dis 2005;191:907-16.

[14] Stamm WE. *Chlamydia trachomatis* infections: progress and problems. J Infect Dis. 1999;179 Suppl 2:S380-3.

[15] Stamm WE. Lymphogranuloma venereum. In: Holmes KK, Sparling FP, Mardh PA, (editors). Sexually Transmitted Diseases. 4th ed: McGraw Hill Professional; 2008. p. 505-605.

[16] Hafner L. M. and Pelzer, E.S.Tubal Damage, Infertility and Tubal Ectopic Pregnancy: *Chlamydia trachomatis* and Other Microbial Aetiologies, Ectopic Pregnancy - Modern Diagnosis and Management, Dr. Michael Kamrava (Ed.), ISBN: 978-953-307-648-5, Rijeka:InTech, 2011 DOI: 10.5772/21555. Available from: http://www.intechopen.com/books/ectopic-pregnancy-modern-diagnosis-and-management/tubal-damage-infertility-and-tubal-ectopic-pregnancy-*Chlamydia-trachomatis*-and-other-microbial-aetio (acessed 14 September, 2013)

[17] Haggerty CL, Gottlieb SL, Taylor BD, Low N, Xu F, Ness RB. Risk of sequelae after *Chlamydia trachomatis* genital infection in women. J Infect Dis. 2010 ;201 Suppl 2:S134-55.

[18] RoursIG, Hammerschlag, MR., Ott,A., DeFaber, TJ, VerbrughHA, deGroot R et al.*Chlamydia trachomatis* as a cause of neonatal conjunctivitis in Dutch infants. Pediatrics 2008; 121:e321-326.

[19] Rours, GI, Hammerschlag, MR, Van Doornum, GJ, Hop WC, de Groot, R, Willemse HF et al., *Chlamydia* trachomais respiratory infection in Dutch infants. Arch Dis Child. 2009; 94: 705-707.

[20] World Health Organization. Global prevalence and incidence of selected curable sexually transmitted infections. Geneva: World Health Organization,2008.

[21] Chesson, H. W., Gift, T. L., Owusu-Edusei, K. Jr., et al. A Brief Review of the Estimated Economic Burden of Sexually Transmitted Diseases in the United States: Inflation-Adjusted Updates of Previously Published Cost Studies Sexually Transmitted Diseases 2011; 38(10): 889-891.

[22] Reckart,M.L., Gilbert, M., Meza, R., Kim, P.H., Chang, M., Money, D.M. and Brunham, RC. *Chlamydia* public health programs and the epidemiology of pelvic inflammatory disease and ectopic pregnancy. J.Infect.Dis., 2013; 207: 30-8.

[23] Centers for Disease Control (CDC) Sexually disease treatment guidelines. MMWR Moribid Mortal Wkly Rep. 2006 51:1-78.

[24] Brunham, RC and Reckart ML. The arrested immunity hypothesis and the epidemiology of *Chlamydia* control. Sex. Transm. Dis.2008; 35: 53-54.

[25] Geisler, W.M., Lensing, S.Y., Press, C.G., and Hook, E.W. Spontaneous resolution of genital *Chlamydia trachomatis* infection in women and protection from re-infection. J. Infect. Dis.2013; 207: 1850-6.

[26] World Health Organisation (WHO) Initiative for Vaccine Research. SexuallyTransmitted Diseases. *Chlamydia trachomatis.*WorldHealthOrganisation.Available at http://www.who.int/vaccine_research/diseases/soa_std/en/index1.html (accessed September 1, 2013).

[27] Hafner LM, Wilson DP, Timms P. Development status and future prospects for a vaccine against *Chlamydia trachomatis* infection. Vaccine. 2013b doi:pii: S0264-410X(13)01111-0. 10.1016/j.vaccine.2013.08.020.

[28] Elwell, C. A., Jiang, S., Kim, J.H., et al. *Chlamydia trachomatis* Co-opts GBF1 and CERT to Acquire Host Sphingomyelin for Distinct Roles during Intracellular Development PLoS Pathog. 2011: 7(9):e1002198.

[29] Stamm, W. E. *Chlamydia trachomatis* infections in adults. In: Holmes KK, Sparling PF, Mardh, P-A et al., (editors). Sexually Transmitted Diseases. 4th edition. New York, NY McGraw-Hill Companies Inc. 2008. 575-594.

[30] Collingro, A., Tischler, P., Weinmaier, T., Penz, T., Heinz, E., Brunham, R.C., Read, TD., Bavoil, PM., Saschse, K., Kahane, S., et al., Unity in variety-the pan-genome of the Chlamydiae. Molec. Biol Evol. 2011; 28: 3253-3270.

[31] Hammerschlag, M.R. The intracellular life of Chlamydiae. Semin Pediatr Infect Dis. 2002; 13(4):239-48.

[32] Stephens, R.S., Wagar, E.A. and Schoolnik, G.K. High-resolution mapping of serovar-specific and common antigenic determinants of the major outer membrane protein of *Chlamydia trachomatis*. J.Exp.Med.1988; 167:817-831.

[33] Stephens, R.S., Sanchez-Pescador, R., Wager, E., et al. Diversity of the major outer membrane proteins of *Chlamydia trachomatis*. J. Bacteriol.,1987;169:3879-3885.

[34] Stephens, R.S., Myers, G., Eppinger, M. et al.Divergence without difference: phylogenetics and taxonomy of *Chlamydia* resolved. FEMS immunology and medical microbiology 2009; 55: 115-119.

[35] Bush, R. M. and Everett, K.D.Molecular evolution of Chlamydiaceae. Int J Syst Evol Microbiol. 2001; 51:203-220

[36] Schachter, J., Stephens, R.S, Timms, P. et al. Radical changes to Chlamydial taxonomy are not necessary just yet. Int J Syst Evol Microbiol 2001; 51:251-253,

[37] Caldwell, H.D., Wood, H., Crane, D., et al. Polymorphisms in *Chlamydia trachomatis* tryptophan synthase genes differentiate between genital and ocular isolates. J Clin Invest.2003; 111:1757–69.

[38] Thomas NS, Lusher M, Storey CC & Clarke IN. Plasmid diversity in *Chlamydia*.Microbiol.1997; 143 (Pt 6): 1847-1854.

[39] Rockey, D.D Unravelling the basic biology and clinical significance of the Chlamydial plasmid J. Exp. Med.2011; 208(11): 2159-2162.

[40] Russell, M., T. Darville, K. Chandra-Kuntal, B. Smith, C.W. Andrews Jr., and C.M. O'Connell. Infectivity acts as in *vivo* selection for maintenance of the Chlamydial cryptic plasmid. Infect. Immun.2011; 79:98–107.

[41] O'Connell, C.M., Ingalls, R.R., Andrews, C.W. Jr, et al. Plasmid deficient *Chlamydia muridarum* fails to induce immune pathology and protect against oviduct disease. J Immunol.2007; 179: 4027–4034.

[42] Ripa, T., Nilsson, P. A variant of *Chlamydia trachomatis* with deletion in cryptic plasmid: implications for use of PCR diagnostic tests. Eur Sureveill 2006; 11: E061109.

[43] Farencena, A., M. Comanducci, M. Donati, G. Ratti, and R. Cevenini. Characterization of a new isolate of *Chlamydia trachomatis* which lacks the common plasmid and has properties of biovar trachoma. Infect. Immun.1997; 65:2965-2969.

[44] Peterson, E. M., B. A. Markoff, J. Schachter, and L. M. De La Maza. The 7.5-kbplasmid present in *Chlamydia trachomatis* is not essential for the growth of this microorganism. Plasmid 1990; 23:144-148

[45] Stothard, D. R., J. A. Williams, B. Van Der Pol, and R. B. Jones. Identification of a *Chlamydia trachomatis* serovar E urogenital isolate which lacks the cryptic plasmid. Infect. Immun. 1998; 66:6010-6013.

[46] Sigar,I.M., Justin H. Schripsema, Yibing Wang, Ian N. Clarke, Lesley T. Cutcliffe, Helena M.B. Seth-Smith, Nicholas R. Thomson, Carina Bjartling, Magnus Unemo, Kenneth Persson and Kyle H. Ramsey. Plasmid deficiency in urogenital isolates of *Chlamydia trachomatis* reduces infectivity and virulence in a mouse model. Pathogens and Disease. Accepted manuscript online: 23 AUG 2013 09:02AM EST | DOI: 10.1111/2049-632X.12086

[47] Hatch, TP Developmental biology. In: RS Stephens, (ed.) *Chlamydia*: Intracellular biology, pathogenesis, and immunity. American Society for Microbiology, Washington, DC. 1999 p 29-68.

[48] Schachter, J. and Stephens, R.S. Biology of *Chlamydia trachomatis*. In: Sexually Transmitted Diseases. 4th edition. Edited by: Holmes KK, Sparling PF, Stamm WE, Piot P, Wasserheit JN, Corey L, Cohen MS, Watts C. The McGraw-Hill Companies.New York; 2008 p555-574.

[49] Schoborg, R.V.*Chlamydia* persistence – a tool to dissect *Chlamydia*-host interactions. Microb. and Infect.2011; 13: 649-662.

[50] Hafner, L.M. and Timms, P. *Chlamydia* In: Stanberry, L.R. and Rosenthal, S. L (eds.) Sexually Transmitted Diseases, 2nd edition, Elsevier (Academic Press) Ltd., Waltham, MA, USA, 2013: p369-410.

[51] Saka, H.A., and Valdivia, R.H.Acquisition of nutrients by Chlamydiae: unique challenges of living in an intracellular compartment. Curr Opin Microbiol.2010; 13(1): 4-10.

[52] Abdelrahman, Y.M. and Belland, R.J.The Chlamydial developmental cycle. FEMS Microbiol.Rev.2005; 29, 949-959.

[53] Hackstadt, T., Fischer, ER., Scidmore MA, Rockey DD, Heinzen RA. Origins and functions of the Chlamydial inclusion. Trends in Microbiol.1997; 5: 288-293.

[54] Wyrick, P.B. *Chlamydia trachomatis* persistence *in vitro*: an overview.J Infect Dis. 2010;201 Suppl 2:S88-95.

[55] Brunham, RC and Rey-Ladino,J. Immunology of *Chlamydia* infection: implications for a *Chlamydia trachomatis* vaccine. Nature Rev. Immunol. 2005; 5(2):149–61.

[56] Zhong G, Liu L, Fan T, Fan P, Ji H. Degradation of transcription factor RFX5 during the inhibition of both constitutive and interferon gamma-inducible major histocom-

patibility complex class I expression in *Chlamydia*-infected cells. J Exp Med. 2000;191(9):1525-34.

[57] Ibana, JA, Schust, DJ, Sugimato, J., Nagamatsu, T., Greene, SJ. and Quayle, AJ *Chlamydia trachomatis* Immune Evasion via Downregulation of MHC Class I Surface Expression Involves Direct and Indirect Mechanisms 2011 Inf Dis. Obstet. Gynecol. Volume 2011, Article ID 420905, 8 pages doi:10.1155/2011/420905

[58] Bastidas, R.J., Elwell,C.A., Joanne N. Engel J.N., and Raphael H. Valdivia, R.H. Chlamydial Intracellular Survival Strategies Cold Spring Harb Perspect Med. 2013: doi: 10.1101/cshperspect.a010256.

[59] Betts, H.J., Wolf, K., and Fields, K.A. Effector protein modulation of host cells:examples in the *Chlamydia* spp. Arsenal. Curr. Opin. Microbiol. 2009; 12: 81-87.

[60] Dunn, J.D. and Valdivia, R.H. (2010).Uncivil engineers: *Chlamydia*, Salmonella and Shigella alter cytoskeleton architecture to invade epithelial cells.Fut. Microbiol.2010; 5(8):1219-1232

[61] Soupene, E., Rothschild, J., Kuypers, F.A. and Dean, D. Eukaryotic protein recruitment into the *Chlamydia* inclusion: Implications for survival and growth. PLoS ONE 2012; 7(5): : e36843. Doi: 10.1371/journal.pone.0036843

[62] .Brunham, R., Paavonen, J., Stevens, C.E. et al. Mucopurulent cervicitis – the ignored counterpart in women of urethritis in men. New Eng. J. Med.1984; 311: 1-6.

[63] Marrazzo, J.M., and Martin DH. Management of women with cervicitis. Clin Infect Dis.2007; 44 (Suppl 3):S102-10.

[64] Falk, L. The overall agreement of proposed definitions of mucopurulent cervicitis in women at high risk of Chlamydial infection Acta Derm Venereol, 2010; 90: 506-511.

[65] Lusk, M. J. and Konecny, P. Cervicitis: a review.Curr.Opin.Infect.Dis.2008; 21: 49-55.

[66] Falk, L., Fredlund, H., and Jensen, J.S. Signs and symptoms of urethritis andcervicitis among women with or without Mycoplasma genitalium or *Chlamydia trachomatis* infection. Sex. Trans. Infect. 2005; 81:73-78.

[67] Carvalho JP, Carvalho FM. Is *Chlamydia*-infected tubal fimbria the origin of ovarian cancer? Med Hypotheses. 2008; 71(5):690-3.

[68] Diniz PM, Carvalho JP, Baracat EC, Carvalho FM. Fallopian tube origin of supposed ovarian high-grade serous carcinomas. Clinics (Sao Paulo). 2011; 66(1):73-6.

[69] Taylor-Robinson D, Stacey CM, Jensen JS, Thomas BJ, Munday PE. Further observations, mainly serological, on a cohort of women with or without pelvic inflammatory disease. Int J STD AIDS. 2009 (10):712-8.

[70] World Health Organisation (WHO). Sexually transmitted infections, Fact sheet No. 110, 2011

[71] Bakken IJ and Ghaderi S. Incidence of pelvic inflammatory disease in a large cohort of women tested for *Chlamydia trachomatis*: a historical follow-up study. BMC Infect Dis.2009; 9:130 http://www.biomedcentral.com/1471-2334/9/130

[72] Price MJ, Ades AE, De Angelis D, Welton NJ, Macleod J, Soldan K, Simms I, Turner K, Horner PJ. Risk of Pelvic Inflammatory Disease Following *Chlamydia trachomatis* Infection: Analysis of Prospective Studies With a Multistate Model. Am J Epidemiol. 2013;178(3):484-92.

[73] Shaw JL, Wills GS, Lee KF, Horner PJ, McClure MO, Abrahams VM, Wheelhouse N, Jabbour HN, Critchley HO, Entrican G, Horne AW. *Chlamydia trachomatis* infection increases fallopian tube PROKR2 via TLR2 and NFκB activation resulting in a microenvironment predisposed to ectopic pregnancy. Am J Pathol. 2011;178(1):253-60.

[74] Bebear C, de Barbeyrac B. Genital *Chlamydia trachomatis* infections. Clin Microbiol Infect.2009; 15:4-10.

[75] Shao R, Wang X, Wang W, Stener-Victorin E, Mallard C, Brännström M, Billig H.From mice to women and back again: causalities and clues for *Chlamydia*-induced tubal ectopic pregnancy. Fertil Steril. 2012;98(5):1175-85.

[76] Ness RB, Smith KJ, Chang CC, Schisterman EF, Bass DC; Gynecologic Infection Follow-Through, GIFT, Investigators. Prediction of pelvic inflammatory disease among young, single, sexually-active women. Sex Transm Dis. 2006; 33(3):137-42.

[77] Haggerty CL, Gottlieb SL, Taylor BD, Low N, Xu F, Ness RB. Risk of sequelae after *Chlamydia trachomatis* genital infection in women. J Infect Dis. 2010 15;201 Suppl 2:S134-55.

[78] Hillis SD, Owens LM, Marchbanks PA, Amsterdam LF, Mac Kenzie WR. Chow JM, Yonekura, ML Recurrent Chlamydial infections increase the risks of hospitalization for ectopic pregnancy and pelvic inflammatory disease. Am J Obstet Gynecol. 1997;176(1 Pt 1):103-7.

[79] Chow JM, Yonekura ML, Richwald GA, Greenland S, Sweet RL, Schachter J. The association between *Chlamydia trachomatis* and ectopic pregnancy. A matched-pair, case-control study.JAMA. 1990;263(23):3164-7.

[80] Bakken, IJ, Skjeldestad, FE and Nordbe, SA. *Chlamydia trachomatis* infections increase the risk for ectopic pregnancy: a population-based, nested case-control study. Sex. Trans. Dis.2007; 34: 166-169.

[81] Claman P, Honey L, Peeling RW, Jessamine P, Toye B. The presence of serum antibody to the Chlamydial heat shock protein (CHSP60) as a diagnostic test for tubal factor infertility. Fertil. Steril. 1997; 67:501-4.

[82] Rodgers AK, Wang J, Zhang Y, Holden A, Berryhill B, Budrys NM, Schenken RS, Zhong G. Association of tubal factor infertility with elevated antibodies to *Chlamydia trachomatis* caseinolytic protease P. Am J Obstet Gynecol. 2010 ;203(5):494.e7-494.e14.

[83] Brunham RC, and Peeling RW. *Chlamydia trachomatis* antigens: role in immunity and pathogenesis. Infect Agents Dis. 1994 Oct; 3(5):218-33.

[84] Mårdh PA. Tubal factor infertility, with special regard to Chlamydial salpingitis.Curr Opin Infect Dis. 2004;17(1):49-52.

[85] Ness RB, Soper DE, Richter HE, Randall H, Peipert JF, Nelson DB, Schubeck D, McNeeley SG, Trout W, Bass DC, Hutchison K, Kip K, Brunham RC. *Chlamydia* antibodies, *Chlamydia* heat shock protein, and adverse sequelae after pelvic inflammatory disease: the PID Evaluation and Clinical Health (PEACH) Study.Sex Transm Dis. 2008;35(2):129-35.

[86] Oakeshott P, Kerry S, Aghaizu A, Atherton H, Hay S, Taylor-Robinson D, Simms I, Hay P. Randomised controlled trial of screening for *Chlamydia trachomatis* to prevent pelvic inflammatory disease: the POPI (prevention of pelvic infection) trial. BMJ. 2010 ;340:c1642. doi: 10.1136/bmj.c1642. Neonatal infections

[87] Institute of Medicine (US) Committee to Study Priorities for Vaccine Development (2000).Vaccines for the 21st Century. Washington, DC: National Academy Press

[88] Schachter, J., Grossman, M., Sweet, R.L., et al. Prospective Study of Perinatal Transmission of *Chlamydia trachomatis* JAMA.1986; 255(24):3374-3377.

[89] Rosenman, M.B., Mahon, B.E., Downs, S.M., et al. Oral erythromycin prophylaxis vs watchful waiting in caring for newborns exposed to *Chlamydia trachomatis*. Arch. Pediatr. Adolesc. Med.2003; 157(6):565-71.

[90] Brocklehurst P, Rooney G. Interventions for treating genital *Chlamydia trachomatis* infection in pregnancy. Cochrane Database Syst Rev. 2000; (2):CD000054

[91] Beem, M.O., and Saxon, E.M. Respiratory-tract colonization and a distinctive pneumonia syndrome in infants infected with *Chlamydia trachomatis*. N Engl J Med.1977; 296(6):306-10.

[92] Darville, T.*Chlamydia trachomatis* infections in neonates and young children. Semin.Pediatr. Infect Dis.2005; 16(4):235-44.

[93] Darville T. Recognition and treatment of Chlamydial infections from birth to adolescence. Adv Exp Med Biol. 2013; 764:109-22.

[94] Chandler JW, Alexander ER, Pheiffer TA, Wang SP, Holmes KK, English M. Ophthalmia neonatorum associated with maternal Chlamydial infections. Trans Sect Ophthalmol Am Acad Ophthalmol Otolaryngol. 1977;83(2):302-8.

[95] Chandran, L. and Boykan, R. Chlamydial infections in children and adolescents.Pediatr Rev. 2009; 30(7):243-50.

[96] de Borborema-Alfaia AP, de Lima Freitas NS, Filho SA, Borborema-Santos CM. *Chlamydia trachomatis* infection in a sample of northern Brazilian pregnant women: preva-

lence and prenatal importance. Braz J Infect Dis. 2013; pii: S1413-8670(13)00142-6. doi: 10.1016/j.bjid.2013.01.014.

[97] Schachter J, Lum L, Gooding CA, Ostler B. Pneumonitis following inclusion blennorrhea.J Pediatr1975;87(5):779-80.

[98] Tipple MA, Beem MO, Saxon EM. Clinical characteristics of the afebrile pneumonia associated with *Chlamydia trachomatis* infection in infants less than 6 months of age. Pediatrics.1979; 63(2):192-7.

[99] Mishra KN, Bhardwaj P, Mishra A, Kaushik A. Acute *Chlamydia trachomatis* respiratory infection in infants. J Glob Infect Dis. 2011;3(3):216-20.

[100] Johansson, M and Lycke, N.Y. Immunology of the human genital tract. Curr. Opin. Infect. Dis.2003; 16: 43-49.

[101] Hafner LM, Cunningham K, Beagley KW. Ovarian steroid hormones: effects on immune responses and *Chlamydia trachomatis* infections of the female genital tract. Mucosal Immunol. 2013a;6(5):859-75.

[102] Farage M A, Miller, K.W. and Sobel, J.D. Dynamics of the vaginal ecosystem - hormonal influences.Infectious Diseases Research and Treatment 2010; 3: 1-15.

[103] Cole, A M. Innate host defense of human vaginal and cervical mucosae. Curr Top Microbiol Immunol., 2006;306:199-230.

[104] Wira, C.R., and Fahey, J.V. The innate immune system: gatekeeper to the female reproductive tract. Immunol., 2004; 111: 13-15.

[105] Wira, C.R., Grant-Tschudy, K.S., Crane-Godreau, M,A. Epithelial cells in the female reproductive tract: a central role as sentinels of immune protection. Am. J. Reprod. Immunol.2005;, 53: 65-76.

[106] Horne AW, Stock SJ, King AE. Epithelial cells in the female reproductive tract: a central role as sentinels of immune protection. Reprod. J, 2008; 135(6):739-49.

[107] Ochiel, D.O., Fahey, J.V., Ghosh, M., Haddad, S.N., Wira, C.R. Innate immunity in th female reproductive tract: Role of sex hormones in regulating uterine epithelial cell protection against pathogens.Curr. Womens Health Reviews, 2008;4(2): 102-117.

[108] Hosenfeld, CB, Workowski KA, Berman,S et al., Repeat infection with *Chlamydia* and gonorrhoea among females: a systematic review of the literature. Sex.Transm. Dis. 2009; 36(8): 478-489.

[109] Kumar H, Kawai T, Akira S. Pathogen recognition by the innate immune system. Int Rev Immun.2011; 30(1):16-34.

[110] Bailey RL, Natividad-Sancho A, Fowler A,Peeling RW, Mabey DC, Whittle HC, Jepson AP: Host genetic contribution to the cellular immune response to *Chlamydia tra-*

chomatis :heritability estimate from a Gambian twin study. Drugs Today (Barc) 2009; 45(supplB):45–50.

[111] Malogajski J, Brankovic I, Verweij SP, Ambrosino E, van Agtmael MA, Brand A, Ouburg S, Morré SA. Translational potential into health care of basic genomic and genetic findings for human immunodeficiency virus, *Chlamydia trachomatis,* and human papilloma virus. Biomed Res Int. 2013:892106. doi: 10.1155/2013/892106.

[112] Karimi, O., Ouburg, S. De Vries, HJ., Pena, AS, Pliejster, J., Land, JA et al., TLR2 haplotypes in the susceptibility to and severity of *Chlamydia trachomatis* infections in Dutch women. Drugs Today (Barc)2009; 45 (Suppl B): 67-74.

[113] Den Hartog JE, Lyons JM, Ouburg S, et al. TLR4 in *Chlamydia trachomatis* infections: knockout mice, STD patients and women with tubal factor subfertility. Drugs of Today B. 2009;45: 75–82.

[114] Broeze KA, Opmeer BC, Van Geloven N,Coppus SF, Collins JA, Den Hartog JE, Vander Linden PJ, Marianowski P, Ng EH, Vander Steeg JW, Steures P, Strandell A, Van derVeen F, Mol BW: Are patient characteristics associated with the accuracy of hysterosalpingography in diagnosing tubal pathology? An individual patient data meta-analysis. HumReprod Update 2011; 17: 293–300.

[115] Morré SA, Karimi O, Ouburg S. Review *Chlamydia trachomatis*: identification of susceptibility markers for ocular and sexually transmitted infection by immunogenetics. FEMS Immunol Med Microbiol. 2009 Mar; 55(2):140-53.

[116] Lal JA, Malogajski J, Verweij SP, de Boer P, Ambrosino E, Brand A, Ouburg S, Morré SA. *Chlamydia trachomatis* infections and subfertility: opportunities to translate host pathogen genomic data into public health. Public Health Genomics.2013;16(1-2): 50-61.

[117] Agrawal, T., Vats, V., Salhan, S., and Mittal, A. The mucosal immune response to *Chlamydia trachomatis* infection of the reproductive tract in women. J. Reprod. Immunol.2009; 83(1-2), 173-178.

[118] Agrawal, T., Vats, V., Salhan, S., and Mittal, A. Mucosal and peripheral immune responses to Chlamydial heat shock proteins in women infected with *Chlamydia trachomatis*. Clin. Exp. Immunol. 2007a ; 148(3):461-468.

[119] Cohen CR., Koochesfahani, KM., Meier, AS, Shen, C., Karunakaran, K., Ondondo, B et al Immunoepidemiologic profile of *Chlamydia trachomatis* infection: importance of heat shock protein 60 and interferon-gamma. J. Infect. Dis.2005; 192: 591-599.

[120] Roan, N.R. and Starnbach., M.N. Immune-mediated control of *Chlamydia* infection. Cell.Microbiol.2008;10: 9-19.

[121] Kimani, J., Maclean IW, Bwayo, JJ., MacDonald, K., Oyugi, J., Maitha, GM., et al., Risk factors for *Chlamydia trachomatis* pelvic inflammatory disease among sex workers in Nairobi, Kenya J.Infect.Dis.1996; 173: 1437-1444.

[122] Brunham, RC, Kimani, J, Bwayo, J., Maitha, G., Maclean,I., Yang, C et al. The epidemiology of *Chlamydia trachomatis* within a sexually transmitted core group. J. Infect. Dis.1996; 173: 950-956.

[123] Kaldensjö,T.,Petersson,P.,Tolf,A.,Morgan,G.,Broliden,K., Hirbod T. Detection of intraepithelial and stromal Langerin and CCR5 positive cells in the human endometrium: potential targets for HIV infection. PLoS One. 2011; 6(6): e21344.

[124] Arrivito, L., Sanz, M., Banham, A.H., Fainboim, L. Expansion of CD4+CD25+ and FOXP3+ regulatory T cells during the follicular phase of the menstrual cycle: implications for human reproduction.J. Immunol.2007; 178: 2572-2578.

[125] Ficarra M, Ibana JS, Poretta C, Ma L, Myers L, Taylor SN, Greene S, Smith B, Hagensee M, Martin DH, Quayle AJ. A distinct cellular profile is seen in the human endocervix during *Chlamydia trachomatis* infection. A J Reprod Immunol, 2008; 60:415-425.

[126] Mascellino MT, Boccia P, Oliva A. Immunopathogenesis in *Chlamydia trachomatis* Infected Women. SRN Obstet Gynecol. 2011:436936. doi: 10.5402/2011/436936.

[127] Pudney J, Quayle AJ, Anderson DJ. Immunological microenvironments in the human vagina and cervix: mediators of cellular immunity are concentrated in the cervical transformation zone.Biol Reprod.2005; 73(6):1253-63.

[128] Yeaman, G.R Guyre, P.M., Fanger, M.W., Collins, J.E., White, H.D., Rathbun, W., et al. Unique CD8+ T cell rich lymphoid aggregates in human uterine endometrium. PMCID1997; : 9103229.

[129] Wira, C.R., Fahey, J.V.,Ghosh,M., Patel,V., Hickey D.K. and Ochiel D.O. Sex Hormone Regulation of Innate Immunity in the Female Reproductive Tract: The Role of Epithelial Cells in Balancing Reproductive Potential with Protection against Sexually Transmitted Pathogens Am J Reprod. Immunol. 2010; 63: 544–565.

[130] Bouman A, Heineman MJ, Faas MM. Sex hormones and the immune response in humans Hum Reprod Update.2005; 11(4):411-23.

[131] Wira C, Fahey J, Wallace P, Yeaman G. Effect of the menstrual cycle on immunological parameters in the human female reproductive tract. J Acquir Immune Defic Syndr.2005;38 Suppl 1:S34-6.

[132] Butts, C.L., Sternberg, E.M. Neuroendocrine factors alter host defense by modulating immune function. Cellular Immunology,2008; 252(1-2):7-15.

[133] Aflatoonian R, Tuckerman E, Elliott SL, Bruce C, Aflatoonian A, Li TC, Fazeli A. Menstrual cycle-dependent changes of Toll-like receptors in endometrium. Hum Reprod.2007; 22(2):586-93.

[134] Aflatoonian R, Fazeli A. Toll-like receptors in female reproductive tract and their menstrual cycle dependent expression. J Reprod Immunol. 2008;77(1):7-13.

[135] Wira, C.R., Grant-Tschudy, K.S., Crane-Godreau, M,A. Epithelial cells in the female reproductive tract: a central role as sentinels of immune protection. Am. J Reprod. Immunol.2005;, 53: 65-76.

[136] Kang, L, Zhang, X, Xie, Y, Tu, Y, Wang, D, Liu, ZWang, ZY, Tsai, MJ Involvement of estrogen receptor variant ER-alpha36, not GPR30, in non-genomic estrogen signalling. Mol Endocrinol. 2010; 24(4): 709-730.

[137] Solar, P and Velasquez, T: Consequences of non-genomic actions of estradiol on pathogenic genital tract response. Journal of Molecular Signaling 2013 8:1. doi: 10.1186/1750-2187-8-1.

[138] Lesmeister, M.J., Jorgensen, R.L., Young, S.L., and Misfeldt, M.L. 17 beta-estradiol suppresses TLR3-induced cytokine and chemokine production in endometrial epithelial cells. Reprod. Biol. Endocrinol.2005;, 3:74-89.

[139] Nalbandian, G and Kovats, S. Understanding sex biases in immunity. Immunologic Research, 2005; 31(2): 91-106.

[140] Hughes GC, Clark EA. Regulation of dendritic cells by female sex steroids: relevance to immunity and autoimmunity. Autoimmunity2007; 40(6):470-81.

[141] Kovats, S., Carreras, E. Regulation of dendritic cell differentiation and function by estrogen receptor ligands. Cell. Immunol.,2008; 252: 81-90.

[142] Heine H, Müller-Loennies S, Brade L, Lindner B, Brade H. Endotoxic activity and chemical structure of lipopolysaccharides from *Chlamydia trachomatis* serotypes E and L2 and *Chlamydophila psittaci* 6BC. Eur J Biochem.2003; 270(3):440-50.

[143] Da Costa CU, Wantia N, Kirschning CJ, Busch DH, Rodriguez N, Wagner H, Miethke T. Heat shock protein 60 from *Chlamydia pneumoniae* elicits an unusual set of inflammatory responses via Toll-like receptor 2 and 4 in vivo. Eur J Immunol.2004; 34(10): 2874-84.

[144] Derbigny WA, Kerr MS, Johnson RM. Pattern recognition molecules activated by *Chlamydia muridarum* infection of cloned murine oviduct epithelial cell lines. J Immunol.2005;175(9):6065-75.

[145] Vabulas RM, Ahmad-Nejad P, da Costa C, Miethke T, Kirschning CJ, Häcker H, Wagner H. Endocytosed HSP60s use toll-like receptor 2 (TLR2) and TLR4 to activate the toll/interleukin-1 receptor signaling pathway in innate immune cells. J Biol Chem.2001; 276(33):31332-9.

[146] Prebeck S, Kirschning C, Dürr S, da Costa C, Donath B, Brand K, Redecke V, Wagner H, Miethke T. Predominant role of toll-like receptor 2 versus 4 in *Chlamydia pneumoniae*-induced activation of dendritic cells. J Immunol. 2001;167(6):3316-23.

[147] Welter-Stahl L, Ojcius DM, Viala J, Girardin S, Liu W, Delarbre C, Philpott D, Kelly KA, Darville T. Stimulation of the cytosolic receptor for peptidoglycan, Nod1, by in-

fection with *Chlamydia trachomatis* or *Chlamydia muridarum*.Cell Microbiol.2006; 8(6): 1047-57.

[148] Kaushic, C. The role of the local microenvironment in regulating susceptibility and immune responses to sexually transmitted viruses in the female genital tract. J. Reprod. Immunol.2009;, 83:168-72.

[149] Keenihan, S.N., and Roberston, A.A. Diversity in phenotype and steroid hormone dependence in dendritic cells and macrophages in the mouse uterus. Biol.Reprod. 2004; 70:1562-1572.

[150] Patton, D.L., Thinn, S.S., Meier, A., Hooton, T.M. Stapleton, A.E., Eschenbach, D.A. Epithelial cell layer thickness and immune cell populations in the normal human vagina at different stages of the menstrual cycle. Am. J. Obstet. Gynecol.2000;183(4): 967-73.

[151] Kaul R, Pettengell C, Sheth PM, Sunderji S, Biringer A, MacDonald K, Walmsley S, Rebbapragada A. The genital tract immune milieu: an important determinant of HIV susceptibility and secondary transmission. J Reprod Immunol.2008; 77(1):32-40.

[152] Fish, E.N. The X-files in immunity: sex-based differences predispose immune responses. Nat. Rev. Immunol.2008; 8 :737-744.

[153] Kelly, K.A. T-lymphocyte trafficking to the female reproductive tract mucosae. In: Editor. P.B. Wyrick (ed.). *Chlamydia*: Genomics and Pathogenesis,. Norfolk, UK.: Horizon Bioscience, 2006. p. 413-435.

[154] Menge AC, Mestecky J. Surface expression of secretory component and HLA class II DR antigen on glandular epithelial cells from human endometrium and two endometrial adenocarcinoma cell lines.J Clin Immunol. 1993; 13(4):259-64.

[155] Wang Y, Ben K, Cao X, Wang Y. Transport of anti-sperm monoclonal IgA and IgG into murine male and female genital tracts from blood. Effect of sex hormones. J Immunol.1996;156(3):1014-9.

[156] Lu, F.X., Ma, Z., Moser, S., Evans, T.G., Miller, C.J. Effects of ovarian steroids on immunoglobulin-secreting cell function in healthy women.Clin. and Diag. Lab. Immunol.2003; 10(5):944-949.

[157] Rank RG. Animal models for urogenital infections. Methods Enzymol.1994;235:83-93.

[158] Rank RG, White HJ, Hough AJ Jr, Pasley JN, Barron AL. Effect of estradiol on Chlamydial genital infection of female guinea pigs. Infect Immun. 1982;38(2):699-705.

[159] Pasley JN, Rank RG, Hough AJ, Jr, Cohen C, Barron AL. Effects of various doses of estradiol on Chlamydial genital infection in ovariectomized guinea pigs. Sex. Transm. Dis.1985; 12:8–13.

[160] Rank RG, Barron AL.Specific effect of estradiol on the genital mucosal antibody response in Chlamydial ocular and genital infections. Infect Immun.1987; 55:2317–2319.

[161] Barron AL, Pasley JN, Rank RG, White HJ, Mrak RE. Chlamydial salpingitis in female guinea pigs receiving oral contraceptives. Sex Transm Dis1988; 15:169–173.

[162] Kaushic C, Murdin AD, Underdown BJ, Wira CR. *Chlamydia trachomatis* infection in the female reproductive tract of the rat: influence of progesterone on infectivity and immune response.Infect Immun.1998 Mar;66(3):893-8.

[163] Kaushic C, Zhou F, Murdin AD, Wira CR. Effects of estradiol and progesterone on susceptibility and early immune responses to *Chlamydia trachomatis* infection in the female reproductive tract. Infect Immun. 2000;68(7):4207-16.

[164] Bose SK, Goswami PC. Enhancement of adherence and growth of *Chlamydia trachomatis* by estrogen treatment of HeLa cells. Infect Immun. 1986;53(3):646-50.

[165] Agrawal T, Vats V, Wallace PK, Salhan S, Mittal A. Role of cervical dendritic cell subsets, co-stimulatory molecules, cytokine secretion profile and beta-estradiol in development of sequalae to *Chlamydia trachomatis* infection. Reprod Biol Endocrinol.2008; 6:46. doi: 10.1186/1477-7827-6-46.

[166] Amirshahi A, Wan C, Beagley K, Latter J, Symonds I, Timms P. Modulation of the *Chlamydia trachomatis* in vitro transcriptome response by the sex hormones estradiol and progesterone. BMC Microbiol. 2011;25;11:150. doi: 10.1186/1471-2180-11-150.

[167] Hogan RJ, Mathews SA, Mukhopadhyay S, Summersgill JT, Timms P. Chlamydial persistence: beyond the biphasic paradigm. Infect Immun. 2004;72(4):1843-55

[168] Akers JC, Tan M. Molecular mechanism of tryptophan-dependent transcriptional regulation in *Chlamydia trachomatis*. J Bacteriol. 2006;188 (12):4236-43.

[169] Schaefer TM, Desouza K, Fahey JV, Beagley KW, Wira CR. Toll-like receptor (TLR) expression and TLR-mediated cytokine/chemokine production by human uterine epithelial cells. Immunol.2004; 112(3):428-36.

[170] Pioli, PA, Amiel E, Schaefer TM, Connolly JE, Wira CR, Guyre PM. Differential expression of Toll-like receptors 2 and 4 in tissues of the human female reproductive tract. Infect Immun., 2004;72(10):5799-806.

[171] Fazeli A, Bruce C, Anumba DO. Characterization of Toll-like receptors in the female reproductive tract in humans. Hum Reprod.2005; 20(5):1372-8.

[172] Agrawal T, Bhengraj AR, Vats V, Salhan S, Mittal A. Expression of TLR 2, TLR 4 and iNOS in Cervical Monocytes of *Chlamydia trachomatis*-infected Women and Their Role in Host Immune Response. Am J Reprod Immunol. 2011 ; 66 (6):534-43.

[173] Agrawal T, Bhengraj AR, Vats V, Mittal A. *Chlamydia trachomatis*: TLR4-mediated recognition by human dendritic cells is impaired following oestradiol treatment. Br J Biomed Sci. 2013;70(2):51-7.

[174] Mahmoud EA, Hamad EE, Olsson SE, Mårdh PA. Anti-Chlamydial activity of cervical secretion in different phases of the menstrual cycle and influence of hormonal contraceptives. Contraception.1994; 49(3):265-74.

[175] Sweet RL, Landers DV, Walker C, Schachter J. *Chlamydia trachomatis* infection and pregnancy outcome. Am J Obstet Gynecol.1987;156(4):824-33.

[176] Agrawal, T., Vats, V., Wallace, P.K., Salhan, S., and Mittal, A. Cervical cytokine reponses in women with primary or recurrent Chlamydial infection. Journal of Interferon and Cytokine Research,2007b 27: 221-226. contraceptives

[177] Washington AE, Gove S, Schachter J, Sweet RL. Oral contraceptives, *Chlamydia trachomatis* infection, and pelvic inflammatory disease. A word of caution about protection. J Am Med Assoc.1985; 253:2246–2250.

[178] Baeten JM, Nyange PM, Richardson BA, Lavreys L, Chohan B, Martin HL Jr, Mandaliya K, Ndinya-Achola JO, Bwayo JJ, Kreiss JK. Hormonal contraception and risk of sexually transmitted disease acquisition: results from a prospective study. Am J Obstet Gynecol. 2001;185(2):380-5.

[179] Morrison CS, Bright P, Wong EL, Kwok C, Yacobson I, Gaydos CA, Tucker HT, Blumenthal PD. Hormonal contraceptive use, cervical ectopy, and the acquisition of cervical infections. Sex Transm Dis. 2004, 31(9):561-7.

[180] Williams DM, Schachter J, Drutz DJ, Sumaya CV. Pneumonia due to *Chlamydia trachomatis* in the immunocompromised (nude) mouse. *J Infect Dis.* 1981 143: 238-41.

[181] Igietseme JU, Eko FO, He Q, Black CM. Antibody regulation of Tcell immunity: implications for vaccine strategies against intracellular pathogens. *Expert Rev Vaccines.* 2004 3: 23-34.

[182] Stephens RS. The cellular paradigm of Chlamydial pathogenesis. *Trends Microbiol.* 2003 11: 44-51.

[183] Rice PA, Westrom LV. Pathogenesis and inflammatory response in pelvic inflammatory disease. In: Berger GS, Westrom LV. eds. *Pelvic Inflammatory Disease*. New York: Raven Press. 1992 35-47.

[184] Oakeshott P, Hay P, Hay S, Steinke F, Rink E, Kerry S. Association between bacterial vaginosis or Chlamydial infection and miscarriage before 16 weeks' gestation: prospective community based cohort study. *BMJ.* 2002 325: 1334.

[185] Molano, M., Meijer, CJ, Weiderpass E et al., The natural course of *Chlamydia trachomatis* infection in asymptomatic Colombian women: a 5-year follow-up study. J. Infect. Dis., 2005, 191: 907-16

[186] Cohen, C.R., Koochesfahani, A.S., Meoer et al., Immunoepidemiologic profile of *Chlamydia trachomatis* infection: importance of heat shock protein 60 and interferon-γ. J.Infect.Dis.;192(4):591-99

[187] Morrison, R.P., et al., 1989. Chlamydial disease pathogenesis. The 57-kDa Chlamydial hypersensitivity antigen is a stress response protein. J. Exp.Med. 170, 1271–1283.

[188] Ault, K.A., et al., 1998. Antibodies to the Chlamydial 60 kilodalton heat shock protein in women with tubal factor infertility. Infect. Dis. Obstet. Gynecol. 6, 163–167

[189] Bax, C.J., et al., 2004. *Chlamydia trachomatis* heat shock protein 60 (cHsp60) antibodies in women without and with tubal pathology using a new commercially available assay. Sex. Transm. Infect. 80, 415–416.

[190] Dapontea,A, Pournarasb,, S., Deligeoroglouc,E., Skentoua,H., Messinisa, I.E. Serum interleukin-1_, interleukin-8 and anti-heat shock 60 *Chlamydia trachomatis* antibodies as markers of ectopic pregnancy. J.Reprod. Immunol. 2012; 93: 102-108

[191] Taylor BD, Darville T, Ferrell RE, Kammerer CM, Ness RB, Haggerty CL. Variants in toll-like receptor 1 and 4 genes are associated with *Chlamydia trachomatis* among women with pelvic inflammatory disease. J Infect Dis. 2012 Feb 15;205(4):603-9. doi: 10.1093/infdis/jir822. Epub 2012 Jan 11

[192] Haggerty, C.L., Panum, I., Uldum, S., et al., *Chlamydia trachomatis* infection may increase the risk of preeclampsia Pregnancy Hypertension: An international journal of womens cardiovascular health 3 (2013) 28-33.

[193] Srivastava P, Jha R, Bas S, Salhan S, Mittal A. In infertile women, cells from *Chlamydia trachomatis* infected sites release higher levels of interferon-gamma, interleukin-10 and tumor necrosis factor-alpha upon heat-shock-protein stimulation than fertile women. Reprod Biol Endocrinol. 2008 May 20;6:20. doi: 10.1186/1477-7827-6-20.

[194] Taylor BD, Darville T, Ferrell RE, Ness RB, Haggerty CL. Racial variation in toll-like receptor variants among women with pelvic inflammatory disease. J Infect Dis. 2013 Mar 15;207(6):940-6. doi: 10.1093/infdis/jis922. Epub 2012 Dec 18

[195] Stephens R, Kalman S, Lammel C, et al. Genome sequence of an obligate intracellular pathogen of humans: *Chlamydia trachomatis*. *Science*. 1998;282(5389):754–759

[196] Taylor BD, Darville T, Tan C, Bavoil PM, Ness RB, Haggerty CL. The role of *Chlamydia trachomatis* polymorphic membrane proteins in inflammation and sequelae among women with pelvic inflammatory disease. Infect Dis Obstet Gynecol. 2011;2011:989762. doi: 10.1155/2011/989762. Epub 2011 Oct 19.

[197] Gijsen, A.P., Land, J.A., Goossens, V.J., Slobbe, M.E., Bruggeman, C.A. *Chlamydia* antibody testing in screening for tubal factor subfertility: the significance of IgG antibody decline over time. Hum Reprod. 2002 17:699-703

[198] Veenemans, L.M., van der Linden, P.J. The value of *Chlamydia trachomatis* antibody testing in predicting tubal factor infertility. Hum Reprod. 2002 17:695-98

[199] den Hartog, J.E., Land, J.A., Stassen, F.R., Kessels, A.G., Bruggeman, C.A. Serological markers of persistent *C. trachomatis* infections in women with tubal subfertility. Hum Reprod. 2005 20:986-90

[200] den Hartog, J.E., Morre, S.A., Land, J.A. *Chlamydia trachomatis*-associated tubal factor subfertility: Immunogenetic aspects and serological screening. Hum Reprod Update. 2006 12:719-30

[201] Tiitinen, A., Surcel, H.M., Hlttunen, M., Birkeland, S., Bloigu, A., Christiansen, G., Koskela, P., Morrison, S.G., Morrison, R.P., Paavonen, J. *Chlamydia trachomatis* an Chlamydial heat shock protein 60-specific antibody and cell-mediated responses predict tubal factor infertility. Hum Reprod. 2006 21:151-60

[202] Westrom L, Joesoef R, Reynolds G, Hagdu A, Thompson SE. Pelvic inflammatory disease and fertility. A cohort study of 1,844 women with laparoscopically verified disease and 657 control women with normal laparoscopic results. *Sex Transm Dis.* 1992 19: 185-192.

[203] Ohman H, Tiitinen A, Halttunen M, Lehtinen M, Paavonen J, Surcel HM. Cytokine polymorphisms and severity of tubal damage in women with *Chlamydia*-associated infertility. J Infect Dis. 2009 May 1;199(9):1353-9. doi: 10.1086/597620.

[204] Ohman H, Bailey R, Natividad A, Ragoussis J, Johnson LL, Tiitinen A, Halttunen M, Paavonen J, Surcel HM. Effect of IL12A and IL12B polymorphisms on the risk of *Chlamydia trachomatis*-induced tubal factor infertility and disease severity. Hum Reprod. 2012 Jul;27(7):2217-23. doi: 10.1093/humrep/des136. Epub 2012 May 11.

[205] Ohman H, Tiitinen A, Halttunen M, Paavonen J, Surcel HM. Cytokine gene polymorphism and *Chlamydia trachomatis*-specific immune responses. Hum Immunol. 2011 Mar;72(3):278-82. doi: 10.1016/j.humimm.2010.12.012. Epub 2011 Jan 4.

[206] Rodgers AK, Wang J, Zhang Y, Holden A, Berryhill B, Budrys NM, Schenken RS, Zhong G. Association of tubal factor infertility with elevated antibodies to *Chlamydia trachomatis* caseinolytic protease P. Am J Obstet Gynecol. 2010 Nov;203(5): 494.e7-494.e14. doi: 10.1016/j.ajog.2010.06.005.

[207] Hjelholt A, Christiansen G, Johannesson TG, Ingerslev HJ, Birkelund S. Tubal factor infertility is associated with antibodies against *Chlamydia trachomatis* heat shock protein 60 (HSP60) but not human HSP60. Hum Reprod. 2011 Aug;26(8):2069-76. doi: 10.1093/humrep/der167. Epub 2011 Jun 4.

[208] Surana A, Rastogi V, Nirwan PS. Association of the Serum Anti-Chlamydial Antibodies with Tubal Infertility. J Clin Diagn Res. 2012 Dec;6(10):1692-4. doi: 10.7860/JCDR/2012/3771.2632. Epub 2012 Sep 12.

[209] Brunham RC, Rey-Ladino. Immunology of *Chlamydia* infection: implications for a *Chlamydia trachomatis* vaccine. Nat Rev Immunol, 2005 5: 149–16.

[210] Krause W, Bohring C: Male infertility and genital Chlamydial infection: victim or perpetrator? Andrologia 2003; 35:209–216.

[211] Zervomanolakis I, Ott W, Hadziomerovic D, Mattle V, Seeber B, Virgolini I, Heute D, Kissler S, Leyendecker G, Wildt L: Physiology of upward transport in the human female genital tract. Ann NY Acad Sci 2007; 1101:1–20.

[212] Geisler WM, Wang C, Morrison SG, Black CM, Bandea CI, Hook EW 3rd. The natural history of untreated *Chlamydia trachomatis* infection in the interval between screening and returning for treatment. Sex Transm Dis 2008; 35:119–23.

[213] Joyner JL, Douglas JM Jr, Foster M, Judson FN. Persistence of *Chlamydia trachomatis* infection detected by polymerase chain reaction in untreated patients. Sex Transm Dis 2002; 29:196–200.

[214] Kelly K. Cellular immunity and *Chlamydia* genital infection: induction, recruitment and effector mechanisms. Int Rev Immunol 2003;22:2-41.

[215] Hosenfeld CB, Workowski KA, Berman S, et al. Repeat infection with *Chlamydia* and gonorrhea among females: a systematic review of the literature. Sex Transm Dis 2009; 36:478–89)

[216] Xu F, Stoner BP, Taylor SN, et al. Use of home-obtained vaginal swabs to facilitate rescreening for *Chlamydia trachomatis* infections: two randomized controlled trials. Obstet Gynecol 2011; 118(2 Pt 1):231–9.

[217] Dunne EF, Chapin JB, Rietmeijer CA, et al. Rate and predictors of repeat *Chlamydia trachomatis* infection among men. Sex Transm Dis 2008; 35: S40–4.

[218] Yang, X., K.T. HayGlass, and R.C. Brunham, Genetically determined differences in IL-10 and IFN-gamma responses correlate with clearance of *Chlamydia trachomatis* mouse pneumonitis infection. J Immunol, 1996. 156(11): p. 4338-44.

[219] Yang, X., Role of cytokines in *Chlamydia trachomatis* protective immunity and immunopathology. Curr Pharm Des, 2003. 9(1): p. 67-73.

[220] Su H, Caldwell HD., CD4+ T cells play a significant role in adoptive immunity to *Chlamydia trachomatis* infection of the mouse genital tract. Infect Immun., 1995 63: 3302–3308.

[221] Caldwell, H.D. and L.J. Perry, Neutralization of *Chlamydia trachomatis* infectivity with antibodies to the major outer membrane protein, in Infect Immun. 1982. p. 745-54.

[222] Berry LJ, Hickey DK, Skelding KA, Bao S, Rendina AM, et al. (2004) Transcutaneous immunization with combined cholera toxin and CpG adjuvant protects against *Chlamydia* muridarum genital tract infection. Infect Immun 72: 1019–1028

[223] Skelding KA, Hickey DK, Horvat JC, Bao S, Roberts KG, et al. (2006) Comparison of intranasal and transcutaneous immunization for induction of protective immunity against *Chlamydia* muridarum respiratory tract infection. Vaccine 24: 355–366

[224] Pal, S., et al., Monoclonal immunoglobulin A antibody to the major outer membrane protein of the *Chlamydia trachomatis* mouse pneumonitis biovar protects mice against a Chlamydial genital challenge Vaccine. 1997;15(5): 575-82.

[225] Morrison, S.G. and R.P. Morrison, Resolution of secondary *Chlamydia trachomatis* genital tract infection in immune mice with depletion of both CD4+ and CD8+ T cells, in Infect Immun. 2001. p. 2643-9.

[226] (Morrison, S.G. and R.P. Morrison, A predominant role for antibody in acquired immunity to Chlamydial genital tract reinfection, in J Immunol. 2005. p. 7536-42.

[227] (Morrison, S.G., et al., Immunity to murine *Chlamydia trachomatis* genital tract reinfection involves B cells and CD4(+) T cells but not CD8(+) T cells, in Infect Immun. 2000. p. 6979-87.

[228] Igietseme JU, Magee DM, Williams DM, Rank RG: Role for CD8+ T cells in antiChlamydial immunity defined by *Chlamydia*-specific T-lymphocyte clones. Infect Immun. 1994; 62:5195–5197

[229] Barteneva N, Theodor I, Peterson E, de la Maza L: Role of neutrophils in controlling early stages of a *Chlamydia trachomatis* infection. Infect Immun 1996; 64:4830–4833.

[230] Zhang D, Yang X, Lu H, Zhong G, Brunham RC: Immunity to *Chlamydia trachomatis* mouse pneumonitis induced by vaccination with live organisms correlates with early granulocyte-macrophage colony-stimulating factor and interleukin-12 production and with dendritic cell-like maturation. Infect Immun1999; 67:1606–1613.

[231] Agrawal T, Vats V, Wallace PK, Singh A, Salhan S, Mittal A: Recruitment of myeloid and plasmacytoid dendritic cells in cervical mucosa during *Chlamydia trachomatis* infection. Clin Microbiol Infect 2009; 15:50–59.

[232] Hvid M, Baczynska A, Deleuran B, Fedder J, Knudsen HJ, Christiansen G, Birkelund S: Interleukin-1 is the initiator of fallopian tube destruction during *Chlamydia trachomatis* infection. Cell Microbiol 2007; 9:2795–2803.

[233] Rasmussen SJ, Eckmann L, Quayle AJ, Shen L, Zhang Y-X, Anderson DJ, Fierer J, Stephens RS, Kagnoff MF: Secretion of proinflammatory cytokines by epithelial cells in response to *Chlamydia* infection suggests a central role for epithelial cells in Chlamydial pathogenesis. J Clin Invest 1997; 99:77–87.

[234] Horne AW, Stock SJ, King AE. Epithelial cells in the female reproductive tract: a central role as sentinels of immune protection. Reproduction J, 2008; 135(6):739-49.

[235] O'Connell CM, Ionova IA, Quayle AJ, Visintin A, Ingalls RR. Localization of TLR2 and MyD88 to *Chlamydia trachomatis* inclusions. Evidence for signaling by intracellular TLR2 during infection with an obligate intracellular pathogen. J Biol Chem. 2006; 281(3):1652-9.

[236] Darville T, O'Neill JM, Andrews CW Jr, Nagarajan UM, Stahl L, Ojcius DM: Toll-like receptor-2, but not toll-like receptor-4, is essential for development of oviduct pathology in Chlamydial genital tract infection. J Immunol 2003; 171:6187–6197.

[237] Buchholz, K.R. and Stephens, R.S. The Cytosolic Pattern Recognition Receptor NOD1 Induces Inflammatory.Infection and Immunity, 2008; 76(7):3150–3155.

[238] Buchholz, K. R. and Stephens, R.S. Activation of the host cell proinflammatory interleukin-8 response by *Chlamydia trachomatis*. Cell. Microbiol.2006; 8:1768–1779.

[239] Tseng C-TK, Rank RG: Role of NK cells in early host response to Chlamydial genital infection. Infect Immun.1998; 66:5867–5875.

[240] Rank RG, Bowlin AK, Kelly KA. Characterization of lymphocyte re- sponse in the female genital tract during ascending Chlamydial genital infection in the guinea pig model. Infect Immun 2000;68(9): 5293–5298).

[241] Carey, A. J., & Beagley, K. W. (2010). *Chlamydia trachomatis*, a hidden epidemic: effects on female reproduction and options for treatment. *American journal of reproductive immunology (New York, N.Y. : 1989)*, *63*(6), 576–586.

[242] Patton DL, Sweeney YT, Kuo CC: Demonstration of delayed hypersensitivity in *Chlamydia trachomatis* salpingitis in monkeys: a pathogenic mechanism of tubal damage. J Infect Dis 1994; 169:680–683

[243] Watkins NG Hadlow WJ, Moos AB, Caldwell HD: Ocular delayed hypersensitivity: a pathogenetic mechanism of Chlamydial-conjunctivitis in guinea pigs. Proc Natl Acad Sci USA 1986; 83: 7480–7484

[244] Taylor H, Johnson S, Schachter J, Caldwell H, Prendergast R: Pathogenesis of trachoma: the stimulus for inflammation. J Immunol 1987;138:3023–3027.

[245] Kinnunen A, Paavonen J, Surcel HM: Heat shock protein 60 specific T-cell response in Chlamydial infections. Scand J Immunol 2001; 54:76–81.

[246] Campanella C, Marino Gammazza A, Mularoni L, Cappello F, Zummo G, Di Felice V: A comparative analysis of the products of GROEL-1 gene from *Chlamydia trachomatis* serovar D and the HSP60 var1 transcript from Homo sapiens suggests a possible autoimmune response. Int J Immunogenet 2009; 36:73–78

[247] Yi Y, Yang X, Brunham RC: Autoimmunity to heat shock protein 60 and antigen-specific production of interleukin-10. Infect Immun 1997; 65:1669–1674.

[248] Peeling RW, Kimani J, Plummer F, Maclean I, Cheang M, Bwayo J, Brunham RC: Antibody to Chlamydial hsp60 predicts an increased risk for Chlamydial pelvic inflammatory disease. J Infect Dis 1997; 175:1153–1158)

[249] Ness,RB, Soper, DE,Richter, HE,et al. *Chlamydia* antibodies, *Chlamydia* heat shock protein, and adverse sequelae after pelvic inflammatory disease: the PID Evaluation and Clinical Health (PEACH) Study. Sex Transm Dis 2008;35(2):129–135

[250] Cohen CR, Koochesfahani KM, Meier AS, et al. Immunoepidemiologic profile of *Chlamydia trachomatis* infection: importance of heat-shock protein 60 and interferon-gamma. J Infect Dis 2005; 192(4):591–599

[251] O'Connell, C. M., AbdelRahman, Y. M., Green, E., Darville, H. K., Saira, K., Smith, B., et al. (2011). Toll-like receptor 2 activation by *Chlamydia trachomatis* is plasmid dependent, and plasmid-responsive chromosomal loci are coordinately regulated in response to glucose limitation by C. trachomatis but not by C. muridarum. *Infection and immunity*, *79*(3), 1044–1056.

[252] Frazer, L. C., Darville, T., Chandra-Kuntal, K., Andrews, C. W., Zurenski, M., Mintus, M., et al. (2012). Plasmid-cured *Chlamydia* caviae activates TLR2-dependent signaling and retains virulence in the guinea pig model of genital tract infection. *PloS one*, *7*(1), e30747.

[253] Kari, L., M.M. Goheen, L.B. Randall, L.D. Taylor, J.H. Carlson, W.M. Whitmire, D. Virok, K. Rajaram, V. Endresz, G. McClarty, et al. 2011. Generation of targeted *Chlamydia trachomatis* null mutants. *Proc. Natl. Acad. Sci. USA.* 108:7189–7193

[254] Zimmerman HL, Potterat JJ, Dukes RL, Muth JB, Zimmerman HP, Fogle JS, Pratts CI. Epidemiologic differences between *Chlamydia* and gonorrhea. Am J Public Health. 80(11):1338-42 (1990)

[255] Stamm WE, Wagner KF, Amsel R, Alexander ER, Turck M, Counts GW, Holmes KK. Causes of the acute urethral syndrome in women. N Engl J Med.;303(8):409-15(1980)

[256] Centers for Disease Control and Prevention. Sexually transmitted Disease Treatment Guideline.Morbid Mortal Wkly Rep.;55:79-85 (2010)

[257] Lau CY, Qureshi AK. Azithromycin versus doxycycline for genital Chlamydial infections: a meta-analysis of randomized clinical trials. Sex Transm Dis ;29:497e502 (2002)

[258] Centers for Disease Control and Prevention. Sexually Transmitted Diseases Treatment Guidelines. 2010. http://www.cdc.gov/std/treatment/2010/STD- Treatment-2010-RR5912.pdf

[259] Horner P, Boag F. 2006 UK National Guideline for the Management of Genital Tract Infection with *Chlamydia trachomatis*. 2006. http://www.bashh.org/guidelines

[260] Handsfield HH. Questioning Azithromycin for Chlamydial Infection. Sex Transm Dis 2011;38: 1028–1029.

[261] Hosenfeld CB, Workowski KA, Berman S, Zaidi A, Dyson J, Mosure D, Bolan G, Bauer HM. Repeat infection with *Chlamydia* and gonorrhea among females: a systematic review of the literature.Sex Transm Dis. 2009 Aug;36(8):478-89. doi: 10.1097/OLQ.0b013e3181a2a933.

[262] Gaydos CA. Nucleic acid amplification tests for gonorrhea and *Chlamydia*: Practice and applications. Infect Dis Clin North Am 2005; 19:367–386

[263] Batteiger BE, Tu W, Ofner S, et al. Repeated *Chlamydia trachomatis* genital infections in adolescent women. J Infect Dis 2010; 201:42–51

[264] Golden MR, Whittington WL, Handsfield HH, Hughes JP, Stamm WE, Hogben M, Clark A, Malinski C, Helmers JR, Thomas KK, Holmes KK. Effect of expedited treatment of sex partners on recurrent or persistent gonorrhea or Chlamydial infection N Engl J Med. 2005 Feb 17;352(7):676-85.

[265] Kelsi M Sandoz and Daniel D Rockey, Antibiotic resistance in Chlamydiae, Future Microbiology. 2010 September; 5(9): 1427-1442

[266] Horner PJ (2012) Azithromycin antimicrobial resistance and genital *Chlamydia trachomatis* infection: duration of therapy may be the key to improving efficacy. Sex Transm Infect 88: 154–156

[267] Drummond F, Ryder N, Wand H, et al. Is azithromycin adequate treatment for asymptomatic rectal *Chlamydia*? Int J STD AIDS 2011;22:478e80.

[268] Thejls H, Gnarpe J, Lundkvist O, Heimer G, Larsson G, Arne V. Diagnosis and prevalence of persistent *Chlamydia* infection in infer- tile women: tissue culture, direct antigen detection, and serology. Fertil Steril 1991; 55:304–310

[269] Campbell LA, Patton DL, Moore DE, Cappuccio AL, Mueller BA, Wang SP. Detection of *Chlamydia trachomatis* deoxyribonucleic acid in women with tubal infertility. Fertil Steril 1993; 59:45–50

[270] Patton DL, Askienazy-Elbhar BD, Henry-Suchet J, et al. Detection of *Chlamydia trachomatis* in fallopian tube tissue in women with post infectious tubal infertility. Am J Obstet Gynecol 1994; 171:95– 101

[271] Beatty WL, Byrne GI, Morrison RP (1994) Repeated and persistent infection with *Chlamydia* and the development of chronic inflammation and disease.
Trends Microbiol 2: 94–98

[272] Wiggins R, Graf S, Low N, et al; *Chlamydia* Screening Studies (ClaSS) Study Group. Real-time quantitative PCR to determine Chlamydial load in men and women in a community setting. J Clin Microbiol 2009;47:1824e9

[273] Michel CE, Sonnex C, Carne CA, et al. *Chlamydia trachomatis* load at matched anatomic sites: implications for screening strategies. J Clin Microbiol 2007;45:1395e402

[274] West ES, Munoz B, Mkocha H, et al. Mass treatment and the effect on the load of *Chlamydia trachomatis* infection in a trachoma-hyperendemic community.Invest Ophthalmol Vis Sci 2005;46:83–7

[275] Westrom LV. Sexually transmitted diseases and infertility. Sex Transm Dis 1994;21:S32–7

[276] Centers for Disease control and Prevention, 2011 Sexually transmitted Disease surveillance. Atlanta, GA: US Department of Health and Human Services

[277] Centers for Disease control and Prevention, Sexually transmitted Disease surveillance 2008. Atlanta, GA: US Department of Health and Human Services 2009

[278] Health protection agency, Sexually transmitted infections and young people in the united kingdom: 2008 Report, July 2008

[279] European Centre for Disease Prevention and Control. *Chlamydia* Control in Europe. Stockholm 2009

[280] British Columbia Centre for Disease Control. STI Prevention & Control: Annual Reports 1997 – 2011, March 2013

[281] 2008 Annual Surveillance Report: HIV/AIDS, Viral Hepatitis and Sexually Transmissible Infections in Australia

[282] Brunham RC, Pourbohloul B, Mak S, White R, Rekart ML (2005) The unexpected impact of a *Chlamydia trachomatis* infection control program on susceptibility to reinfection. J Infect Dis 192: 1836–1844

[283] Farris CM, Morrison RP.Vaccination against *Chlamydia* genital infection utilizing the murine C. muridarum model. Infect Immun. 2011 Mar;79(3):986-96. doi: 10.1128/IAI.00881-10. Epub 2010 Nov 15

[284] Longbottom. Chlmaydial vaccine development. J Med Microbiology 2003;52(July (Pt 7)):537-40

[285] Mitzel, Vaccination against feline pneumonitis. Am J Vet Res.1977 Sep;38(9):1361-3

[286] Grayston JT, Woolridge RL, Wang S. Trachoma Vaccine studies in Taiwan. Ann. N.Y. Acad. Sci. (1962) 98, 352-367

[287] Poland GA, Kennedy RB, Ovsyannikova IG (2011) Vaccinomics and Personalized Vaccinology: Is Science Leading Us Toward a New Path of Directed Vaccine Development and Discovery? PLoS Pathog 7(12): e1002344

[288] Caldwell HD, Ku CC, Kenny GE. Antigenic analysis of Chlamydiae by two-dimensional immunoelectrophoresis. II A trachoma-LGV-specific antgen. Journal of Immunology (1975). 115, 969-975

[289] Sanchez-Campillo M, Bini L, ComanducciM et al. Identificationof immunoreactive proteins of a two dimensional electroporesis map with patient sera. Electrophoresis (1999). 20(11), 2269-2279

[290] Murphey C, Murthy AK, Meier PA, Neal Guentzel M, Zhong G, Arulanandam BP. The protective efficacy of Chlamydial protease-like activity factor for vaccination is dependent on CD4+ T cells. (2006).242, 110-117

[291] Stemke-Hale K, Kaltenboeck B, Degraves FJ at al. Screening the whole genomeof a pthogen in vivo for individual protective antigens (2005) Vaccine 23(23), 3016-3025

[292] Starnbach MN, Loomis WP, Ovendale P, Regan D, Hess B, Alderson MR, Fling SP. An inclusion membrane protein from *Chlamydia trachomatis* enters the MHC class I pathway and stimulates a CD8+ T cell response. J Immunol. 2003 Nov 1;171(9):4742-9

[293] Karunakaran KP, Rey-Ladino J, Stoynov N, Berg K, Shen C, Jiang X, Gabel BR, Yu H, Foster LJ, Brunham RC. Immunoproteomic discovery of novel T cell antigens from the obligate intracellular pathogen *Chlamydia*. J Immunol. 2008 Feb 15;180(4):2459-65

[294] Brunham, R.C. and R.W. Peeling, *Chlamydia trachomatis* antigens: role in immunity and pathogenesis, in Infectious agents and disease. 1994. p. 218-33.

[295] Sanchez-Campillo, M., et al., Identification of immunoreactive proteins of *Chlamydia trachomatis* by Western blot analysis of a two-dimensional electrophoresis map with patient sera, in Electrophoresis. 1999. p. 2269-79.

[296] Taylor, H.R. and R.A. Prendergast, Attempted oral immunization with Chlamydial lipopolysaccharide subunit vaccine., in Invest Ophthalmol Vis Sci. 1987.

[297] Pal S, Theodor I, Peterson EM, de la Maza LM. Immunization with the *Chlamydia trachomatis* mouse pneumonitis major outer membrane protein can elicit a protective immune response against a genital challenge. Infect Immun, 2001. 69(10): p. 6240-7.

[298] Pal, S., E.M. Peterson, and L.M. de la Maza, Vaccination with the *Chlamydia trachomatis* major outer membrane protein can elicit an immune response as protective as that resulting from inoculation with live bacteria. Infect Immun, 2005. 73(12): p. 8153-60.

[299] Caldwell, H.D. and R.C. Judd, Structural analysis of Chlamydial major outer membrane proteins. Infect Immun, 1982. 38(3): p. 960-8.

[300] Caldwell, H.D. and J. Schachter, Antigenic analysis of the major outer membrane protein of *Chlamydia* spp, in Infect Immun. 1982. p. 1024-31.

[301] Crane DD, Carlson JH, Fischer ER, Bavoil P, Hsia RC, Tan C, et al. *Chlamydia trachomatis* polymorphic membrane protein D is a species-common pan-neutralizing antigen. Proc Natl Acad Sci U S A 2006;103(February (6)):1894–9

[302] Yu H, Jiang X, Shen C, Karunakaran KP, Brunham RC. Novel *Chlamydia* muridarum T cell antigens induce protective immunity against lung and genital tract infection in murine models. J Immunol 2009;182(February (3)):1602–8

[303] Tan C, Hsia RC, Shou H, Haggerty CL, Ness RB, Gaydos CA, et al. *Chlamydia trachomatis*-infected patients display variable antibody profiles against the nine-member polymorphic membrane protein family. Infect Immun 2009;77 (August (8)):3218–26

[304] Murphey C, Murthy AK, Meier PA, Neal Guentzel M, Zhong G, Arulanandam BP The protective efficacy of Chlamydial protease-like activity factor vaccination is dependent upon CD4+ T cells. Cell Immunol. 2006 Aug;242(2):110-7. Epub 2006 Nov 20.

[305] Meoni E, Faenzi E, Frigimelica, Zedda L,Skibinski Giovinazzi S,Bonci A,Petracca R,1 Bartolini E, Galli G, Agnusdei M, Nardelli F, Buricchi F, Norais N, Ferlenghi I, Dona-

ti, Cevenini R, Finco O,Grandi G, and Grifantini R. CT043, a Protective Antigen That Induces a CD4+ Th1 Response during *Chlamydia trachomatis* Infection in Mice and Humans. Infect Immun. 2009 September; 77(9): 4168–4176

[306] Sharma J, Bosnic AM, Piper JM, Zhong G. Human Antibody Responses to a *Chlamydia*-Secreted Protease Factor. Infection and Immunity, Dec. 2004, p. 7164–7171

[307] He Q, Martinez-Sobrido L, Eko FO, Palese P, Garcia-Sastre A, Lyn D, et al. Live-attenuated influenza viruses as delivery vectors for *Chlamydia* vaccines. Immunology 2007;122:28–37

[308] Karunakaran KP, Yu H, Foster LJ, Brunham RC. Development of a *Chlamydia trachomatis* T cell vaccine. Hum Vaccin 2010;6:676–80

[309] Dong-Ji Z, Yang X, Shen C, Lu H, Murdin A, Brunham RC. Priming with *Chlamydia trachomatis* major outer membrane protein (MOMP) DNA fol- lowed by MOMP ISCOM boosting enhances protection and is associated with increased immunoglobulin A and Th1 cellular immune responses. Infect Immun 2000;68:3074–8

[310] Hansen J, Jensen KT, Follmann F, Agger EM, Theisen M, Andersen P. Liposome delivery of *Chlamydia* muridarum major outer membrane protein primes a Th1 response that protects against genital Chlamydial infection in a mouse model. J Infect Dis 2008;198:758–67

[311] Pal S, Peterson EM, Rappuoli R, Ratti G, de la Maza LM. Immunization with the *Chlamydia trachomatis* major outer membrane protein, using adjuvants developed for human vaccines, can induce partial protection in a mouse model against a genital challenge. Vaccine 2006;24:766–75

[312] Hickey DK, Aldwell FE, Beagley KW (2010) Oral immunization with a novel lipid-based adjuvant protects against genital *Chlamydia* infection. Vaccine 28: 1668–1672

[313] Hickey DK, Aldwell FE, Beagley KW (2009) Transcutaneous immunization with a novel lipid-based adjuvant protects against *Chlamydia* genital and respiratory infections. Vaccine 27: 6217–6225

[314] Macmillan L, Ifere GO, He Q, Igietseme JU, Kellar KL, Okenu DM, et al. A recombinant multivalent combination vaccine protects against *Chlamydia* and genital herpes. FEMS Immunol Med Microbiol 2007;49:46–55

[315] Hickey DK, Bao S, Ikeda LT, Carey AJ, Beagley KW (2005) Induction of anti-Chlamydial mucosal immunity by transcutaneous immunization is enhanced by topical application of GM-CSF. Curr Mol Med 5: 599–605).

[316] Eko FO, Ekong E, He Q, Black CM, Igietseme JU (2011) Induction of immune memory by a multisubunit Chlamydial vaccine. Vaccine 29: 1472–1480

[317] Manam S, Chaganty BK, Evani SJ, Zafiratos MT, Ramasubramanian AK, Arulanandam BP, Murthy AK. Intranasal vaccination with *Chlamydia* pneumoniae induces

cross-species immunity against genital *Chlamydia* muridarum challenge in mice. PLoS One. 2013 May 31;8(5):e64917. doi: 10.1371/journal.pone.0064917.

[318] Marks E, Helgeby A, Andersson JO, Schön K, Lycke NY (2011) CD4+ T-cell immunity in the female genital tract is critically dependent on local mucosal immunization. Eur J Immunol 41: 2642–2653)

[319] R. T. Gray, K. W. Beagley, P. Timms, and D. P. Wilson, "Modeling the impact of potential vaccines on epidemics of sexually transmitted *Chlamydia trachomatis* infection," Journal of Infectious Diseases, vol. 199, no. 11, pp. 1680–1688, 2009

[320] Carey A, Cunningham K, Andrew D, Hafner L, Timms P, Beagley K. A comparison of the effects of a Chlamydial vaccine administered during or after a C. muridarum urogenital infection of female mice. Vaccine 2011;29: 6505–13

Chapter 8

The Roles of Invariant NKT Cells in Bowel Immunity — Suppression of Tumor Progression and Rejection of Intestinal Transplants

Tatsuaki Tsuruyama and Wulamujiang Aini

Additional information is available at the end of the chapter

http://dx.doi.org/10.5772/57588

1. Introduction

The roles of natural killer (NK)T cells in intestinal immunity have not been sufficiently investigated. The bowel possesses its own unique mucosal immune system, the gut-associated lymphoepithelial tract (GALT). In this review, we focused on CD1d-independent invariant type NKT (iNKT) cells as modulators of GALT. iNKT cells have a restricted invariant T-cell receptor (TCR) Vα24 chain paired with Vβ11 chain. In addition to T helper (Th)1 cytokines, such as IFN-γ, iNKT cells can produce anti-inflammatory Th2 cytokines, such as interleukin (IL)-4.

Although invariant NKT cells are rare in normal small-intestine mucosa, they have been observed in intestinal allografts during rejection. Infiltrating iNKT cells release IL-4 and IL-5, Th2-related cytokines that antagonize the Th1 responses that induce acute cellular rejection. Also, iNKT cells form an immunological barrier against parasite infection. We found that CD1d +cells are actually localized in the lamina propria of the villi in the human intestine and they may present the antigen for the recruited iNKT cells.

On the other hand, a small number of invariant NKT cells are resident in the normal colorectal mucosa. iNKT cells are involved in defense against colorectal tumor progression and metastasis through the apoptosis-inducing molecule Fas ligand (FasL). Their numbers increase markedly in colorectal carcinomas. Increased iNKT cell infiltration in colorectal carcinomas is an independent favorable prognostic factor. iNKT cells probably play an important role in the pathogenesis of ulcerative colitis.

Thus, iNKT cells are modulators of bowel mucosal immunity.

2. Background

2.1. Gut-associated lymphoepithelial tract (GALT)

The bowel possesses a distinct mucosal immune system, known as the gut-associated lymphoepithelial tract (GALT), which is comprised of high endothelial venules (HEVs) located in the inter-follicular region (IFR) around the Peyer's patches (PPs). GALT-associated immunity involves an exquisite balance between activation and suppression mediated through the release of cytokines [1] (Figure 1). The GALT contains the largest collection of lymphocytes in the body. Physiologic and barrier functions of GALT against bacterial infection are associated with mucosal surfaces and are essential; therefore, only limited damage can be tolerated. The mucosa is continuously exposed to a vast array of antigens, necessitating the distinguishing of self from non-self/infectious antigens. Infectious agents, malignant tumors such as adenocarcinomas, and immune and inflammatory bowel diseases of the gut all contribute to morbidity and mortality.

The lymphocytes in the bowel are believed to play pivotal roles in bowel immunity. Two types of lymphocytes are found in the bowel: intra-epithelial lymphocytes (IELs) and lamina propria (LP) lymphocytes (LPLs). In addition, the PPs are comprised of B cells and T cells, unique lymphocyte subsets that interact with M epithelial cells. Antigens are taken up by the PPs through the M-cell layer, inducing an immune reaction (Figure 1).

In addition, lymphocytes from the GALT circulate in the common mucosal immune system, including the mesenteric lymph nodes.

LPLs play important roles in immune homeostasis. Although these cells function in mucosal defense against pathogens, they ignore non-pathogenic bacteria and foods, a phenomenon known as oral tolerance. LPLs also play a supporting role in barrier defenses and are involved in the pathogenesis of inflammatory intestinal diseases. At the onset of Crohn's disease, mucosal T cells appear to mount a typical T helper (Th)1 response that resembles an acute infectious process, but this response is lost with progression to later stages of Crohn's disease. Such polarization of bowel cytokines is believed to be responsible for inflammatory bowel diseases (IBD).

2.2. Natural killer T cells

NKT cells are associated with both innate and adaptive immunity due to their ability to interact with a broad spectrum of antigens.

NKT cells are currently classified into three types classical NKT cells (non-classical NKT cells); and NKT-like cells, or CD1d-independent NK1.1+T cells [2]. Classical NKT cells express CD161 [2, 3]. Human classical NKT cells express an invariant TCR, Vα24, whereas mouse NKT cells express TCRVα14 [4, 5]. In contrast, the T-cell receptor V regions expressed by non-classical NKT cells and NKT-like cells are highly diverse. CD56-NKT cells are believed to function as effector or regulatory cells in innate immunity.

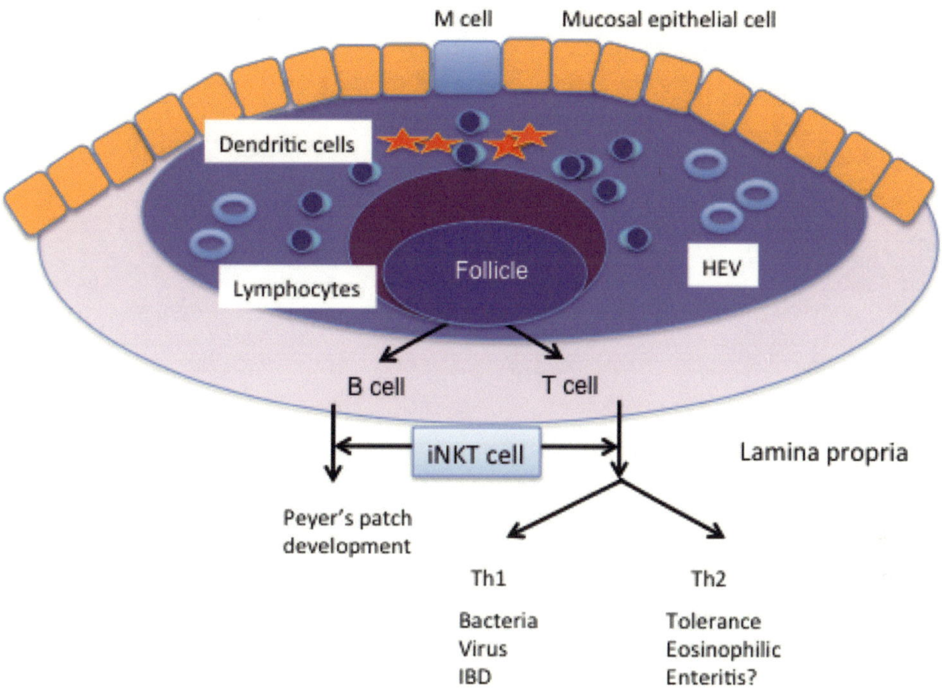

Figure 1. GALT and iNKT cells. M cells and mucosal epithelial cells cover the lamina propria of the bowel. HEV: high endothelial venules, Th1 & Th2, helper T cell Type 1 & 2. iNKT cells relate to the development of B cells and T cells in the lamina propria by release of cytokines such as IL-4, IL-5, IFN-γ.

2.3. Invariant natural killer T (iNKT) cells

Among these NK cells, iNKT cells have a very restricted TCR repertoire, which in human peripheral blood consists of an invariant Vα24-Ja18 chain (formerly Vα24-JaQ) paired with a Vβ11 chain [4, 6]. Therefore, this classical type is termed "invariant" NKT (iNKT) cells (Figure 2). Human iNKT cells can be activated by glycolipid antigens such as beta-galactosylceramide and iGb3, which are presented by CD1d expressed on dendritic cells [7]. When activated, iNKT cells immediately produce pro-inflammatory Th1 cytokines such as IFN-γ and tumor necrosis factor (TNF)-α as well as anti-inflammatory Th2 cytokines, such as IL-4, IL-10, and IL-13. Thus, iNKT cells are capable of bidirectional differentiation, which is probably directed by the immunological environment.

iNKT cells are localized primarily in the thymus, bone marrow, liver, and spleen, and they are rare in the lymph nodes [8]. Bannai et al. [9] reported that mouse colon contains a considerable number of NKT cells. More recently, O'Keeffe et al. reported that T cells expressing CD161+(a phenotypic marker of NK cells) are the major natural killer receptor–positive cell population in the intestine. Although the intestines harbor a diverse array of NKT cells, iNKT cells are rare in the small intestine [10].

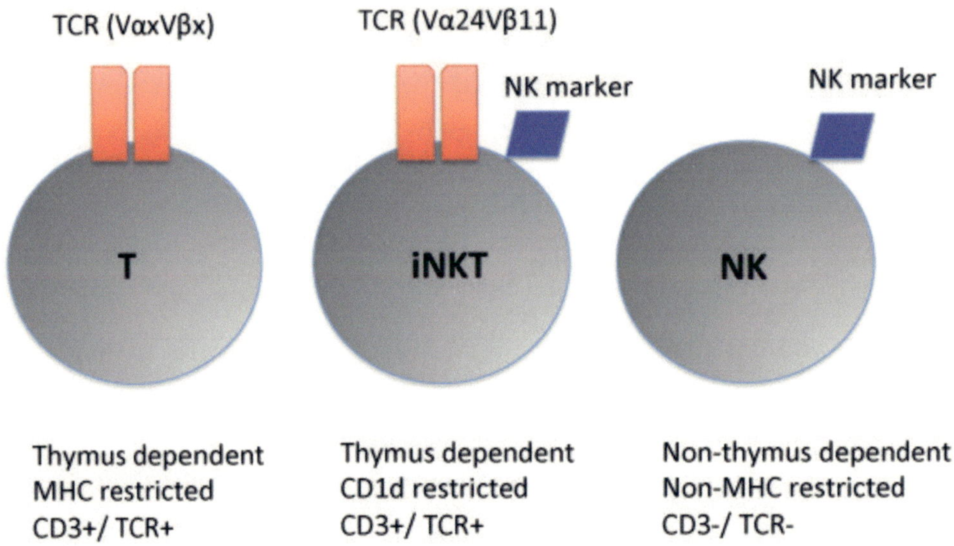

Figure 2. T, invariant natural killer (NK)T, and NK cells. The phenotypic surface antigens are shown. The T cell receptor (TCR) is variable in T cells; the TCR on the invariant type of human NKT cells is restricted to the Vα24β11 type. NK cells do not carry a TCR and express CD161, CD56, or CD57 NK markers, which are also expressed by NKT cells.

2.4. Invariant natural killer T (iNKT) cells in diseases

iNKT cells have been implicated as playing roles in infection control [11, 12], inflammatory bowel diseases [13], abortion [14], transplantation tolerance [15, 16], suppression of autoimmune diseases [17-20], psoriasis and atopic dermatitis [21], and the regulation of allergic disorders [22, 23]. iNKT cells have the potential to activate or suppresses immune system by release of variable cytokines including IFN-γ, IL-4, IL-10, and IL-17.

Moreover, a number of reports have suggested that iNKT cells play protective as well as tolerogenic roles in tumor immunity [24-29]. In addition, infiltration of iNKT cells is a prognostic indicator for colorectal cancer metastasis [29].

3. iNKT cells in the small intestine

3.1. Mucosal immunity of the small intestine

The mucosal immune system of the small intestine is unique. Mucosal barrier damage and inflammation have been associated with high levels of flagellin protein in the lumen. One of the roles of intestinal immunity is defense against pathogens within the bacterial flora. The mucosa is covered by mucin, which is one of the central determinants of gut immune specificity and immune tolerance.

The LP, located beneath the mucosa, includes various types of immune cells that form the GALT. The PP is a predominant immune apparatus that is covered by M cells and is capable of controlling mucosal immunity. In addition to the lymph apparatus and lymphocytes, the intestinal immune system contains dendritic cells (DCs) that interact with goblet cells. Mucus sensing enhances DC tolerogenic functions, including the release of TGF-β and suppressive IL-10, which are factors that induce FoxP3+regulatory T (T_{reg}) cell production. Populations of CD3+TCR-γδ cells are also observed [29]. CD56+NK cells are classically viewed as lymphocytes that provide innate immunity against virus-infected cells and tumor cells through the release of cytolytic mediators and IFN-γ.

3.2. iNKT cells in the small intestine and coeliac disease

Intestinal iNKT cells are rare in the normal status [10], but small population is observed in the villi of the small intestine [30]. Although they have not been considered as minor participants in the control of GALT. However, iNKT cells are found to decrease in the celiac disease without affecting development of classical T cells. Coeliac disease is one of the autoimmune disorders of the small intestine. This disease occurs in genetically predisposed people of all ages from middle infancy. Symptoms include pain, chronic constipation and diarrhea in children. Diagnoses are occasionally being made in asymptomatic persons in the screening examination. Importantly, coeliac disease is not allergic disease, but caused by a reaction to a gluten protein in wheat. When the small intestine is exposed to gluten, the tissue transglutaminase modifies the protein, and the GALT autoimmunologically cross-reacts with the small intestinal tissue, causing an inflammatory reaction. As a result, villous atrophy is observed histologically and endoscopically. The absorption of nutrients is significantly affected. The effective treatment is a lifelong gluten-free diet. The deficiency of Vα24+ cells in coeliac disease was independent of age, gluten status of diet or duration of gluten-free diet. Probably, T cells are selected by glycolipids on CD1d expressing CD4+CD8+thymocytes [30].

3.3. Small-intestine allograft immunity

3.3.1. Background on intestinal transplantation

Intestinal transplantation is a commonly accepted standard therapy for patients with irreversible parenteral nutrition complications associated with short-bowel syndrome, [31-33], Hirschsprung and related diseases, chronic idiopathic intestinal pseudo-obstruction syndrome, and megacystis-microcolon-intestinal hypoperistalsis syndrome [34, 35]. Acute cellular rejection (ACR) remains the major cause of intestinal graft failure after transplantation. Diagnosis of ACR requires detection by histopathologic evaluation [35-38] as well as clinical examination and laboratory data [38].

3.3.2. Histologic criteria for diagnosis of ACR of small-intestine transplants

Pathologists have diagnosed acute rejection based on the finding of crypt apoptosis in the intestinal mucosa upon histologic examination of the graft [36-38], rather than lymphocytic infiltrates. The number of apoptotic bodies is certainly augmented during the acute rejection; however, the mechanism underlying this phenomenon has not been determined.

Mucosal damage cannot be prevented once crypt apoptosis has become evident [38]. It is possible that apoptosis of crypt cells is induced by direct attack by cytotoxic T-lymphocytes (CTLs), but such a finding has not been reported. Therefore, it remains unclear whether CTL infiltration is necessary for ACR. Humoral factors may also play a role in crypt apoptosis.

Although there are reports describing T-cell apoptosis in the intestine in ongoing ACR, its clinical significance has not been determined [39]. T cells interact with Fas on other T cells to induce their apoptosis [40]. The apoptotic T cells are then phagocytosed by macrophages in the small-intestine allografts. Similar findings in a liver allograft has been reported by us [41]. Thus, these phagocytic findings may be common to various allografts in ACR. The phagocytosing macrophages form granulomas. Furthermore, apoptotic bodies are also positive for Fas, which is a surface antigen of activated T lymphocytes. Treatment with a steroid pulse significantly diminishes the apoptotic and phagocytotic responses that are indicative of ACR [42]. Although it is possible that both recipient and donor lymphocytes interact with each other via Fas and FasL molecules to induce apoptosis, a study using animal models reported that TNF-α (rather than interaction between Fas and FasL) is the primary factor for induction of lymphocytic apoptosis [39].

3.3.3. iNKT cells infiltrate during acute rejection of the allograft

Using systematic immunohistochemical analysis of an intestinal allograft, we assessed the behavior of iNKT cells during acute rejection of the intestinal allograft [38]. In practice, the diagnosis of intestinal rejection is difficult, particularly due to the complicated interactions between lymphocytes and other immunological cells resulting from the transient coexistence of donor-derived and recipient-derived cells in the graft.

iNKT cells are transiently recruited to the intestinal LP (Figure 3), but immunosuppressive therapy significantly decreased iNKT cells in number (Figure 4&5). The infiltrating intestinal iNKT cells have the potential to produce IL-4, which antagonizes IFN-γ and contributes to the development of Th2 cells. Higher levels of IL-4 prior to and shortly after kidney transplantation have been reported, and IL-4 may have a protective effect on renal graft survival [43]. Indeed, iNKT cells have been implicated in tolerance in experimental mouse models, in induction of chimerism in allogenic cardiac transplant models [44], and in acceptance of rat-islet xenografts in mice [16]. IFN-γ production remains low relative to normal donor intestine and does not change during the course of ACR development. Therefore, infiltration of iNKT cells implies that they are involved in the response to rejection. Asaoka et al. reported the activation of CTLs in granzyme B/perforin-mediated graft injury [45]. Therefore, release of Th2-related cytokines by iNKT cells may antagonize this activation.

3.3.4. PPs and iNKT cells in small-intestine allografts

After transplantation, recipient-derived T cells traffic into the allograft across the HEVs located in the IFR around the PPs. Therefore, the PP serves as the interface through which the allograft

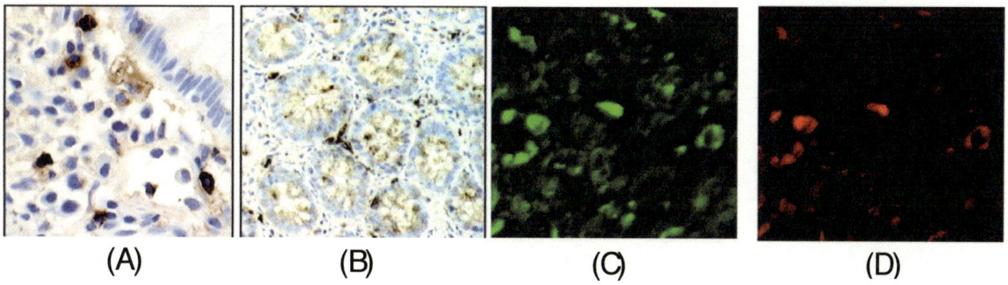

Figure 3. Immunohistochemistry of iNKT cells: (A) TCRVα24 (left) and (B) TCRVβ11 stained cells in brown. Fluorescent immunostaining of TCRVα24 (C), IL-4 (D).

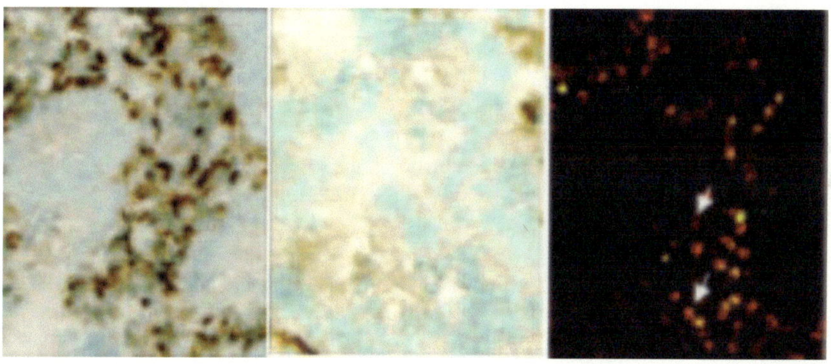

Figure 4. Time-course analyses using allograft tissues showed a significant decrease in the number of iNKT cells after immunosuppressant administration. The left photo illustrates the significant decrease in the number of iNKT cells after administration. Immunostaining of iNKT cells at the onset of ACR (left) and 48 hrs after administration of steroids (middle) is shown. Brown cells are iNKT cells in the allograft mucosa. Counterstaining was performed using methyl-green. iNKT cells underwent apoptosis in the graft. The right photo below shows TUNEL-positive (yellow) iNKT cells. Non-iNKT cells were stained red (phycoerythrin-labeled). This photo is the serial section of the left section [39].

encounters recipient-derived cells. Although, few studies have examined injury to the PPs during rejection, histology of PP showed the hyperplastic change of PP with an increase in expression of CD20, a mature B cell marker at the onset of rejection (Figure 6).

PPs consist primarily of B cells, T cells and DCs. In general, B cells carry out a variety of immune functions, including immunoglobulin production, cytokine release, antigen presentation, regulation of DC activity, and participation in the induction of immune tolerance [46]. A large number of T cells and B cells are present in the intestinal LP. The majority of T cells in the LP express the TCR$\alpha\beta$, and the proportion of CD8+T cells to CD4+T cells ranges from 2:1 to 3:1. The production of IL-4 and IL-5 by CD4+T cells in the LP promotes IgA production in the intestinal tract. Furthermore, CD8+T cells in the LP are responsible for damage by recognizing and activating macrophages. The primary antibodies secreted into the intestinal tract mucus are IgA. A number of IgA-producing cells distribute in the LP, and IgA molecules that are secreted into the intestinal tract are transported to the gut luminal side by binding to multi-meric antibody receptors that are retained on the intestinal epithelial cells.

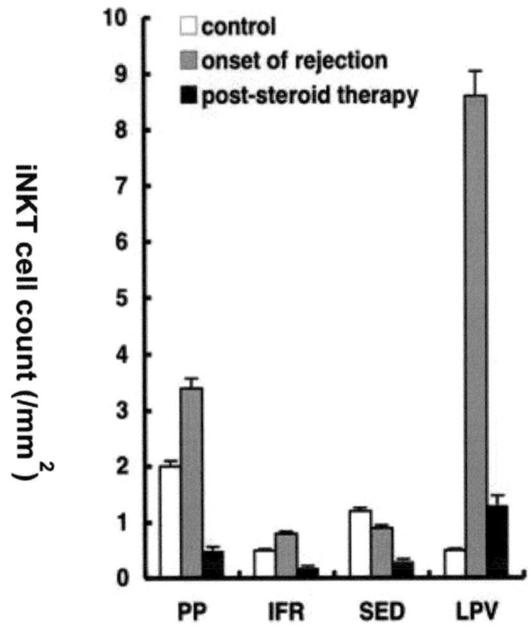

Figure 5. Distribution of iNKT cells in six intestinal allografts. The count of iNKT cells was evaluated by their number per 1mm^2 of a section. PP, Peyer's patch; IFR, inter-follicular region; SED, mucosal sub-epithelial dome; LPV, lamina propria of the villi. Individual bars of intact, onset, and post-administration display the TCRVα24+T cell counts in the intact mucosa, in the mucosa with rejection, and in the mucosa 48 hours after >30mg of steroid administration (post-steroid therapy).

Both B-1 and B-2 cells produce IgA. B-2 cells are derived from PP B cells and exhibit a CD23+, CD11b-, CD5-, and CD19^{low} phenotype. Follicular B cells in the PPs are stimulated by antigen in the intestinal lumen and differentiate from IgM+to IgA+cells by class switching. IgA+cells in the PPs circulate throughout the body via the thoracic duct and differentiate into IgA-producing cells by the effect of IL-6 produced by intestinal epithelial cells. B-1 cells, in contrast, are derived from B cells of the abdominal cavity and exhibit a CD19+, CD23-, and CD11b+ (B-1a, CD5+; B-1b, CD5-) phenotype. Whereas B-2 cell-derived secretory IgA recognizes foreign antigens with high affinity, B-1 cell-derived secretory IgA recognizes common bacterial phosphorylcholine, lipopolysaccharide, and self-antigens with low affinity.

3.3.5. Cytokine production in the intestinal allograft

Cytokine measurements have suggested that the levels of a variety of cytokines are increased at the onset of ACR and that TNF-α contributes to mucosal damage in graft-versus-host disease [47]. The graph below shows the production of various cytokines in graft mucosal tissues without PPs before transplantation, during ACR, and 72 hrs after administration of a steroid pulse. The data show that production of both IL-4 and IL-5 increase significantly relative to other cytokines in the allograft tissue during ACR, suggesting that ACR involves hypercytokinemia (Figure 7)[38].

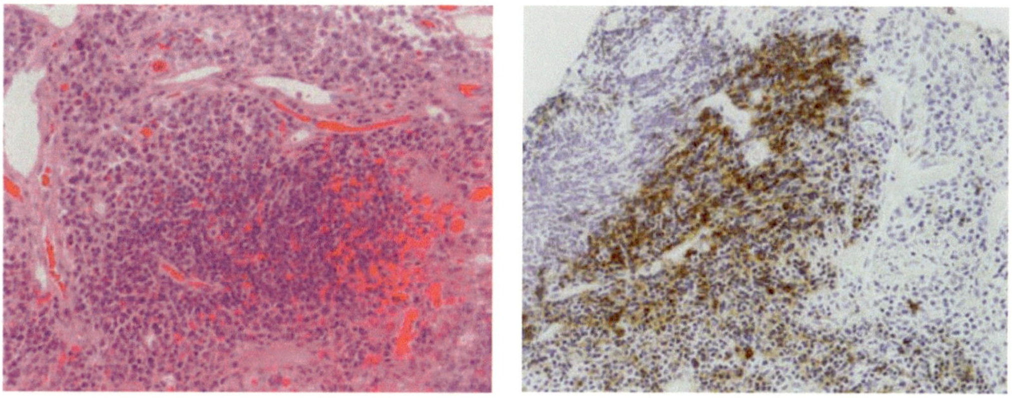

Figure 6. Peyer's patch (PP) hyperplasia in acute rejection of small intestinal allograft. Left photo shows an H&E stained hyperplastic PP in the graft at the onset of rejection. Right photo shows the CD20+ stained hyperplastic PP.

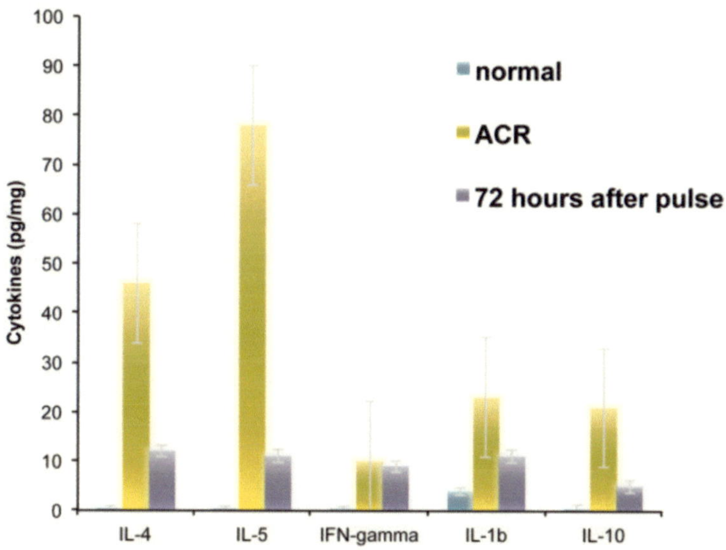

Figure 7. Cytokine concentration in the histologic normal allograft, at the onset of acute cellular rejection (ACR) and 72 hours after steroid pulse. Error bars indicate S.D. [38].

3.3.6. Activated iNKT cells may damage the small-intestine allograft by release of IL-4/IL-5

Cytokine production by iNKT cells was observed in grafts and total cytokine concentration in sampled tissue was measured. Graphs show plots of the concentrations of IL-4, IL-5, IL-10, and IFN-γ (pg/mg in graft tissue) versus the mean number of IL-4+-, IL-5+-, IFN-γ+-, and IL-10+-iNKT cells (per 10 high-power foci [HPF]). Linear regression lines and correlation coefficient (R^2) values are also shown (Figure 8).

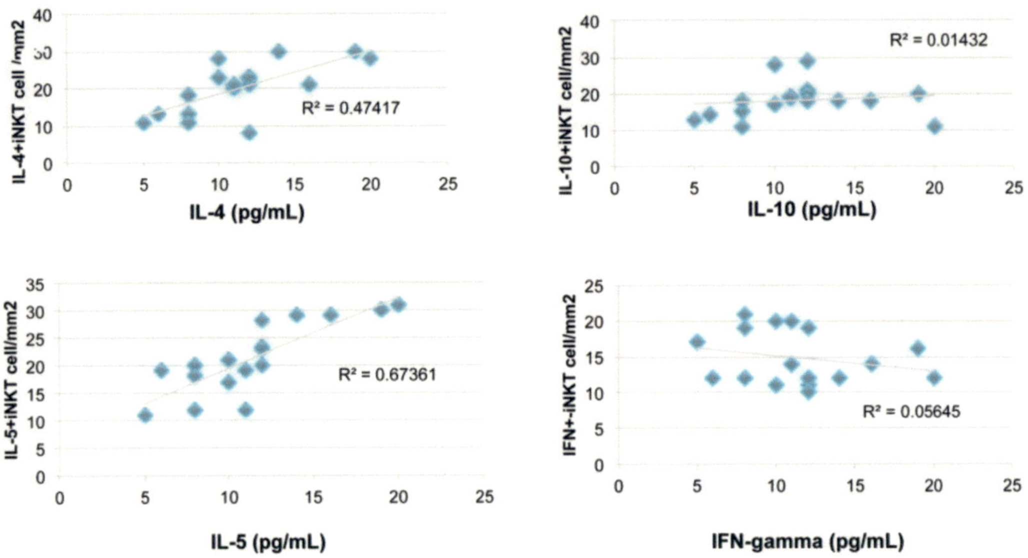

Figure 8. Regression analysis of cytokine concentration and counts of iNKT cells. IL-4 and IL-5 iNKT cell count correlate with total concentration of IL-4 and IL-5 in the graft.

It is likely that as yet unknown humoral factors recruit iNKT cells to the graft mucosa in order to suppress allograft rejection. iNKT cells have the ability to release IL-4 and antagonize Th1 and CTL responses [48]. However, because the released IL-4 and IL-5 may damage the allograft via eosinophilic enteritis, appropriate immunosuppression is necessary for recovery. We therefore investigated humoral rejection. iNKT cells may modulate such ACR via the release of cytokines.

3.4. NKT cells in intestinal inflammation caused by parasites

iNKT cells can also modulate mucosal immunity through the release of IL-4 and IL-5 in response to parasite infection. A previous study showed that NKT cells play a critical role in the lethal ileitis induced in C57BL/6 mice after infection with *Toxoplasma gondii* [49]. This intestinal inflammation is caused by overproduction of IFN-γ by iNKT cells in the LP. This detrimental activity of iNKT cells can be blocked by treatment with alpha-galactosylceramide, which induces a shift in cytokine production by iNKT cells toward a Th2 profile. iNKT cells participate in the clearance of parasites by shifting the cytokine profile toward a Th1 pattern. Another study using CD1d-deficient mice lacking iNKT cells showed that iNKT cells are critical for the elimination of *T. gondii* [50]. Thus, iNKT cells may form an immunological barrier against parasite infection.

4. iNKT cells in large-intestine immunity

4.1. NKT cells in the large intestine

Unlike the small intestine, a considerable number of NKT cells reside intra-epithelially in the colon of mice [9]. CD161+T cells are the major natural killer receptor-positive cell population in the intestine [10]. On the other hand, few reports have been published regarding human NKT cells, particularly iNKT cells, in the normal and neoplastic colon.

Our previous study was the first report the presence of TCRVα24+ iNKT cells in the colon [29]. In that study, a small number of Vα24+NKT cells were observed in the normal colorectal mucosa (2.6 ± 3.7 cells/5 HPF), unlike the small intestine, which contained few resident NKT cells.

4.2. Intra-colorectal tumor iNKT cells

Furthermore, we investigated intra-tumor TCRVα24-positive cells in 103 primary colorectal carcinoma samples [29]. The observation that intra-tumor Vα24+T cells invariably coexpress TCRVβ11 and other NK cell markers indicates that they are iNKT cells. The density of iNKT cells in colorectal carcinomas increased significantly. iNKT cells were actually found in the luminal space of tumor-infiltrating vessels. iNKT cells could migrate from the peripheral blood to the tumors. A higher fraction of iNKT cells express the activation marker CD69 in colorectal carcinomas than in normal mucosa, and these cells are probably involved in local cytotoxicity against tumor cells through secretion of IFN-γ and apoptosis-inducing molecules such as FasL, perforin, and granzyme B. In this way, iNKT cells may play a role in the primary defense against colorectal carcinoma by induction of tumor cell death. Alternatively, the increase in the number of NKT cells in tumors may represent a surrogate marker of antitumor activity.

Coca et al. reported that colorectal carcinomas with a higher degree of CD57+NK cell infiltration have better prognosis [51]. Because the CD57+cell population includes NKT cells, the present observation agrees in part with their conclusion. Another interesting feature of our study was the finding that iNKT cells play a role in the inhibition of lymph node metastasis of colorectal carcinomas [29]. Although iNKT cells are normally rare in lymph nodes, a large number of these cells appear in the metastasis-free swollen lymph nodes of colorectal carcinoma patients. The precise mechanism through which iNKT cells inhibit lymph node metastasis remains unclear. Activated iNKT cells may migrate to regional lymph nodes, where they may prevent metastasis by inducing apoptosis of the colorectal carcinoma cells. A recent study reported that chemokine CXCL16 suppresses liver metastasis of colorectal cancer via augmentation of tumor-infiltrating iNKT cells in a murine model [52].

Patients with a higher degree of intra-tumor NKT-cell infiltration show significantly higher rates of overall and disease-free survival. This is consistent with the fact that these patients exhibit much less lymph node metastasis. The degree of NKT cell infiltration in tumors was evaluated as low degree (<7 NKT cells/five x400 foci) or high degree (≥7 NKT cells/ five x400 foci). The number of iNKT cells increased markedly in colorectal carcinomas, and a majority of these cells showed a phenotype of activation expressing FasL or CD69. A higher degree of iNKT cell infiltration correlated with lower lymph node metastasis (P=0.042). Patients with a high degree of iNKT cell infiltration showed higher overall (P=0.018) as well as disease-free (P=0.0006) survival rates. Intra-tumor iNKT cell infiltration was an independent prognostic factor for overall (P=0.033) and disease-free (P=0.0064) survival. A higher degree of iNKT infiltration in colorectal carcinomas is therefore an independent indicator of a favorable prognosis [29] (Figure 9).

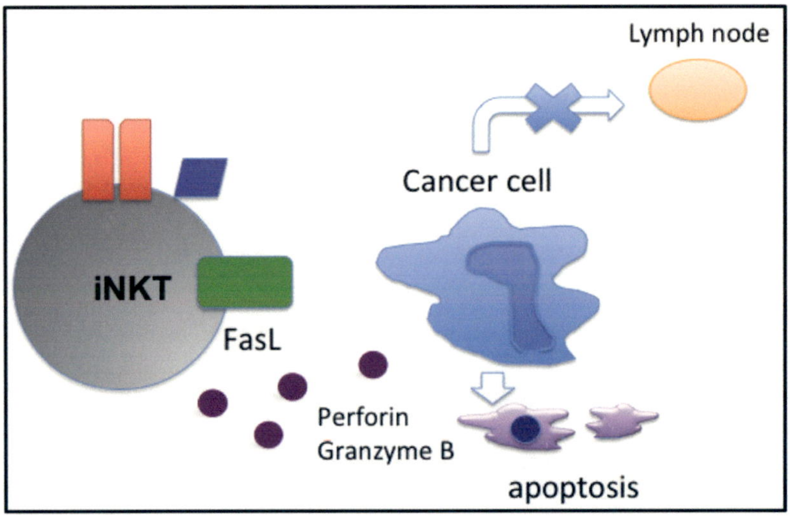

Figure 9. iNKT cells and apoptosis of tumor cells. FasL, perforin, and granzyme B are apoptosis-inducing molecules. iNKT cells may contribute to apoptosis of the cancer cell by release of these molecules and prevent the metastasis to the lymph node.

4.3. IBD and iNKT cells

The relevance of iNKT cells in IBD has also been examined. iNKT cells probably play an important role in the pathogenesis of ulcerative colitis [13, 22, 52]. Although our immunohistochemical data indicated that iNKT cells certainly contribute to inflammation, their influence is limited in the initial phase of IBD (data not shown). Several reports have indicated that iNKT cells secrete abundant amounts of IL-4 upon activation [53]. There has been a report that oxazolone colitis, a Th2 colitis model resembling ulcerative colitis, is mediated by IL-13-producing NK-T cells [54].

Important data regarding the role of iNKT cells in IBD were recently reported [31]. iNKT cells accumulate in the colonic lamina propria in germ-free mice, resulting in increased morbidity in models of IBD as compared with specific pathogen-free mice. The chemokine ligand CXCL16 is associated with an increase in the number of mucosal iNKT cells and consequently an increase in susceptibility to tissue inflammation. Age-sensitive contact with commensal microbes is critical for establishing mucosal iNKT cell tolerance to later environmental exposures. Microbial exposure early in life elicits long-lasting effects on iNKT cells, and in the absence of early exposure, exposure later in life to factors that stimulate these cells may induce an auto-inflammatory response.

In a related report, a profound loss of CD56 expression by all lymphocyte populations was noted in the coeliac gut. Adult coeliac disease expanded populations of CD3+TCRγδ cells and decreased populations of NK, NKT, and iNKT cells [30].

4.4. Microbial infection and iNKT cells

The relevance of iNKT cells against microbial infection has also been examined. CD1d-dependent antigen presentation and microbial killing by iNKT cells are critical for host defense [55]. The host defense against microbial infection depends upon cargo trafficking into lysosomes. The mechanism has been reported [56]. Arf-like GTPase Arl8b is one of the critical regulators of cargo delivery to lysosomes. The formation of CD1 antigen-presenting complexes in lysosomes and phagosome-lysosome fusion depends on Arl8b. Subsequently the delivered CD1 antigen-presenting complexes to the plasma membrane activate iNKT cells in microbial killing [56].

5. Methods

5.1. Quantitative morphometry

The quantitative morphometry method to study iNKT cells was applied (Figure 10). Multivariate morphometric analysis images were obtained by microscopy (PROVIS-AX80; Olympus, Tokyo, Japan) and saved as TIF files. Data were analyzed using CELAVIEW software (Olympus), with individual cell signals expressed in terms of relative fluorescent unit. Morphometric data were displayed according to stained area and circularity. Individual cells were represented by the pixel intensities of the nucleus and cytoplasm. Data sets for individual cells on a single slide were represented by two-dimensional scatter plots based on flow cytometry. Gated cells were further analyzed using antibodies for surface antigens. Plots were further gated according to fluorescence intensity, size, and circularity on the scattergram. Circularity was calculated based on the Heywood circularity factor using the following formula:

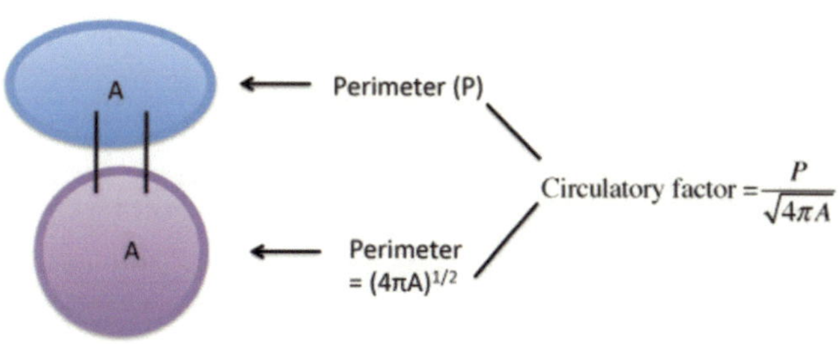

where the perimeter (P) of individual cells was divided by the circumference of a circle with the same area (A), with the real circle factor being equivalent to 1.0. As the boundary of a binary image is composed of discrete pixels, IMAQ Vision (National Instruments Corporation, Austin, TX, USA) was used to sub-sample the boundary [21, 39]. The scheme of quantitative morphometry is shown below.

Lymphocytes are oval or circular and the circulatory factor is nearly to 1.0. Therefore, the subjects of which circulatory factor is nearly to to 1.0 is gated for subsequent analysis using immunostaining. iNKT cells were actually gated for subsequent analysis using antibodies for CD56 and TCRVα24. In the first gating, the area was also analyzed [42] (Figure 10).

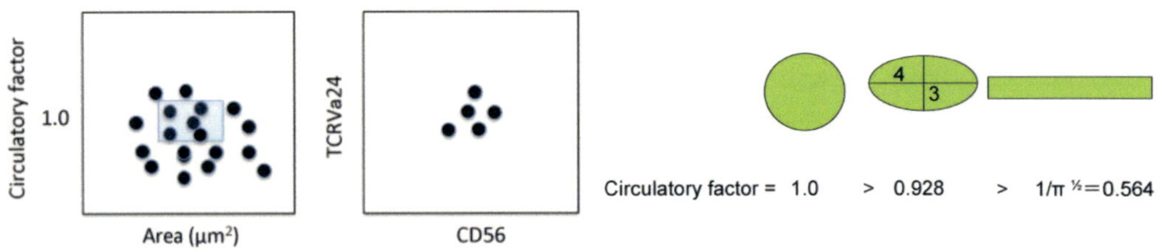

Figure 10. A scheme of two dimensional plots of the morphometric analysis for analysis of surface antigens CD56 and TCRVα24 on the iNKT cells. The gating shown in the left graph shows an example of selection of the analyzed lymphocytes for analysis of the surface antigens shown in the right graph. The similarity to the circle is evaluated by the circulatory factor near 1.0. The right figures the factor values of various shapes.

5.2. Immunohistochemistry

The fluorescent staining method for iNKT cells was as reported using the CSA system (DAKO, Gostrup, Denmark). Frozen section samples and paraffin embedded specimens were used. For primary reagents, we used monoclonal antibody C15 (TCRVα24; Immunotech SA, Marseilles, France). Antibodies against CD3, CD4 and CD8 were purchased from DAKO, and DAB staining was performed for signal visualization. Negative controls for primary antibodies were IgG1, IG2a and IgG2b (Cat No. X0931, X0943 and X0944; DAKO) [29, 38].

6. Conclusion

The mucosa is exposed to an extremely wide variety of antigens in food, and iNKT cells within the mucosa are responsible for mounting immune responses to these antigens. The cytokines released during these responses may damage the small intestine. In the case of small-intestine transplantation, the response of iNKT cells during ACR indicates that iNKT cells may be recruited to the transplant to repress rejection. iNKT cells probably contribute to the suppression of ACR by releasing IL-4, an antagonist of IFN-γ. On the other hand, iNKT cells normally reside within the large intestine, where they also play a pivotal role in immunity. iNKT cells can be activated to express apoptosis-inducing molecules and may induce cytolysis of tumor cells. Thus, iNKT cells have two roles; they can upregulate or downregulate the mucosal

http://dx.doi.org/10.5772/57588

immune response through the release of opposite-acting cytokines. iNKT cells thus play a pivotal role in modulating mucosal immunity in the intestine.

Acknowledgements

This work was supported by a Grant-in-Aid (Synergy of Fluctuation and Structure: Quest for Universal Laws in Non-Equilibrium Systems 2013-2017 Grant-in-Aid for Scientific Research on Innovative Areas, MEXT, Japan; http://sfs-dynamics.jp/eng/index.html). The funding agencies played no role in study design, data collection and analysis, in the decision to publish, or in preparation of the manuscript.

We thank Professor Shinji Uemoto and Dr. Shinya Okamoto of the Departments of Surgery and Pediatric Surgery at Kyoto University Hospital, respectively. Also we thank for Dr. Hisashi Onodera of the Department of Surgery at St. Luke's International Hospital of Tokyo, Japan. We dedicate this chapter to our great teacher, Professor Hirohiko Yamabe, Department of Diagnostic Pathology, Kyoto University Hospital. It was Professor Yamabe who established the pathologic diagnosis of organ transplantation in Japan.

Author details

Tatsuaki Tsuruyama and Wulamujiang Aini

Department of Diagnostic Pathology, Graduate School of Medicine, Kyoto University Hospital, Kyoto City, Japan

References

[1] Neurath, M.F.; Finotto, S.; Glimcher, L.H. (2002). The role of Th1/Th2 polarization in mucosal immunity. Nat Med 8:567-573.

[2] Godfrey, D.I.; MacDonald, H.R.; Kronenberg M.; et al. (2004). NKT cells: what's in a name? Nat Rev Immunol 4:231-237.

[3] Exley, M.; Porcelli, S.; Furman, M.; et al. (1998). CD161 (NKRP1A) costimulation of CD1d-dependent activation of human cells expressing invariant Va24JaQT-cell receptor a chains. J Exp Med 188:867-876.

[4] Taniguchi, M.; Harada, M.; Kojo, S.; Nakayama, T.; Wakao, H. (2003). The regulatory role of Valpha14 NKT cells in innate and acquired immune response. Annu Rev Immunol 21:483-513.

[5] Cui, J.; Shin, T.; Kawano, T.; et al. (1997). Requirement for Valpha14 NKT cells in IL-12-mediated rejection of tumors. Science 278: 1623-1626.

[6] Lee, P.T.; Benlagha, K.; Teyton, L.; Bendelac, A. (2002). Distinct functional lineages of human Va24 natural killer T cells. J Exp Med 195:637-641.

[7] Kawakami, K.; Yamamoto, N.; Kinjo, Y.; et al. (2003). Critical role of Valpha14+ natural killer T cells in the innate phase of host protection against *Streptococcus pneumonia* infection. Eur J Immunol 33:3322-3330.

[8] Kronenberg, M.; Gapin, L. (2002). The unconventional lifestyle of NKT cells. Nat Rev Immunol 2:557-568.

[9] Bannai, M.; Kawamura, T.; Naito T.; et al. (2001). Abundance of unconventional CD8+ natural killer T cells in the large intestine. Eur J Immunol 31:3361-3369.

[10] O'Keeffe, J.; Doherty, D.G.; Kenna, T.; et al. (2004). Diverse populations of T cells with NK cell receptors accumulate in the healthy human intestine and in colorectal cancer. Eur J Immunol 34:2110-2118.

[11] Kawakami, K.; Kinjo, Y.; Uezu, K.; et al. (2001). Monocyte chemoattractant protein-1-dependent increase of Valpha14 NKT cells in lungs and their roles in Th1 response and host defense in cryptococcal infection. J Immunol 167: 6525-6532.

[12] Grubor-Bauk, B.; Simmons, A.; Mayrhofer, G.; Speck, P.G. (2003). Impaired clearance of herpes simplex virus type 1 from mice lacking CD1d or NKT cells expressing the semivariant Valpha14-Ja281 TCR. J Immunol 170:1430-1434.

[13] Fuss, I.J.; Heller, F.; Boirivant, M.; et al. (2004). Nonclassical CD1d-restricted NK T cells that produce IL-13 characterize an atypical Th2 response in ulcerative colitis. J Clin Invest 113:149.

[14] Ito, K.; Karasawa, M.; Kawano, T.; et al. (2000). Involvement of decidual Valpha14 NKT cells in abortion. Proc Natl Acad Sci USA 97:740-744.

[15] Seino, K.; Fukao, K.; Muramoto, K.; et al. (2001). Requirement for natural killer T (NKT) cells in the induction of allograft tolerance. Proc Natl Acad Sci USA 98:2577-2581. Kugathasan, S.; Saubermann, L.J.; Smith, L.; et al. (2007).

[16] Ikehara, Y.; Yasunami, Y.; Kodama, S.; et al. (2000). CD4+ Valpha14 natural killer T cells are essential for acceptance of rat islet xenografts in mice. J Clin Invest 105:1761-1767.

[17] Hammond, K.J.L.; Godfrey, D.I. (2002). NKT cells: Potential targets for autoimmune disease therapy? Tissue Antigens 59:353-363.

[18] Beaudoin, L.; Lalouz, V.; Novak, J.; et al. (2002). NKT cells inhibit the onset of diabetes by impairing the development of pathogenic T cells specific for pancreatic B cells. Immunity 17:725-736.

[19] Hong, S.; Wilson, M.T.; Serizawa, I.; et al. (2001). The natural killer T-cell ligand a-galactosylceramide prevents autoimmune diabetes in non-obese diabetic mice. Nat Med 7:1052-1056.

[20] Kita, H.; Naidenko, O.V.; Kronenberg, M.; et al. (2002). Quantitation and phenotypic analysis of natural killer T cells in primary biliary cirrhosis using a human CD1d tetramer. Gastroenterology 123: 1031-1043.

[21] Kono, F.; Honda, T.; Aini, W.; Manabe, T.; Haga, H.; Tsuruyama T. (2013) IFN-γ/CCR5 expression in invariant NKT cells and CCL5 expression in capillary veins of dermal papillae correlate with development of psoriasis vulgaris. Br J Dermatol. doi: 10.1111/bjd.12812 (in press).

[22] Akbari, O.; Stock, P.; Meyer, E.; et al. (2003). Essential role of NKT cells producing IL-4 and IL-13 in the development of allergen-induced airway hyperreactivity. Nat Med 9:582-588.

[23] Araujo, L.M.; Lefort, J.; Nahori, M.A.; et al. (2004). Exacerbated Th2-mediated airway inflammation and hyperresponsiveness in autoimmune diabetes-prone NOD mice: a critical role for CD1d-dependent NKT cells. Eur J Immunol 34:327-335.

[24] Terabe, M.; Matsui, S.; Noben-Trauth, N.; et al. (2000). NKT cell-mediated repression of tumor immunosurveillance by IL-13 and the IL-4R-STAT6 pathway. Nat Immunol 1:515-520.

[25] Smyth, M.J.; Crowe, N.Y.; Hayakawa, Y.; et al. (2002). NKT cells: conductors of tumor immunity? Curr Opin Immunol 14:165-171.

[26] [26]Tahir, S.M.A.; Cheng, O.; Shaulov, A. (2001). Loss of IFN-gamma production by invariant NK T cells in advanced cancer. J Immunol 167:4046-4050.

[27] Kikuchi, A.; Nieda, M.; Schmidt, C.; et al. (2001). In vitro antitumor activity of a-galactosylceramide-stimulated human invariant Valpha24+ NKT cells against melanoma. Br J Cancer 85:741-746.

[28] Crowe, N.Y.; Smyth, M.J.; Godfrey, D.I.; (2002). A critical role for natural killer T cells in immunosurveillance of methylcholanthrene-induced sarcomas. J Exp Med 196:119-127.

[29] Tachibana, T.; Onodera, H.; Tsuruyama, T.; et al. (2005). Increased intratumor Valpha24-positive natural killer T cells: a prognostic factor for primary colorectal carcinomas. Clin Cancer Res 11: 7322–7327.

[30] Grose, R.H., Cummins, A.G., Thompson, F.M.; Deficiency of invariant natural killer T cells in coeliac disease. Gut. (2007); 790-795.

[31] Avitzur, Y.; Grant, D. (2010). Intestine transplantation in children: update 2010. Pediatr Clin North Am 57:415–431.

[32] Goulet, O.; Sauvat, F. (2006). Short bowel syndrome and intestinal transplantation in children. Curr Opin Clin Nutr Metab Care 9:304–313.

[33] Pirenne, J.; Hoffman, I.; Miserez, M.; et al. (2006). Selection criteria and outcome of patients referred to intestinal transplantation: a European center experience. Transplant Proc 38:1671–1672.

[34] Bond, G.J.; Reyes, J.D.; (2004). Intestinal transplantation for total/near-total aganglionosis and intestinal pseudo-obstruction. Semin Pediatr Surg 13:286–292.

[35] Sharif, K.; Beath, S.V.; Kelly, D.A.; et al. (2003). New perspective for the management of near-total or total intestinal aganglionosis in infants. J Pediatr Surg 38:25–28.

[36] Ruiz, P.; Takahashi, H.; Delacruz, V.; et al. (2010). International grading scheme for acute cellular rejection in small-bowel transplantation: single-center experience. Transplant Proc 42:47–53.

[37] Wu, T.; Abu-Elmagd, K.; Bond, G.; et al. (2003). A schema for histologic grading of small intestine allograft acute rejection. Transplantation 75: 1241–1248.

[38] Tsuruyama, T.; Fujimoto, Y.; Yonekawa, Y.; et al. (2012). Invariant natural killer T cells infiltrate intestinal allografts undergoing acute cellular rejection. Transpl Int 25: 537–544.

[39] Merger, M.; Viney, J.L.; Borojevic, R.; et al. (2002). Defining the roles of perforin, Fas/FasL, and tumour necrosis factor alpha in T cell induced mucosal damage in the mouse intestine. Gut 51:155–163.

[40] [40]Suda, T.; Hashimoto, H.; Tanaka, M.; et al. (1997). Membrane Fas ligand kills human peripheral blood T lymphocytes, and soluble Fas ligand blocks the killing. J Exp Med 186: 2045–2050.

[41] Miyagawa-Hayashino, A.; Tsuruyama, T.; Egawa, H.; et al. (2007). FasL expression in hepatic antigen-presenting cells and phagocytosis of apoptotic T cells by FasL+ Kupffer cells are indicators of rejection activity in human liver allografts. Am J Pathol 171:1499–1508.

[42] Tsuruyama, T.; Okamoto, S.; Fujimoto, Y.; Yoshizawa, A.; Yoshitoshi, E.; Egawa, H.; Nakase, H.; Aini, W.; Miyao, M.; Tamaki, K.; Uemoto, S.; Haga, H. (2013). Histology of intestinal allografts: lymphocyte apoptosis and phagocytosis of lymphocytic apoptotic bodies are diagnostic findings of acute rejection in addition to crypt apoptosis. American J Surg Pathol 37:178-184.

[43] Karczewski, J.; Karczewski, M.; Glyda, M.; Wiktorowicz, K. (2008). Role of TH1/TH2 cytokines in kidney allograft rejection. Transplant Proc 40:3390-3392.

[44] McNerney M,E.; Lee KM;Zhou P; Molinero L; Mashayekhi M; Guzior, Sattar H, Kuppireddi S, Wang CR, Kumar V, Alegre ML. (2006). Role of natural killer cell subsets in cardiac allograft rejection. Am J Transplant. 6: 505-513.

[45] Asaoka, T.; Island, E.R.; Tryphonopoulos, P.; et al. (2011). Characteristic immune, apoptosis and inflammatory gene profiles associated with intestinal acute cellular

rejection in formalin-fixed paraffin-embedded mucosal biopsies. Transpl Int 24:697-707.

[46] Gonnella, PC.; Waldner, H.P.; Weiner, H.L. (2001). B cell-deficient (mMT) mice have alterations in the cytokine microenvironment of the gut-associated lymphoid tissue (GALT) and a defect in the low dose mechanism of oral tolerance. J Immunol 166:4456-4464.

[47] Stuber, E.; Buschenfeld, A.; von Freier, A.; et al. (1999). Intestinal crypt cell apoptosis in murine acute graft versus host disease is mediated by tumour necrosis factor alpha and not by the FasL-Fas interaction: effect of pentoxifylline on the development of mucosal atrophy. Gut 45:229–235.

[48] Kim, C.H.; Johnston, B.; Butcher, E.C. (2002). Trafficking machinery of NKT cells: shared and differential chemokine receptor expression among V alpha 24(+)V beta 11(+) NKT cell subsets with distinct cytokine-producing capacity. Blood 100:11-16.

[49] Ronet, C.; Darche, S.; Leite de Moraes, M.; Miyake, S.; Yamamura, T.; Louis, J.A.; Kasper, L.H.; Buzoni-Gatel, D. (2005). NKT cells are critical for the initiation of an inflammatory bowel response against Toxoplasma gondii. J Immunol 15:175:899-908.

[50] Olszak, T.; An, D.; Zeissig, S.; Vera, M.P.; Richter, J.; Franke A.; Glickman, J.N.; Siebert, R.; Baron R.M.; Kasper, D.L.; Blumberg, R.S. (2012). Microbial exposure during early life has persistent effects on natural killer T cell function. Science; 336:489-493.

[51] Coca, S.; Perez-Piqueras, J.; Martinez, D. (1997). The prognostic significance of intratumoral natural killer cells in patients with colorectal carcinoma. Cancer 79: 2320-2328.

[52] Kee, J.Y.; Ito, A.; Hojo, S.; Hashimoto, I.; Igarashi, Y.; Tsukada, K.; Irimura, T.; Shibahara, N.; Nakayama, T.; Yoshie, O.; Sakurai, H.; Saiki, I.; Koizumi, K. (2013). Chemokine CXCL16 suppresses liver metastasis of colorectal cancer via augmentation of tumor-infiltrating natural killer T cells in a murine model. Oncol Rep 29:975-982.

[53] Kronenberg, M. (2005). Toward an understanding of NKT cell biology: Progress and paradoxes. *Annu Rev Immunol* 26:877-900.

[54] Heller, F.; Fuss, I.J.; Nieuwenhuis, E.E.; Blumberg, R.S.; Strober, W. (2002). Oxazolone colitis, a Th2 colitis model resembling ulcerative colitis, is mediated by IL-13-producing NK-T cells. Immunity 17: 629-638.

[55] Cohen, N.R.; Garg, S.; Brenner, M.B. (2009). Antigen Presentation by CD1 lipids, T cells, and NKT cells in microbial immunity. *Adv Immunol* 102:1-94.

[56] Garg S, Sharma M, Ung C, Tuli A, Barral DC, Hava DL, Veerapen N, Besra GS, Hacohen N, Brenner MB. Lysosomal trafficking, antigen presentation, and microbial killing are controlled by the Arf-like GTPase Arl8b. Immunity (2011) 35; 182-193.

Section 4

Autoimmune Disregulation

Immunostimulation by Silica Particles and the Development of Autoimmune Dysregulation

Suni Lee, Hiroaki Hayashi, Megumi Maeda,
Hidenori Matsuzaki, Naoko Kumagai-Takei,
Ying Chen, Kozo Urakami, Masayasu Kusaka,
Yasumitsu Nishimura and Takemi Otsuki

Additional information is available at the end of the chapter

http://dx.doi.org/10.5772/57544

1. Introduction

Immunostimulation by environmental and occupational factors has been shown to cause various human diseases such as allergy and autoimmune diseases [1,2]. For example, solvents such as vinyl chloride have been linked to the development of scleroderma (SSc) [3-5], and previous studies reported the relationship between exposure to solvents and rheumatoid arthritis (RA) [6] or multiple sclerosis [7,8]. Another typical substance is silica. Patients exposed to silica particles were shown to develop not only pulmonary fibrosis, known as silicosis [9,10], one of the typical forms of pneumoconiosis, but also various autoimmune diseases [11,12] such as RA (historically known as Caplan syndrome) [13,14], SSc [15-17], systemic lupus erythematous (SLE) [18,19], and anti-neutrophil cytoplasmic antibody (ANCA)-related vasculitis/nephritis [20-22]. Many epidemiological reports have demonstrated that silica exposure is a risk factor of autoimmune diseases [11,12].

The mechanism of silica-induced autoimmune dysregulation has been attributed to silica acting as an adjuvant [23,24]. However, silica particles may directly stimulate circulating peripheral immune cells and cause certain alterations in the cellular or molecular functions of these cells because these particles may be retained in pulmonary lesions as well as the lymph nodes after they are inhaled into the body [9-12]. Therefore, if the direct effects of these particles change the characteristics of immune cells leading to the dysregulation of immune tolerance, clarifying these cellular and molecular mechanisms may be useful in preventing immune disorders in silicosis patients as well as providing an insight into the etiology of various autoimmune diseases.

We previously investigated the immunological effects of silica using human peripheral blood immune cells derived from healthy donors and silicosis patients [25-27]. In this review, we summarized our findings, in which silica was shown to be an environmental immunostimulator and the chronic activation of immune cells by recurrent and chronic exposure to silica was demonstrated to cause an imbalance in the regulation of T cell responses.

2. Autoantibodies detected in silicosis patients and their relationship with HLA phenotypes

We previously measured autoantibodies in silicosis patients, all of whom were Japanese brickyard workers in Bizen city, Okayama prefecture, Japan. All patients were diagnosed with silicosis based on their radiological findings in accordance with the ILO 2000 guidelines. The amount of free silica inhaled by these patients was estimated to be from 40 to 60%, as determined by their work environment. No subjects exhibited any symptoms of autoimmune diseases such as sclerotic skin, Raynaud's phenomenon, facial erythema, or cancer.

We demonstrated that the overall titer of anti-nuclear antibodies (ANA) was higher in these patients than in healthy volunteers [28]. In addition, silicosis patients without bullous diseases tested positive for anti-desmoglein autoantibodies and the frequencies of HLA-DRB1*04, HLA-DQB1*03, *0303, and *05, and HLA-DPB1*0402 and *0501 alleles were higher in these patients than in a healthy Japanese control population in the literature [29,30]. Moreover, the relationship between the autoantibodies in silicosis patients and HLA phenotypes was also analyzed in silicosis patients with anti-topoisomerase I autoantibodies [30-34], and the results obtained revealed that the allelic frequency of HLA-DQB1*0402 was significantly higher in anti-topoisomerase I positive Japanese silicosis patients than in anti-topoisomerase I negative patients or healthy donors [30-34].

We also assessed autoantibodies against Fas/CD95 [35], the cell death receptor, which plays an important role in the apoptosis of lymphocytes, and caspase-8 [36,37]. This anti-Fas autoantibody, in particular, was shown to induce apoptosis in Fas-expressing cells [35].

Even silicosis patients without any clinical symptoms of autoimmune diseases have various inapparent alterations in self-tolerance depending on individual factors, such as HLA phenotypes. In addition, when both respiratory and immunological factors were analyzed using factor analysis, this immunological progression was not concomitant with the development of respiratory disease [38]. Respiratory and immunological factors were shown to deteriorate to varying degrees in more than half of silicosis patients; however, a subpopulation was classified as a better respiratory and worse immunological group, while the opposite group was also reported [38].

Therefore, we attempted to confirm whether silica particles directly stimulated human immune cells, particularly T cells, with experimental evidence.

3. Schematic summary of the chronic activation of T cells by silica particles

A summary of the findings obtained and considerations are schematically presented in Figure 1. Silica particles were shown to chronically activate various T cells. Previous studies reported that effector T cells expressed various activation markers such as PD-1 and CD25 and produced many molecular markers for chronic T cell activation such as soluble Fas (sFas), decoy receptor 3 (DcR3), and soluble interleukin (IL)-2 receptor (sIL-2R) [39,40].

On the other hand, silica particles were also shown to activate CD4+CD25+FoxP3+regulatory T cells (Treg). However, this chronic activation caused the enhanced expression of Fas/CD95 on the surface of Treg, which induced early apoptosis [41]. Therefore, Treg may be lost from the peripheral blood, with the resulting imbalance between Treg and effector T cells subsequently leading to autoimmune dysregulation.

Detailed explanations of these findings are presented below.

4. Immune stimulation of effector T cells by silica particles

Freshly isolated peripheral blood mononuclear cells (PBMCs) obtained from healthy donors were incubated with silica particles. The CD69 expression on the membrane surface was examined as a marker, demonstrating gradual activation of T lymphocytes during 10-day incubation [42].

Other activation markers were examined in serum derived from silicosis patients and compared with those from healthy donors [43]. The results showed that sIL-2R levels were slightly higher in silicosis patients than in healthy donors. sIL-2R levels were also examined in serum derived from SSc patients, and correlations between sIL-2R levels and the immunological status of healthy donors, silicosis patients, and SSc patients as 1, 2 and 3 for continuous variables were analyzed. The correlation coefficient was shown to be 0.575 with $p=0.0008$, which indicated that, from the viewpoint of immunological alterations based on serum sIL-2R levels, silicosis patients were located between healthy donors and SSc patients. Elevated sIL-2R levels may be a pathophysiological marker for hematological malignancies such as human T lymphotropic retrovirus type-1 (HTLV-1) associated with adult T cell leukemia (ATL) and hairy cell leukemia, which reflects the increased production of cells leading to an elevation in serum titers [44-47]. Elevated sIL-2R levels have recently been reported in various autoimmune or inflammatory diseases, suggesting that the immune response is activated by chronic stimulation of T cells with an auto-or foreign antigen [48-51]. Therefore, the moderate, chronic activation status of the immune system may play a role in silicosis.

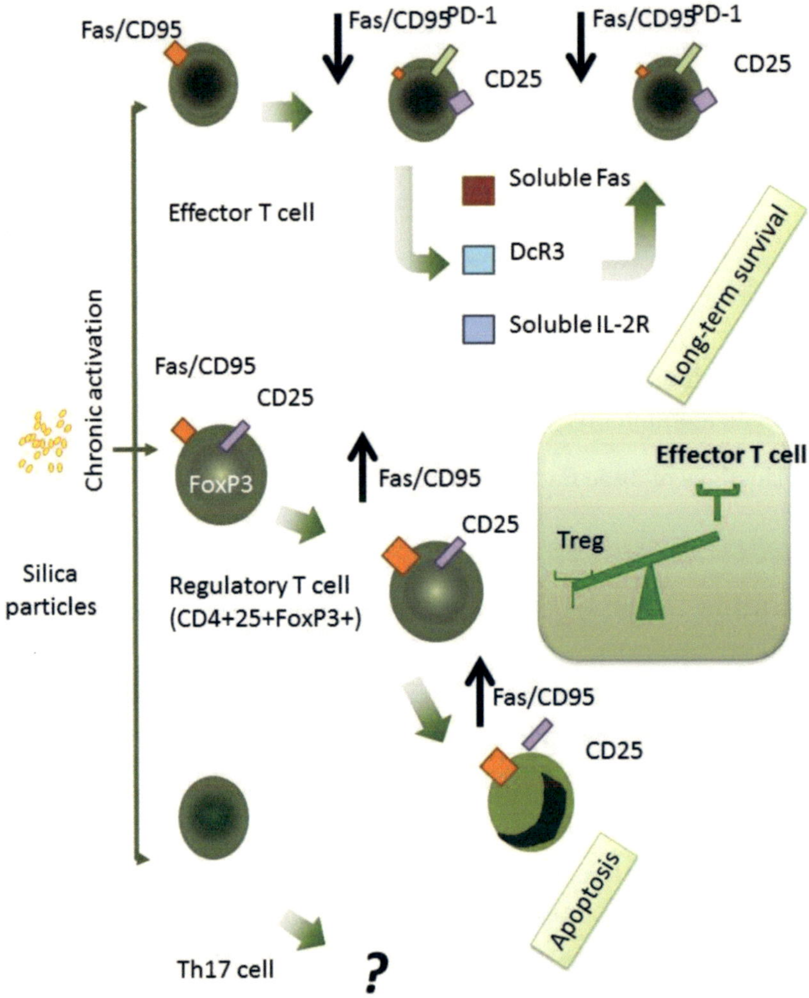

Figure 1. Schematic summary of the chronic activation of effector T cells, regulatory T cells (Treg; CD4+25+FoxP3+), and Th17 caused by exposure to silica particles. The chronic activation of effector T cells caused these cells to express activation surface markers such as CD25 and PD-1 with a decrease in the expression of the Fas/CD95 molecule. Instead of a reduction in membrane Fas, these cells produced soluble Fas, an alternative spliced form of wild-type Fas, and DcR3 as well as the soluble IL-2 receptor (sIL-2R). sFas and DcR3 prevented fas-ligand/Trail-induced apoptosis, leading to longer survival. sIL-2R and DcR3 as well as sFas were markers for the chronic activation of effector T cells. These might be explained by autoantigen-recognizing cells contaminating the long-term surviving cells. Treg enhanced expression of the surface Fas receptor and become prone to Fas-mediated apoptosis as a result of chronic activation. Treg may die quickly in silicosis patients (even when repeatedly recruited from the bone marrow). The overall balance between Treg and reactive T cells moves toward decreased Treg, resulting in the subsequent aberrant regulation of autoimmunity.

http://dx.doi.org/10.5772/57544

Similar to sIL-2R, DcR3 has been identified as a chronic activation marker for the human immune response [52]. DcR3 was initially discovered in malignant cells such as lung and colon cancers [53], and its role was considered to be that of a protective molecule binding with the TNF-related apoptosis-inducing ligand (TRAIL) or the Fas ligand secreted from tumor-attacking T cells [54]. These functions are similar to the soluble Fas molecule, which is an alternative splicing form of wild-type membrane Fas secreted from lymphocytes due to the absence of a transmembrane domain. Soluble Fas has also been shown to bind to the Fas ligand in extracellular areas, which prevented Fas ligand-inducing and Fas–mediated apoptosis in T cells [55-58].

Elevated DcR3 levels were recently reported in the serum or pathological lesions of patients with various autoimmune diseases such as RA and SLE, and these findings indicated that the production of high levels of DcR3 may reflect chronic activation of the immune system [52,59-62], particularly antigen-recognizing T cells.

We previously demonstrated that the expression of DcR3 mRNA in PBMCs was higher in silicosis patients than in healthy donors [63]. Although the expression of DcR3 mRNA was only examined in whole PBMCs including lymphocytes and monocytes, taken together with recent findings showing elevated DcR3 levels in autoimmune diseases, these results suggest that examining serum DcR3 levels in silicosis patients is of importance. We have started this analysis and will report our findings in the near future.

sFas has been shown to have a similar role to that of lymphocytes. Although its molecular function is to prevent apoptosis, elevations in sFas levels have been reported in serum from patients with various autoimmune diseases [62-64] as well as silicosis patients [67]. Using PBMCs, the sFas and membrane (wild-type) Fas message expression ratio was also shown to be higher in silicosis patients than in healthy donors [68]. Our findings also revealed that peripheral T cells, which produce lower levels of surface membrane Fas, were the producers/ expressers of sFas, whereas normal (relatively higher) surface membrane Fas-expressing T cells produced lower levels of sFas [25]. Fas-mediated apoptosis may proceed more easily in the latter fraction due to various stimuli by self-or foreign antigens or the anti-Fas autoantibody, which we discovered in the serum of silicosis patients, and repeated recruitment from the bone marrow. Peripheral T cells derived from silicosis patients were shown to be the dominant sFas producer with a smaller fraction of apoptosis-prone T cells than that from healthy donors [25-27]. The sFas-producing fraction may survive longer and retain a chronically activated status. Thus, this fraction may be stimulated and respond to autoantigens.

Similar to DcR3, the higher expression and production of sFas suggest that the peripheral blood of silicosis patients frequently includes a chronically activated and self-antigen recognizing T cell fraction.

These findings are summarized in Figure 2.

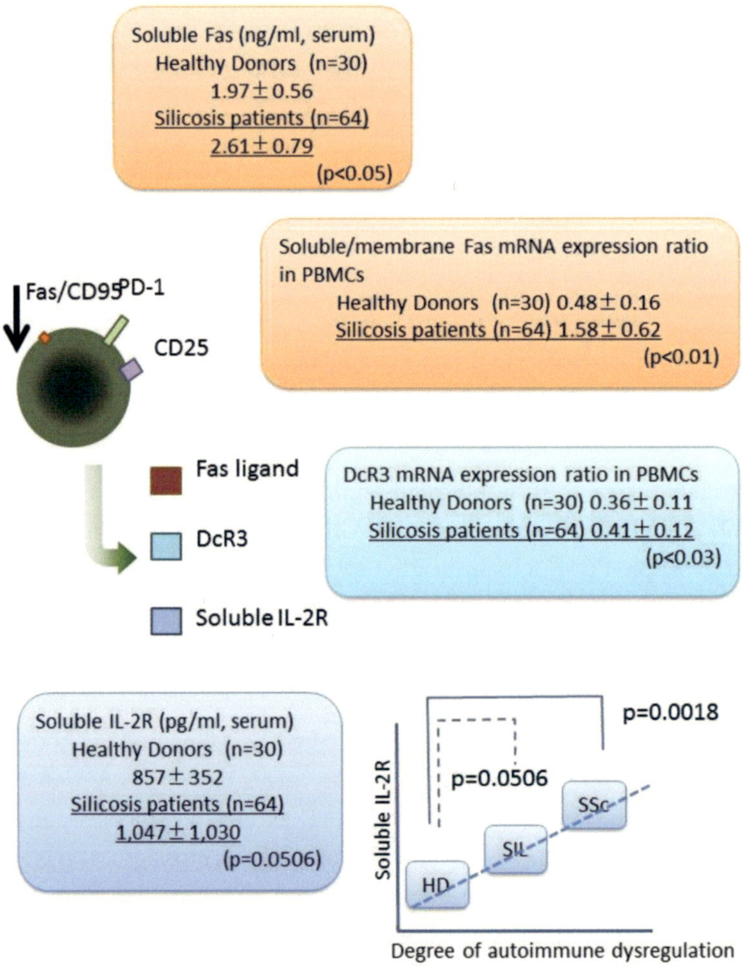

Figure 2. Evidence of chronically-activated effector T cells in silicosis patients. Serum soluble Fas, the soluble/membrane Fas mRNA expression ratio in PBMCs, and DcR3 expression and serum sIL-2R levels were higher in silicosis patients than in healthy donors. In addition, immunological abnormality levels in silicosis patients were determined to be 1, 2, and 3 (normal individuals and silicosis and SSc patients) as continuous variables between healthy donors and SSc patients. Then, the serum sIL-2R levels were positively correlated with these immunological scores. All of these findings indicate that effector T cells chronically and recurrently exposed become activated and their cellular features proceed to autoimmune dysregulation.

5. Immune stimulation of regulatory T cells by silica particle

From the beginning of Treg analysis in silicosis patients, the CD4+CD25+ fraction from PBMCs derived from these patients was shown to be less functional than that from healthy donors [28].

However, FoxP3-positive cells cannot be used in the experiment, since the use of the collected cells in the subsequent cell biological experiment precludes the permeabilization of the cell membrane because of the staining of nuclear molecules, such as FoxP3. Thus, it is unknown whether the CD4+25+ fraction used in the experiment was pure Treg or a mixture of chronically-activated reactive T cells. In other words, it is unknown whether the reduced functions of the Treg fraction with peripheral CD4+25+ in the silicosis patients was caused by the impurity of the Treg cells or the contamination of chronically-activated CD4+25+reactive T cells.

Therefore, we examined the expression of surface Fas in peripheral CD4+FoxP+ T cells derived from both silicosis patients and healthy donors [41], as shown in Figure 3. The results obtained revealed that the expression of Fas was higher in Treg from silicosis patients than in those from healthy donors. Since when Treg is stimulated, Fas expression was shown to be one of the markers for activated Treg; therefore, Treg may be a self-limited inhibitor for the immune response [69,70] and should be terminated by activation-induced cell death. Taken together, these results indicate that exposure to silica may activate Treg as well as effector T cells and induce the higher production of Fas by Treg.

PBMCs from healthy donors and silicosis patients were incubated with silica particles for four days and the percentage of CD4+FoxP3+ cells was then measured [41]. As shown in Figure 3 and reported previously, the frequency of apoptosis-induced Treg cell death during cultivation with silica particles was higher in PBMCs from silicosis patients than in that from healthy donors.

These results demonstrated that silica activated Treg, which then produced higher levels of surface Fas. Apoptosis then occurred in activated Treg. This cascaded reaction can continue for a long time in silicosis because of recurrent encounters between silica particles and T cells. The early loss of Treg may cause T cell recruitment. However, the overall balance between long-surviving reactive T and Treg cells will move toward predominance of reactive T cells [41].

5. Current issues in immune stimulation by silica

The mechanism by which silica affects Th17 cells has not yet been established. Th17 cells are considered to play an important role in the autoimmune reaction and increases in the Th17 cell population or typical cytokines produced by Th17 cells, including IL-17A, may be related to autoimmune reactions [71,72]. However, the microenvironment surrounding the development of T lymphocytes, defined by cytokine profiles such as IL-6 and TGF-β, may affect the developmental direction of both Treg and Th17 cells. Therefore, importance needs to be placed on investigations of how silica particles cause changes in the cellular and molecular characteristics of Th17 cells, and what the link is between these alterations and autoimmune dysregulation in silicosis patients.

6. Immunological effects of asbestos, a mineral silicate

Asbestos is a mineral silicate, in which the chemical core atom is Si and O, and various metals such as iron, magnesium or calcium have been shown to bind to asbestos to chemically form asbestos fibers [73]. However, the physical properties of silica and asbestos are different. The former is particulate matter while the latter is a fibrous mineral. Although silica has been shown to have an effect on the human immune system, as mentioned above, asbestos fibers may also have immunological effects on human lymphocytes, which may alter human anti-tumor immunity because the most important clinical complication in patients exposed to asbestos is malignant tumors.

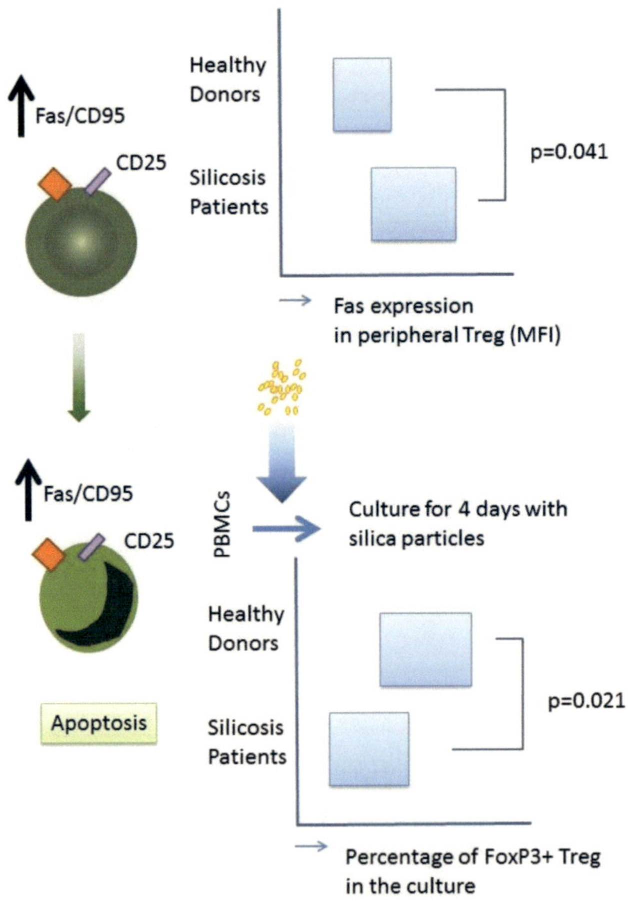

Figure 3. Surface Fas expression in peripheral CD4+FoxP+ T cells (Treg) derived from both silicosis patients and healthy donors. The expression of Fas was higher in the Treg of silicosis patients than in those of healthy donors. PBMCs from healthy donors and silicosis patients were incubated with silica particles for four days and the percentage of CD4+FoxP3+ cells was then measured. The frequency of apoptosis-induced Treg cell death during cultivation with silica particles was higher in PBMCs from silicosis patients than in that from healthy donors.

Although reports of autoimmune diseases in asbestos-exposed patients are rare [74,75], the main complication noted in these patients is malignancies such as mesothelioma and lung cancer [76,77]. In addition, the incidence of cancer in the larynx, GI-tract, and bladder was shown to be high in asbestos-exposed patients [76,77].

We previously examined the immunological effects of asbestos [78,79], and demonstrated that temporary and relatively high-dose exposure to asbestos caused apoptosis in T cells as well as alveolar epithelial cells and mesothelial cells, whereas low-dose and continuous exposure to asbestos caused the acquisition of resistance to asbestos-caused apoptosis in T cells with the activation of Scr-family kinase, IL-10, l STAT3, and Bcl-2 [80]. The expression of CXCR3, one of the chemokine receptors related to the anti-tumor immunity, as well as IFNγ was also reduced in these cells [81,82]. Asbestos exposure also induced the impaired differentiation and proliferation of CD8+ cytotoxic T cells [83], and the reduced expression of NKp46 activating receptor in NK cells [84,85]. Taken together, these findings indicate that asbestos causes a reduction in anti-tumor immunity.

7. Conclusions

Even if core chemical substances, Si and O_2, are identical, the immunological effects of silica seem to be completely opposite to those of asbestos. Silica is a chronic stimulator of T cells, with chronic exposure leading to autoimmune dysregulation due to the chronic activation of responder T cells as well as Treg, resulting in an imbalance in the regulation of T cell responses. On the other hand, asbestos reduces anti-tumor immunity. Therefore, asbestos is not a stimulator, but can alter the function of immune cells.

Acknowledgements

The authors express special thanks to Prof. Ayako Ueki, former professor of the Department of Hygiene, Kawasaki Medical School, and Drs. Fuminori Hyodoh, Akiko Takata-Tomokuni, Yoshie Miura, and Shuko Murakami, Ping Wu, Chen Ying, former members, who assisted in achieving the presented experimental findings. In addition, the authors wish thank to Ms. Tamayo Hatayama, Shoko Yamamoto, Haruko Sakaguchi, Satomi Hatada, Yumika Isozaki, Yoshiko Yamashita, Keiko Kimura, Tomoko Sueishi, Misao Kuroki, Minako Katoh, and Naomi Miyahara, present and former technical assistants. The experimental studies performed by the authors were supported in part by Special Coordination Funds for Promoting Science and Technology (H18-1-3-3-1, Comprehensive approach on asbestos-related diseases), KAKENHI grants (18390186, 19659153 and 20390178), Kawasaki Medical School Project Grants (23S5, 23S6, 23B66, 23P3, 24S4,24S6, 24B39, 25B41, 25B65, 25B67 and 25B82), a Sumitomo Foundation Grant (053027), a Yasuda Memorial Foundation Grant (H18), and funding from the Takeda Science Foundation (I-2008).

Author details

Suni Lee[1], Hiroaki Hayashi[2], Megumi Maeda[3], Hidenori Matsuzaki[1], Naoko Kumagai-Takei[1], Ying Chen[4], Kozo Urakami[5], Masayasu Kusaka[6], Yasumitsu Nishimura[1] and Takemi Otsuki[1*]

*Address all correspondence to: takemi@med.kawasaki-m.ac.jp

1 Department of Hygiene, Kawasaki Medical School, Kurashiki, Japan

2 Department of Dermatology, Kawasaki Medical School, Kurashiki, Japan

3 Department of Biofunctional Chemistry, Division of Bioscience, Okayama University Graduate School of Natural Science and Technology, Okayama, Japan

4 Division of Pneumoconiosis, School of Public Health, China Medical University, Shenyang, China

5 Hinase Urakami Iin, Bizen, Japan

6 Kusaka Hospital, Bizen, Japan

References

[1] Cooper GS, Miller FW, Germolec DR. Occupational exposures and autoimmune diseases. International Immunopharmacology 2002;2(2-3) 303-13.

[2] Pollard KM. Gender differences in autoimmunity associated with exposure to environmental factors. Journal of Autoimmunity 2012;38(2-3) J177-86.

[3] Haustein UF, Ziegler V. Environmentally induced systemic sclerosis-like disorders. International Journal of Dermatology 1985; 24(3) 147-51.

[4] Fox RI, Kang HI. Genetic and environmental factors in systemic sclerosis. Current Opinion in Rheumatology 1992;4(6) 857-61.

[5] Nietert PJ, Silver RM. Systemic sclerosis: environmental and occupational risk factors. Current Opinion in Rheumatology 2000;12(6) 520-6.

[6] Lundberg I, Alfredsson L, Plato N, Sverdrup B, Klareskog L, Kleinau S. Occupation, occupational exposure to chemicals and rheumatological disease. A register based cohort study. Scandinavian Journal of Rheumatology 1994;23(6) 305-10.

[7] Landtblom AM, Flodin U, Söderfeldt B, Wolfson C, Axelson O. Organic solvents and multiple sclerosis: a synthesis of the current evidence. Epidemiology 1996;7(4) 429-33.

[8] Mortensen JT, Brønnum-Hansen H, Rasmussen K. Multiple sclerosis and organic solvents. Epidemiology 1998;9(2) 168-71.

[9] World Health Organization. Silica, Some Silicates, Coal Dust and Para-Aramid Fibrils (IARC Monographs No. 68), 1997. ISBN: 978-9-2832126-83.

[10] Leung CC, Yu IT, Chen W. Silicosis. Lancet 2012;379(9830) 2008-18.

[11] Uber CL, McReynolds RA. Immunotoxicology of silica. Critical Reviews in Toxicology 1982;10(4) 303-19.

[12] Steenland K, Goldsmith DF. Silica exposure and autoimmune diseases. American Journal of Industrial Medicine 1995;28(5) 603-8.

[13] Caplan A. Rheumatoid disease and pneumoconiosis (Caplan's syndrome). Proceedings of the Royal Society of Medicine 1959;52 1111-3.

[14] Sluis-Cremer GK, Hessel PA, Hnizdo E Churchill AR. Relationship between silicosis and rheumatoid arthritis. Thorax 1986;41(8) 596-601.

[15] Sluis-Cremer, G.K., Hessel, P.A., Nizdo, E.H., Churchill, A.R. and Zeiss, E.A. Silica, silicosis, and progressive systemic sclerosis. British Journal of Industrial Medicine 1985;42(12) 838-43.

[16] Barnadas MA, Tuneu A, Rajmil HO, Abud O, de Moragas JM. Impotence in silicosis-associated scleroderma. Journal of the American Academy of Dermatology 1986;15(6) 1294-6.

[17] Cowie RL. Silica-dust-exposed mine workers with scleroderma (systemic sclerosis). Chest 1987;92(2) 260-2.

[18] Sanchez-Roman J, Wichmann I, Salaberri J, Varela JM, Nuñez-Roldan A. Multiple clinical and biological autoimmune manifestations in 50 workers after occupational exposure to silica. Annals of the Rheumatic Diseases 1993;52(7) 534-8.

[19] Brown LM, Gridley G, Olsen JH, Mellemkjaer L, Linet MS, Fraumeni JF. Jr. Cancer risk and mortality patterns among silicotic men in Sweden and Denmark. Journal of Occupational and Environmental Medicine 1997;39(7) 633-8.

[20] Gregorini G, Ferioli A, Donato F, Tira P, Morassi L, Tardanico R, Lancini L, Maiorca R. Association between silica exposure and necrotizing crescentic glomerulonephritis with p-ANCA and anti-MPO antibodies: a hospital-based case-control study. Advances in Experimental Medicine and Biology 1993;336 435-40.

[21] Gregorini G, Tira P, Frizza J, D'Haese PC, Elseviers MM, Nuyts G, Maiorca R, De Broe ME. ANCA-associated diseases and silica exposure. Clinical Reviews in Allergy and Immunology 1997;15(1) 21-40.

[22] Wichmann I, Sanchez-Roman J, Morales J, Castillo MJ, Ocaña C, Nuñez-Roldan A. Antimyeloperoxidase antibodies in individuals with occupational exposure to silica. Annals of the Rheumatic Diseases 1996;55(3) 205-7.

[23] Stratta P, Messuerotti A, Canavese C, Coen M, Luccoli L, Bussolati B, Giorda L, Malavenda P, Cacciabue M, Bugiani M, Bo M, Ventura M, Camussi G, Fubini B. The role of metals in autoimmune vasculitis: epidemiological and pathogenic study. Science of the Total Environment 2001;270(1-3) 179-90.

[24] Cooper GS, Gilbert KM, Greidinger EL, James JA, Pfau JC, Reinlib L, Richardson BC, Rose NR. Recent advances and opportunities in research on lupus: environmental influences and mechanisms of disease. Environmental Health Perspectives 2008;116(6) 695-702.

[25] Otsuki T, Miura Y, Nishimura Y, Hyodoh F, Takata A, Kusaka M, Katsuyama H, Tomita M, Ueki A, Kishimoto T. Alterations of Fas and Fas-related molecules in patients with silicosis. Experimental Biology and Medicine (Maywood) 2006;231(5) 522-33.

[26] Otsuki., Maeda M, Murakami S, Hayashi H, Miura Y, Kusaka M, Nakano T, Fukuoka K, Kishimoto T, Hyodoh F, Ueki A, Nishimura Y. Immunological effects of silica and asbestos. Cellular and Molecular Immunology 2007;4(4) 261-8.

[27] Kumagai N, Hayashi H, Maeda M, Miura Y, Nishimura Y, Matsuzaki H, Lee S, Fujimoto W, Otsuki T. Immunological effects of silica and related dysregulation of autoimmunity. In Autoimmune Disorder Pathogenetic Aspects. (ed: Mavragani, C.P.) Intech Open Access Publisher, Rijeka: InTech; 2011 http://www.intechopen.com/books/autoimmune-disorders-pathogenetic-aspects/immunological-effects-of-silica-and-related-dysregulation-of-autoimmunity (accessed 22 November 2013).

[28] Wu P, Miura Y, Hyodoh F, Nishimura Y, Hatayama T, Hatada S, Sakaguchi H, Kusaka M, Katsuyama H, Tomita M, Otsuki T. Reduced function of CD4+25+regulatory T cell fraction in silicosis patients. International Journal of Immunopathology and Pharmacology 2006;19(2) 357-68.

[29] Akaza T, Imanishi T, Fujiwara K, Tokunaga K, Yashiki S, Fujiyoshi T, Sonoda S, Tsuji T. HLA alleles and haplotypes of Japanese population, MHC IRS 1994;1 (Suppli) 219-26.

[30] Ueki H, Kohda M, Nobutoh T, Yamaguchi M, Omori K, Miyashita Y, Hashimoto T, Komai A, Tomokuni A, Ueki A. Antidesmoglein autoantibodies in silicosis patients with no bullous diseases. Dermatology 2001:202(1) 16-21.

[31] Ueki A, Isozaki Y, Tomokuni A, Tanaka S, Otsuki T, Kishimoto T, Kusaka M, Aikoh T, Sakaguchi H, Hydoh F. Autoantibodies detectable in the sera of silicosis patients. The relationship between the anti-topoisomerase I antibody response and HLA-DQB1*0402 allele in Japanese silicosis patients. Science of the Total Environment 2001;270(1-3) 141-8.

[32] Ueki A, Isozaki Y, Tomokuni A, Otsuki T, Hydoh F, Sakaguchi H, Tanaka S, Kusaka M. Is the anti-topoisomerase I autoantibody response associated with a distinct amino acid sequence in the HLA-DQbeta1 domain? Arthritis and Rheumatism 2001;44(2) 491-2.

[33] Ueki A, Isozaki Y, Tomokuni A, Ueki H, Kusaka M, Tanaka S, Otsuki T, Sakaguchi H, Hyodoh F. Different distribution of HLA class II alleles in anti-topoisomerase I autoantibody responders between silicosis and systemic sclerosis patients, with a common distinct amino acid sequence in the HLA-DQB1 domain. Immunobiology 2001;204(4) 458-65.

[34] Tomokuni A, Otsuki T, Sakaguchi H, Isozaki Y, Hyodoh F, Kusaka M, Ueki A. Detection of anti-topoisomerase I autoantibody in patients with silicosis. Environmental Health and Preventive Medicine 2002;7(1) 7-10.

[35] Takata-Tomokuni A, Ueki A, Shiwa M, Isozaki Y, Hatayama T, Katsuyama H, Hyodoh F, Fujimoto W, Ueki H, Kusaka M, Arikuni H, Otsuki T. Detection, epitope-mapping and function of anti-Fas autoantibody in patients with silicosis. Immunology 2005;116(1) 21-9.

[36] Ueki A, Isozaki Y, Tomokuni A, Hatayama T, Ueki H, Kusaka M, Shiwa M, Arikuni H, Takeshita T, Morimoto K. Intramolecular epitope spreading among anti-caspase-8 autoantibodies in patients with silicosis, systemic sclerosis and systemic lupus erythematosus, as well as in healthy individuals. Clinical and Experimental Immunology 2002;129(3) 556-61.

[37] Ueki A, Isozaki Y, Kusaka M. Anti-caspase-8 autoantibody response in silicosis patients is associated with HLA-DRB1, DQB1 and DPB1 alleles. Journal of Occupational Health 2005;47(1) 61-7.

[38] Otsuki T, Ichihara K, Tomokuni A, Sakaguchi H, Aikoh T, Matsuki T, Isozaki Y, Hyodoh F, Kusaka M, Kita S, Ueki A. Evaluation of cases with silicosis using the parameters related to Fas-mediated apoptosis. International Journal of Molecular Medicine 1999;4(4) 407-11.

[39] Maeda M, Nishimura Y, Kumagai N, Hayashi H, Hatayama T, Katoh M, Miyahara N, Yamamoto S, Hiratsuka J, Otsuki T. Dysregulation of the immune system caused by silica and asbestos. Journal of Immunotoxicology 2010;7(4) 268-78.

[40] Lee S, Hayashi H, Maeda M, Chen Y, Matsuzaki H, Takei-Kumagai N, Nishimura Y, Fujimoto W, Otsuki T. Environmental factors producing autoimmune dysregulation--chronic activation of T cells caused by silica exposure.. Immunobiology 2012;217(7) 743-8.

[41] Hayashi H, Miura Y, Maeda M, Murakami S, Kumagai N, Nishimura Y, Kusaka M, Urakami K, Fujimoto W, Otsuki T. Reductive alteration of the regulatory function of the CD4(+)CD25(+) T cell fraction in silicosis patients. International Journal of Immunopathology and Pharmacology 2010;23(4) 1099-109.

[42] Wu P, Hyodoh F, Hatayama T, Sakaguchi H, Hatada S, Miura Y, Takata-Tomokuni A, Katsuyama H, Otsuki T. Induction of CD69 antigen expression in peripheral blood mononuclear cells on exposure to silica, but not by asbestos/chrysotile-A. Immunology Letters 2005;98(1) 145-52.

[43] Hayashi H, Maeda M, Murakami S, Kumagai N, Chen Y, Hatayama T, Katoh M, Miyahara N, Yamamoto S, Yoshida Y, Nishimura Y, Kusaka M, Fujimoto W, Otsuki T. Soluble interleukin-2 receptor as an indicator of immunological disturbance found in silicosis patients. International Journal of Immunopathology and Pharmacology 2009;22(1) 53-62.

[44] Zerler B. The soluble interleukin-2 receptor as a marker for human neoplasia and immune status. Cancer Cells 1991;3(12) 471-9.

[45] Murakami S. Soluble interleukin-2 receptor in cancer. Frontiers in Bioscience 2004;9, 3085-90

[46] Witkowska, A.M. On the role of sIL-2R measurements in rheumatoid arthritis and cancers. Mediators of Inflammation Mediators of Inflammation 2005;2005(3) 121-30. http://dx.doi.org/10.1155/MI.2005.121 (accessed 22 November 2013).

[47] Bien E, Balcerska A. Serum soluble interleukin 2 receptor alpha in human cancer of adults and children: a review. Biomarkers 2008;13(1) 1-26.

[48] Bleesing J, Prada A, Siegel DM, Villanueva J, Olson J, Ilowite NT, Brunner HI, Griffin T, Graham TB, Sherry DD, Passo MH, Ramanan AV, Filipovich A, Grom AA. The diagnostic significance of soluble CD163 and soluble interleukin-2 receptor alpha-chain in macrophage activation syndrome and untreated new-onset systemic juvenile idiopathic arthritis. Arthritis and Rheumatism 2007;56(3) 965-71.

[49] Coaccioli S, Pinoca F, Giuliani M, Landucci P, Sabatini C, Puxeddu A. Definition of adult-onset rheumatoid arthritis from elderly-onset rheumatoid arthritis by studying T-lymphocyte subpopulations, their soluble receptors and soluble receptor of interleukin-2. Clinica Terapeutica 2007;158(4) 303-6.

[50] Suh CH, Kim HA. Cytokines and their receptors as biomarkers of systemic lupus erythematosus. Expert Review of Molecular Diagnostics 2008;8(2) 189-98.

[51] Maier LM, Anderson DE, Severson CA, Baecher-Allan C, Healy B, Liu DV, Wittrup KD, De Jager PL, Hafler DA. Soluble IL-2RA levels in multiple sclerosis subjects and the effect of soluble IL-2RA on immune responses. Journal of Immunology 2009;182(3) 1541-47.

[52] Lin WW, Hsieh SL. Decoy receptor 3: a pleiotropic immunomodulator and biomarker for inflammatory diseases, autoimmune diseases and cancer. Biochemical Pharmacology 2011;81(7) 838-47.

[53] Pitti RM, Marsters SA, Lawrence DA, Roy M, Kischkel FC, Dowd P, Huang A, Donahue CJ, Sherwood SW, Baldwin DT, Godowski PJ, Wood WI, Gurney AL, Hillan KJ,

Cohen RL, Goddard AD, Botstein D, Ashkenazi A. Genomic amplification of a decoy receptor for Fas ligand in lung and colon cancer. Nature 1998;396(6712) 699-703.

[54] Green DR. Apoptosis. Death deceiver. Nature 1998;396(6712) 629-30.

[55] Cheng J, Zhou T, Liu C, Shapiro JP, Brauer MJ, Kiefer MC, Barr PJ, Mountz JD. Protection from Fas-mediated apoptosis by a soluble form of the Fas molecule. Science 1994;263(5154) 1759-62.

[56] Orlinick JR, Chao MV. TNF-related ligands and their receptors. Cellular Signalling 1998;10(8) 543-51.

[57] Nagata, S. (1994) Fas and Fas ligand: a death factor and its receptor. Adv Immunol. 57, 129-144, ISSN: 0065-2776

[58] Nagata S, Golstein P. The Fas death factor. Science 1995;267(5203) 1449-56.

[59] Chen CC, Yang YH, Lin YT, Hsieh SL, Chiang BL. Soluble decoy receptor 3: increased levels in atopic patients. Journal of Allergy and Clinical Immunology 2004;114(1) 195-7.

[60] Hayashi S, Miura Y, Nishiyama T, Mitani M, Tateishi K, Sakai Y, Hashiramoto A, Kurosaka M, Shiozawa S, Doita M. Decoy receptor 3 expressed in rheumatoid synovial fibroblasts protects the cells against Fas-induced apoptosis. Arthritis and Rheumatism 2007;56(4) 1067-75.

[61] Lee CS, Hu CY, Tsai HF, Wu CS, Hsieh SL, Liu LC, Hsu PN. Elevated serum decoy receptor 3 with enhanced T cell activation in systemic lupus erythematosus. Clinical and Experimental Immunology 2008;151(3) 383-90.

[62] Han B, Bojalil R, Amezcua-Guerra LM, Springall R, Valderrama-Carvajal H, Wu J, Luo H. DcR3 as a diagnostic parameter and risk factor for systemic lupus erythematosus. International Immunology 2008;20(8) 1067-75.

[63] Otsuki T, Tomokuni A, Sakaguchi H, Aikoh T, Matsuki T, Isozaki Y, Hyodoh F, Ueki H, Kusaka M, Kita S, Ueki A. Over-expression of the decoy receptor 3 (DcR3) gene in peripheral blood mononuclear cells (PBMC) derived from silicosis patients. Clinical and Experimental Immunology 2000;119(2) 323-7.

[64] Knipping E, Krammer PH, Onel KB, Lehman TJ, Mysler E, Elkon KB. Levels of soluble Fas/APO-1/CD95 in systemic lupus erythematosus and juvenile rheumatoid arthritis. Arthritis and Rheumatism 1995;38(12) 1735-7.

[65] Nozawa K, Kayagaki N, Tokano Y, Yagita H, Okumura K, Hasimoto H. Soluble Fas (APO-1, CD95) and soluble Fas ligand in rheumatic diseases. Arthritis and Rheumatism 1997;40(6) 1126-9.

[66] Sahin M, Aydintug O, Tunc SE, Tutkak H, Naziroğlu M. Serum soluble Fas levels in patients with autoimmune rheumatic diseases. Clinical Biochemistry 2007;40(1-2) 6-10.

[67] Tomokuni A, Aikoh T, Matsuki T, Isozaki Y, Otsuki T, Kita S, Ueki H, Kusaka M, Kishimoto T, Ueki A. Elevated soluble Fas/APO-1 (CD95) levels in silicosis patients without clinical symptoms of autoimmune diseases or malignant tumours. Clinical and Experimental Immunology 1997;110(2) 303-9.

[68] Otsuki T, Sakaguchi H, Tomokuni A, Aikoh T, Matsuki T, Kawakami Y, Kusaka M, Ueki H, Kita S, Ueki A. Soluble Fas mRNA is dominantly expressed in cases with silicosis. Immunology 1998;94(2) 258-62.

[69] Fontenot JD, Rudensky AY. Molecular aspects of regulatory T cell development. Seminars in Immunology 2004;16(2) 73-80.

[70] Hori S, Sakaguchi S. Foxp3: a critical regulator of the development and function of regulatory T cells. Microbes and Infection 2004;6(8) 745-51.

[71] Weaver CT, Harrington LE, Mangan PR, Gavrieli M, Murphy KM. Th17: an effector CD4 T cell lineage with regulatory T cell ties. Immunity 2006;24(6) 677-88.

[72] Korn T, Bettelli E, Oukka M, Kuchroo VK. IL-17 and Th17 Cells. Annual Review of immunology 2009;27 485-517.

[73] Craighead JE, Gibbs AR, Pooley F. Mineralogy of asbestos. In: Craighead JE, Gibbs AR. (ed.) Asbestos and its diseases. New York, Oxford University Press. New York, 2008. p23-38.

[74] Pfau JC, Sentissi JJ, Weller G, Putnam EA. Assessment of autoimmune responses associated with asbestos exposure in Libby, Montana, USA. Environmental Health Perspectives 2005;113(1) 25-30.

[75] Noonan CW, Pfau JC, Larson TC, Spence MR. Nested case-control study of autoimmune disease in an asbestos-exposed population. Environmental Health Perspectives 2006;114(8) 1243-7.

[76] Lemen RA. Epidemiology of asbestos-related diseases and the knowledge that led to what is known today. (2011) In Asbestos. Risk assessment, epidemiology, and health effects. 2nd ed. (eds,: Dodson, R.F. and Hammar, S.P.) CRC press. New York, 131-268, ISBN:978-1-4398-0968-6

[77] Committee on Asbestos: selected health effects, board on population health and public health practices. Asbestos, selected cancers. Washington, D.C., The National Academic Press. 2006. ISBN:0-309-10169-7.

[78] Kumagai-Takei N, Maeda M, Chen Y, Matsuzaki H, Lee S, Nishimura Y, Hiratsuka J, Otsuki T. Asbestos induces reduction of tumor immunity. Clinical and Developmental Immunology 2011;2011:481439. doi: 10.1155/2011/481439. Epub 2011 Oct 4. http://www.hindawi.com/journals/cdi/2011/481439/ (accessed 22November 2013)

[79] Matsuzaki H, Maeda M, Lee S, Nishimura Y, Kumagai-Takei N, Hayashi H, Yamamoto S, Hatayama T, Kojima Y, Tabata R, Kishimoto T, Hiratsuka J, Otsuki T. Asbestos-induced cellular and molecular alteration of immunocompetent cells and their

relationship with chronic inflammation and carcinogenesis. Journal of Biomedicine and Biotechnology. 2012;2012:492608. doi: 10.1155/2012/492608. Epub 2012 Feb 6. http://www.hindawi.com/journals/bmri/2012/492608/ (accessed 22November 2013)

[80] Miura Y, Nishimura Y, Katsuyama H, Maeda M, Hayashi H, Dong M, Hyodoh F, Tomita M, Matsuo Y, Uesaka A, Kuribayashi K, Nakano T, Kishimoto T, Otsuki T. Involvement of IL-10 and Bcl-2 in resistance against an asbestos-induced apoptosis of T cells. Apoptosis 2006;11(10) 1825-35

[81] Maeda M, Nishimura Y, Hayashi H, Kumagai N, Chen Y, Murakami S, Miura Y, Hiratsuka J, Kishimoto T, Otsuki, T. Reduction of CXC chemokine receptor 3 in an in vitro model of continuous exposure to asbestos in a human T-cell line, MT-2. American Journal of Respiratory Cell and Molecular Biology 2011;45(3) 470-9.

[82] Maeda M, Nishimura Y, Hayashi H, Kumagai N, Chen Y, Murakami S, Miura Y, Hiratsuka J, Kishimoto T, Otsuki T. Decreased CXCR3 expression in CD4+T cells exposed to asbestos or derived from asbestos-exposed patients. American Journal of Respiratory Cell and Molecular Biology 2011;45(4) 795-803.

[83] Kumagai-Takei N, Nishimura Y, Maeda M, Hayashi H, Matsuzaki H, Lee S, Hiratsuka J, Otsuki T. Effect of asbestos exposure on differentiation of cytotoxic T lymphocytes in mixed lymphocyte reaction of human peripheral blood mononuclear cells. American Journal of Respiratory Cell and Molecular Biology 2013;49(1) 28-36.

[84] Nishimura Y, Miura Y, Maeda M, Kumagai N, Murakami S, Hayashi H, Fukuoka K, Nakano T, Otsuki T. Impairment in cytotoxicity and expression of NK cell-activating receptors on human NK cells following exposure to asbestos fibers. International Journal of Immunopathology and Pharmacology 2009;22(3) 579-90.

[85] Nishimura Y, Maeda M, Kumagai N, Hayashi H, Miura Y, Otsuki, T. Decrease in phosphorylation of ERK following decreased expression of NK cell-activating receptors in human NK cell line exposed to asbestos. International Journal of Immunopathology and Pharmacology 2009;22(4) 879-88.